Surgery of the Cranial Nerves of the Posterior Fossa

AANS Publications Committee
Daniel L. Barrow, MD, Editor

Neurosurgical Topics

American Association of
Neurological Surgeons

ISBN: 1-879284-02-2

Neurosurgical Topics ISBN: 0-9624246-6-8

Copyright © 1993 by American Association of Neurological Surgeons

Printed in U.S.A.

This publication is published under the auspices of the Publications Committee of the American Association of Neurological Surgeons (AANS). However, this should not be construed as indicating endorsement or approval of the views presented, by the AANS, or by its committees, commissions, affiliates, or staff.

Daniel L. Barrow, MD, Chairman
AANS Publications Committee

Linda S. Miller, AANS Staff Editor

AANS1.5M493

Forthcoming Books in the *Neurosurgical Topics* Series

1993

Spinal Trauma: Current Evaluation and Management
   Edited by Gary L. Rea, MD, and Carole A. Miller, MD

Current Management of Cerebral Aneurysms
   Edited by Issam A. Awad, MD

Spinal Instrumentation
   Edited by Edward C. Benzel, MD

Interactive Image-Guided Neurosurgery
   Edited by Robert J. Maciunas, MD

Neurosurgical Emergencies
   Edited by Christopher M. Loftus, MD

Contents

List of Contributors

Christopher B.T. Adams, MD
Department of Neurosurgery
Radcliffe Infirmary
Oxford University
Oxford, England

Ossama Al-Mefty, MD, FACS
Division of Neurological Surgery
Loyola University Medical Center
Maywood, Illinois

Fred G. Barker II, MD
Neurological Surgery
Massachusetts General Hospital
Department of Surgery
Harvard Medical School
Boston, Massachusetts

Kim J. Burchiel, MD
Professor and Head
Division of Neurosurgery
Oregon Health Science Center
Portland, Oregon

Franco DeMonte, MD, FRCS (C)
Assistant Professor of Neurosurgery
University of Texas, MD Anderson Cancer Center
Clinical Assistant Professor of Neurosurgery
Baylor College of Medicine
Houston, Texas

Patricia M. Fernandez, MD
Skull Base Fellow, Department of Neurosurgery
University of Cincinnati
Cincinnati, Ohio

Steven L. Giannotta, MD
Professor, Department of Neurological Surgery
USC School of Medicine
Los Angeles, California

Aage R. Møller, PhD
Professor of Neurological Surgery
Department of Neurological Surgery
University of Pittsburgh School of Medicine
Pittsburgh, Pennsylvania

Dennis S. Poe, MD, FACS
Department of Otolaryngology
Lahey Clinic Medical Center
Burlington, Massachusetts

Robert G. Ojemann, MD
Neurological Surgery
Massachusetts General Hospital
Department of Surgery, Harvard Medical School
Boston, Massachusetts

Albert L. Rhoton, Jr., MD
R.D. Keene Family Professor and Chairman
Department of Neurological Surgery
University of Florida, College of Medicine
Gainesville, Florida

Daniel C. Rohrer, MD
Senior Resident, Division of Neurosurgery
Oregon Health Science Center
Portland, Oregon

Edward C. Tarlov, MD
Department of Neurosurgery
Lahey Clinic Medical Center
Burlington, Massachusetts

John M. Tew, Jr., MD, FACS
Frank H. Mayfield Professor of Neurosurgery
Chairman, Department of Neurosurgery
University of Cincinnati
Cincinnati, Ohio

Harry Van Loveren, MD
Assistant Professor of Neurosurgery
Department of Neurosurgery
University of Cincinnati Medical Center
Cincinnati, Ohio

Robert H. Wilkins, MD
Professor and Chief
Division of Neurosurgery
Duke University Medical Center
Durham, North Carolina

AANS Publications Committee

Preface

The posterior intracranial fossa includes some of the most complex and crucial anatomy in the human body. Among these critical anatomic structures are the majority of cranial nerves, subserving a myriad of vital functions. When these nerves misfire or malfunction, the disorders that ensue can cause highly painful, disabling, and disfiguring syndromes. Cranial nerve dysfunction syndromes include trigeminal neuralgia (tic douloureux), vagoglossopharyngeal neuralgia, hemifacial spasm, disabling positional vertigo, Meniere's syndrome, and spasmodic torticollis, among others. Patients are often desperate in seeking cures for these ailments. Neoplasms involving the cranial nerves located in the posterior fossa present other unique challenges to the surgeon due to the dense anatomic arena involved in their removal. Surgical problem solving and technical expertise are acutely tested in managing lesions such as meningiomas, acoustic neuromas, glomus tumors, and other neoplasms arising in the region of the brain stem and cerebellopontine angle.

Appropriate treatment can range from simpler percutaneous procedures or medical treatment to the more controversial and risky microvascular decompressions (MVDs) and skull base procedures. Optimizing the operative approaches to the cranial nerves in the posterior cranial fossa requires an understanding of the relationship of these nerves to the cerebellar arteries, brain stem, peduncles, and the cerebellar surfaces and fissures. Dr. Rhoton has provided an outstanding description of these complex relationships in a thorough and well-illustrated opening chapter on the microanatomy of the posterior fossa cranial nerves. Monitoring and operative positioning are also factors in optimizing the outcome of surgery on and around the cranial nerves, and these topics are also detailed in excellent chapters.

The management of lesions affecting the posterior fossa cranial nerves is controversial. From skull base surgery to MVD, conservative versus aggressive and traditional versus radical strategies often come head-to-head. There is much debate on the concept of microvascular compression—whether or not it is of etiologic importance, and on the utility of MVD as an effective treatment. Such opposing views are represented in this volume in an effort to offer a full range of theory and approach. This book is not meant as an endorsement of one technique over another, but rather as a means to better educate neurosurgeons as to the realistic and, ultimately, best options they can offer their patients.

Daniel L. Barrow, MD
Editor

CHAPTER 1

Microsurgical Anatomy of Posterior Fossa Cranial Nerves

Albert L. Rhoton, Jr., MD

Optimizing the operative approaches to the cranial nerves in the posterior cranial fossa requires an understanding of the relationship of these nerves to the cerebellar arteries, brain stem, cerebellar peduncles, fissures between the cerebellum and brain stem, and the cerebellar surfaces.[34] When examining these relationships, three neurovascular complexes can be defined: an upper complex related to the superior cerebellar artery (SCA); a middle complex related to the anterior inferior cerebellar artery (AICA); and a lower complex related to the posterior inferior cerebellar artery (PICA) (Figure 1).

A group of structures occurs in sets of three in the posterior fossa that bear a consistent relationship to the upper, middle, and lower neurovascular complexes. These structures are the parts of the brain stem (midbrain, pons, and medulla); the cerebellar peduncles (superior, middle, and inferior); the fissures between the brain stem and the cerebellum (cerebellomesencephalic, cerebellopontine, and cerebellomedullary); and the surfaces of the cerebellum (tentorial, petrosal, and suboccipital). Each neurovascular complex includes one of the three parts of the brain stem, one of the three surfaces of the cerebellum, one of the three cerebellar peduncles, and one of the three major fissures between the cerebellum and the brain stem. In addition, each neurovascular complex contains a group of cranial nerves.

The upper complex includes the oculomotor (III), trochlear (IV), and trigeminal (V) nerves that are related to the SCA. The oculomotor and trochlear nerves pass above and the trigeminal nerve passes below the SCA. The middle complex includes the abducens (VI), facial (VII), and vestibulocochlear (VIII) nerves that are related to the AICA. The AICA passes above or below or splits the fascicles of the abducens nerve, and then passes above, below, or between the facial and vestibulocochlear nerves. The lower complex includes the glossopharyngeal (IX), vagus (X), spinal accessory (XI), and hypoglossal (XII) nerves that are related to the PICA. The PICA first courses around or between the rootlets of the hypoglossal nerve and then reaches the dorsal surface of the medulla by passing between the rootlets of the glossopharyngeal, vagus, or spinal accessory nerves.

The relationship of the three cerebellar arteries to the three parts of the brain stem and the three cerebellar peduncles is relatively simple. The SCA courses around the midbrain to reach the superior cerebellar peduncle. The AICA courses around the pons to reach the middle cerebellar peduncle. The PICA courses around the medulla to reach the surface of the inferior cerebellar peduncle.

The relationship of the three cerebellar arteries to the fissues between the brain stem and the cerebellum is more complicated. The upper fissure is situated between the cerebel-

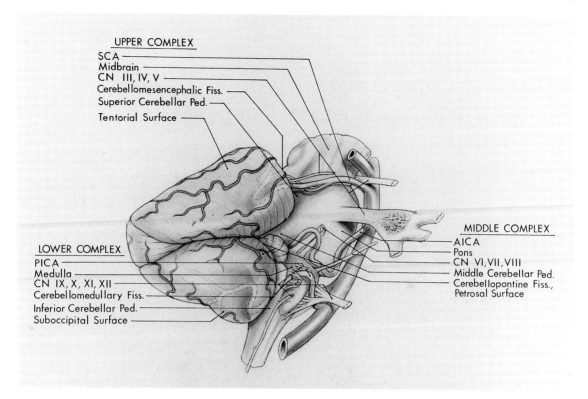

Figure 1. Each of the 3 neurovascular complexes in the posterior fossa includes 1 of the 3 cerebellar arteries, 1 of the 3 parts of the brain stem, 1 of the 3 cerebellar peduncles, 1 of the 3 cerebellar surfaces, 1 of the 3 fissures between the brain stem and the cerebellum, and 1 of the 3 groups of cranial nerves. The upper complex is related to the superior cerebellar artery (S.C.A.); the middle complex is related to the anterior inferior cerebellar artery (A.I.C.A.); and the lower complex is related to the posterior inferior cerebellar artery (P.I.C.A.). The upper complex includes the SCA, midbrain, superior cerebellar peduncle, cerebellomesencephalic fissure, tentorial surface of the cerebellum, and the oculomotor (III), trochlear (IV), and trigeminal (V) nerves. The middle complex includes the AICA, pons, middle cerebellar peduncle, cerebellopontine fissure, petrosal surface of the cerebellum, and the abducens (VI), facial (VII), and vestibulocochlear (VIII) nerves. The lower complex includes the PICA, medulla, inferior cerebellar peduncle, cerebellomedullary fissure, suboccipital surface of the cerebellum, and the glossopharyngeal (IX), vagus (X), spinal accessory (XI), and hypoglossal (XII) nerves.

lum and the midbrain and is called the cerebellomesencephalic fissure. The middle fissure is located between the cerebellum and the pons and is called the cerebellopontine fissure. The lower fissure is located between the cerebellum and the medulla and is called the cerebellomedullary fissure.

The cerebellomesencephalic fissure, in which the SCA courses, extends from the pineal region downward between the cerebellum and the superior half of the roof of the fourth ventricle. The superior cerebellar peduncles are located in the anterior wall of this fissure. The SCA is anchored in this fissure by branches that pass along the superior cerebellar peduncle to reach the dentate nuclei located in the roof of the fourth ventricle.

The cerebellopontine fissure, along which the AICA courses, is an angular V-shaped fissure located between the cerebellum and the lateral part of the pons and middle cerebellar peduncle. The apex of the fissure is located posteriorly. It has a superior limb that is directed upward and forward from the apex and an inferior limb directed inferiorly and forward. The space between the two limbs is referred to as the cerebellopontine angle (CPA). The middle cerebellar peduncle courses in the space between the two limbs. Cranial nerves V through IX arise in the area between the two limbs.

The cerebellomedullary fissure, in which the PICA courses, is located between the medulla and the cerebellum. This fissure extends upward around the cerebellar tonsils into the deep cleft between the tonsils and the lower half of the roof of the fourth ventricle, which is formed by the tela choroidea and the inferior medullary velum. The tela choroidea is the thin arachnoidlike membrane in which the choroid plexus arises. The inferior medullary velum is a thin band of neural tissue that extends from the nodule of the vermis in the midline to the flocculus laterally in the CPA. Together, the flocculus, the nodule, and the group of connecting fibers in the inferior medullary velum form the flocculonodular lobe of the cerebellum.

Three surfaces of the cerebellum (tentorial, suboccipital, and petrosal) have a consistent relationship to the three cerebellar arteries. The tentorial surface, which is supplied by the SCA, is the surface facing the lower margin of the tentorium. This surface is tent shaped, with its apex located below the straight sinus. From the apex, its surface slopes downward and laterally. The highest part of this surface is the vermis. The suboccipital surface, which is supplied by the PICA, is exposed in a wide suboccipital craniectomy. It extends from the transverse sinuses down to the foramen magnum and laterally to the sigmoid sinuses. This surface is different from the tentorial surface because the vermis on this surface is folded into a deep vertical trough, called the posterior cerebellar incisura, rather than located at the apex as it is on the tentorial surface. The petrosal surface, which is supplied by the AICA, is the surface that faces the posterior surface of the temporal bone and is elevated to reach the CPA.

In summary, the upper complex includes the SCA, midbrain, cerebellomesencephalic fissure, superior cerebellar peduncle, tentorial surface of the cerebellum, and the oculomotor, trochlear, and trigeminal nerves (Figures 1 and 2). The SCA arises in front of and

encircles the midbrain, passes below the oculomotor and trochlear nerves and above the trigeminal nerve to reach the cerebellomesencephalic fissure, where it runs on the superior cerebellar peduncle and terminates by supplying the tentorial surface of the cerebellum.

The middle complex includes the AICA, pons, middle cerebellar peduncle, cerebellopontine fissure, petrosal surface of the cerebellum, and the abducens, facial, and vestibulocochlear nerves. The AICA arises at the pontine level, courses in relationship to the abducens, facial, and vestibulocochlear nerves to reach the surface of the middle cerebellar peduncle, where it courses along the cerebellopontine fissure and terminates by supplying the petrosal surface of the cerebellum.

The lower complex includes the PICA, medulla, inferior cerebellar peduncle, cerebellomedullary fissure, suboccipital surface of the cerebellum, and the glossopharyngeal, vagus, spinal accessory, and hypoglossal nerves. The PICA arises at the medullary level, encircles the medulla passing in relationship to the glossopharyngeal, vagus, spinal accessory, and hypoglossal nerves to reach the surface of the inferior cerebellar peduncle, where it dips into the cerebellomedullary fissure and terminates by supplying the suboccipital surface of the cerebellum.

Upper Neurovascular Complex

The most common operation directed through the posterior cranial fossa to the upper neurovascular complex is the exposure of the posterior root of the trigeminal nerve. The posterior trigeminal root joins the brain stem about halfway between the lower and upper borders of the pons (Figure 3).[14] Frequently, a lobule of cerebellum projects forward and obscures the course of the posterior root through the middle cerebellar peduncle into the pons. In its intradural course, the trigeminal nerve uniformly runs obliquely upward from the lateral part of the pons

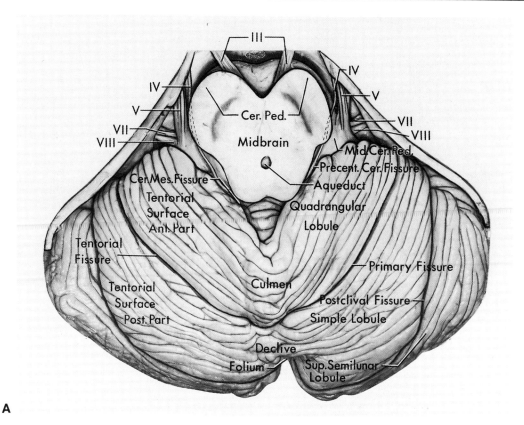

A

B

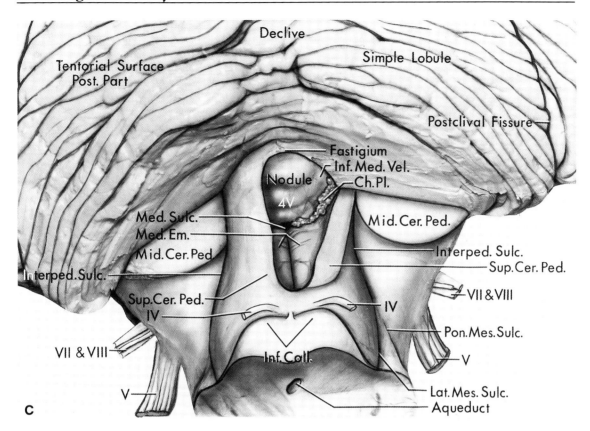

Figure 2A. *Superior views of the tentorial surface of the cerebellum and the cerebellomesencephalic fissure. The cerebellomesencephalic fissure (Cer. Mes. Fissure) extends downward between the midbrain and the cerebellum. It also has been called the precentral cerebellar fissure (Precent. Cer. Fissure). The traditional nomenclature applied to the vermian and hemispheric subdivisions of the tentorial surface is listed on the right, and the author's simplified nomenclature is listed on the left. The culmen and quadrangular lobules correspond to the anterior part (Ant. Part) of the tentorial surface, and the declive, simple lobule, and part of the superior semilunar lobule correspond to the posterior part (Post. Part) of the tentorial surface. The tentorial fissure, which also is called the primary fissure, separates the tentorial surface into anterior (Ant.) and posterior (Post.) parts. Other structures in the exposure include the oculomotor (III), trochlear (IV), trigeminal (V), facial (VII), and vestibulocochlear (VIII) nerves and the cerebral (Cer. Ped.) and middle cerebellar (Mid. Cer. Ped.) peduncles.*

Figure 2B. *Part of the cerebellum has been removed to expose the brain stem side of the cerebellomesencephalic fissure. This fissure extends inferiorly between the cerebellum and the roof of the fourth ventricle. The fissure has the inferior colliculi (Inf. Coll.), trochlear nerves, lingula of the vermis, and superior cerebellar peduncles (Sup. Cer. Ped.) on its anterior margin. Other structures include the lateral mesencephalic sulcus (Lat. Mes. Sulc.) and the middle cerebellar peduncle (Mid. Cer. Ped.).*

Figure 2C. *The left half of the roof of the fourth ventricle has been removed. The nodule and the inferior medullary velum (Inf. Med. Vel.) are seen in the inferior part of the fourth ventricle (4V). The choroid plexus (Ch. Pl.) projects into the ventricle from the tela choroidea. The median sulcus (Med. Sulc.) divides the floor longitudinally, and the medial eminences (Med. Em.) are longitudinal strips on either side of the median sulcus. Other structures include the pontomesencephalic (Pon. Mes. Sulc.) and interpeduncular (Interped. Sulc.) sulci.*

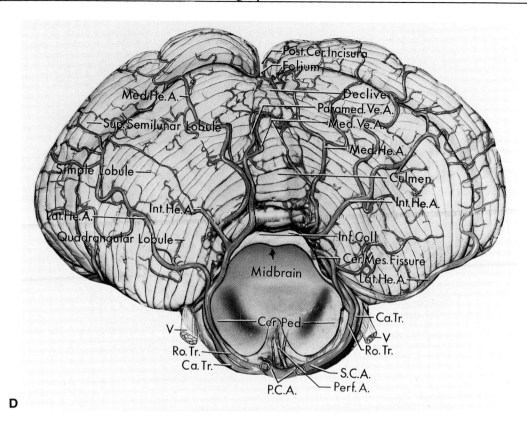

D

E

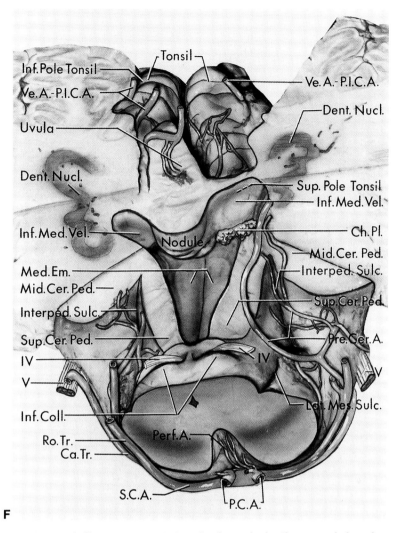

F

Figure 2D. *The superior cerebellar arteries (S.C.A.) arise from the basilar artery below the posterior cerebral arteries (P.C.A.) and supply the tentorial surface of the cerebellum. The SCAs bifurcate into rostral (Ro. Tr.) and caudal (Ca. Tr.) trunks. The rostral trunk supplies the vermis, and the caudal trunk passes to the hemispheric surface. The SCA's terminal branches are the lateral (Lat. He. A.), intermediate (Int. He. A.), and medial (Med. He. A.) hemispheric, and the median (Med. Ve. A.) and paramedian vermian (Paramed. Ve. A.) arteries. The posterior cerebellar incisura (Post. Cer. Incisura) is located at the posterior margin of the tentorial surface. Perforating arteries (Perf. A.) enter the interpeduncular fossa.*

Figure 2E. *Part of the cerebellum and the roof of the fourth ventricle have been removed to expose the SCA within the cerebellomesencephalic fissure. Precerebellar branches (Pre. Cer. A.) of the SCAs pass along the superior cerebellar peduncles (Sup. Cer. Ped.)*

Figure 2F. *The dorsal half of the cerebellum has been removed. The precerebellar arteries pass along the superior cerebellar peduncles to reach the dentate nuclei (Dent. Nucl.). The superior poles of the tonsils (Sup. Pole Tonsil) protrude into the roof of the fourth ventricle. The cerebellomedullary fissure extends upward between the tonsils and the inferior medullary velum. The dentate nuclei are located lateral to the superior pole of the tonsils. Other structures include the inferior pole of the tonsil (Inf. Pole Tonsil) and the vermian branches of the PICA (Ve. A.-P.I.C.A.).*[34]

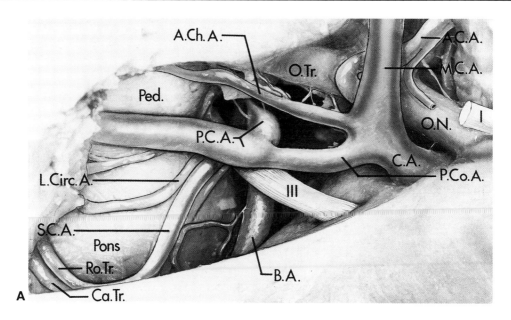

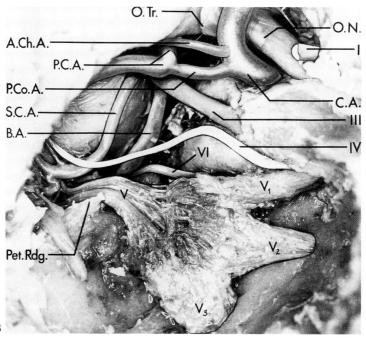

Figure 3A. *Right lateral views. The superior cerebellar artery (S.C.A.) arises from the basilar artery (B.A.) and dips below the free edge of the tentorium cerebelli. The rostral (Ro. Tr.) and caudal (Ca. Tr.) trunks arise near the free edge of the tentorium. Other structures in the exposure include the anterior (A.C.A.), middle (M.C.A.), and posterior cerebral (P.C.A.), posterior communicating (P. Co. A.), anterior choroidal (A. Ch. A.), long circumflex (L. Circ. A.) and carotid (C.A.) arteries; olfactory tract (I), optic (O.N.), and oculomotor (III) nerves; cerebral peduncle (Ped.); and optic tract (O. Tr.).*

Figure 3B. *The dura mater lining the middle fossa has been removed to show the caudal dip of the SCA toward the trigeminal nerve (V). Other structures in the exposure include the petrous ridge (Pet. Rdg.), ophthalmic (V₁), maxillary (V₂), and mandibular (V₃) divisions of the trigeminal nerve, and the abducens (VI) and trochlear (IV) nerves.*

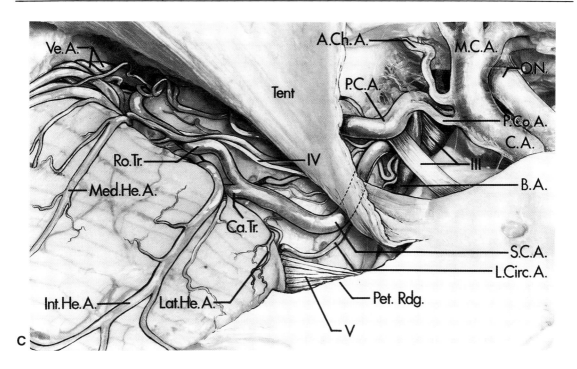

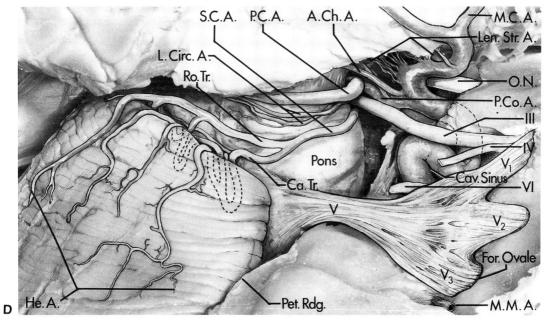

Figure 3C. Lateral view of another dissection with the lateral part of the tentorium cerebelli (Tent.) divided near the petrous ridge and elevated to expose the trigeminal and trochlear nerves. The rostral trunk gives rise to vermian (Ve. A.) and medial hemispheric (Med. He. A.) arteries; and the caudal trunk gives rise to intermediate (Int. He. A.) and lateral hemispheric (Lat. He. A.) arteries. (D) The tentorium has been removed in another specimen. The SCA passes around the brain stem above the trigeminal nerve. Other structures include the cavernous sinus (Cav. Sinus), middle meningeal (M.M.A.) and lenticulostriate (Len. Str. A) arteries, and foramen ovale (For. Ovale).[17]

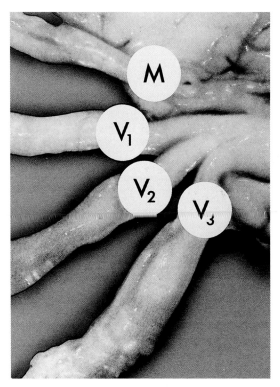

Figure 4. *Lateral view of the left trigeminal nerve at its junction with the pons. Each division was identified at the foramen of exit from the skull and the cleavage plane between the divisions was extended to the pons. In all dissections, the first-division fibers (V_1) entered the pons in the dorsomedial portion of the root and in a location adjacent to the motor root (M). The third-division fibers (V_3) were caudolateral with the second-division fibers (V_2) in an intermediate location.[14]*

toward the petrous apex. It exits the posterior fossa to enter the middle cranial fossa by passing forward beneath the tentorial attachment to enter Meckel's cave.

Trigeminal Root Anatomy

The fibers from the third division remain in a caudolateral position in the posterior root throughout the interval from the ganglion to the pons, the first division rostromedial, with second-division fibers in an intermediate position (Figures 4 and 5). Conclusions that the third-division fibers remain caudolateral and that the first-division fibers remain rostromedial from the pons to the ganglion agree with

data from clinical and laboratory studies.[6,10,40] There are anastomoses between the fibers from each division in the area posterior to the ganglion (Figure 6). Results of selective rhizotomy of the posterior root in human beings indicate that somatotopic localization with the third division inferolaterally and the ophthalmic division dorsomedially is well maintained posterior to, and despite the prominent retrogasserian anastomoses.[6]

A cross section of the sensory root between the pons and the petrous apex is elliptical. In most nerves, the angle between the longest diameter of this cross section and the long axis of the body is 40° to 50°; the angle, however, can vary from 10° to 80° (Figure 7).[14] An angle of 80° places the third-division fibers almost directly lateral to those of the first

Figure 5. *(Opposite page) Diagrams of 12 trigeminal nerves showing the relationship of the trigeminal sensory root, motor rootlets, and aberrant sensory rootlets at the site of entry into the pons. The central diagrams are for orientation and show the elliptical cross-section of the sensory root. The large ovals (A-F) represent the sensory root and are oriented in the same manner as the sensory root in the central diagram. The sites of origin of the motor rootlets are black. **Upper:** Nerves on the right. Only 5 motor rootlets are present in B, but 13 are seen in F. The aberrant sensory rootlets are shown by the dark outline with clear center. None are present in D and F. In C and E, some aberrant rootlets arose farther from the sensory root than some of the motor rootlets. **Lower:** Nerves on the left. Only 4 motor rootlets are present in A, but there are 10 in B and C. Aberrant sensory rootlets are shown by the dark outline with clear center. None are present in B and C. In A, D, E, and F, some aberrant rootlets arose farther from the sensory root than some of the motor rootlets.*

Lines through the oval representing the main sensory root show portions of the nerve from each of the three divisions. In all diagrams, the rostromedial portion was from the first division, the caudolateral portion was from the third division, and the second division was in an intermediate position. In all these nerves, except A and B in the left nerve, the second-division fibers made up a greater portion of the medial than the lateral portion of the sensory root. Small arteries or veins coursing between the rootlets at the level of entry into the pons are shown in all diagrams of both nerves except D in the right nerve (upper).[14]

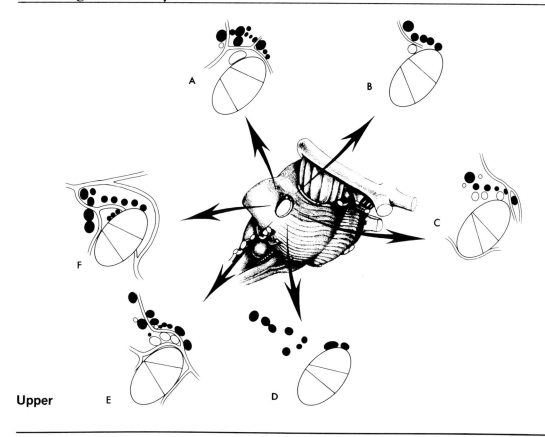

Upper

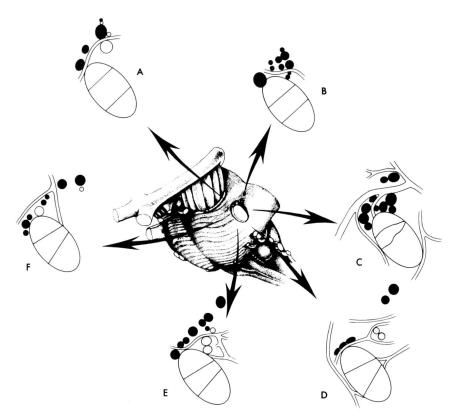

Lower

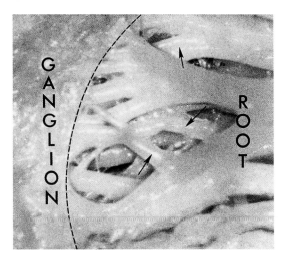

Figure 6. Magnified lateral view of the left trigeminal ganglion and root. The ganglion is to the left and the posterior root to the right. The dotted line marks the junction between the root and the ganglion. There are numerous anastomoses (arrows) between the filaments immediately posterior to the ganglion.[14]

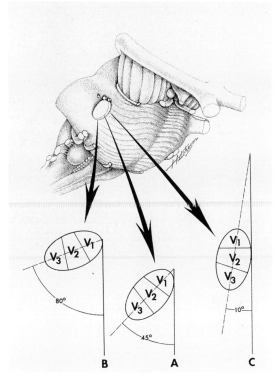

Figure 7. Variability of the longest axis of the elliptical cross section of the trigeminal nerve at the pons (broken line) to the longitudinal axis of the body (solid line). The long axis of most nerves makes a 40° to 50° angle with the longitudinal axis of the body (A); however, this can vary from 10° (C) to 80° (B). In B, the third division (V₃) is almost directly lateral to the first division (V₁), and in C, it is almost directly caudal.[14]

division; but an angle of 10° places the third-division fibers almost directly caudal to those of the first division. The variability in the degree of rotation of the sensory root entering the pons may explain some differences in the quantity of sensation retained after partial section of the nerve in the posterior cranial fossa. The most frequent pattern is for the third-division fibers to be caudolateral to the first-division fibers; some nerves, however, are rotated so that third-division fibers will be almost directly lateral to the first division; others are rotated nearly 70° away from this so that the third-division fibers will be directly caudal to those of the first division. Cutting into the nerve partially from a caudolateral direction would give a significantly different pattern of sensory loss if the nerve is rotated with the third division lateral to the first, than if the third division is almost directly caudal to the first division.

At the junction of the nerve with the pons, as many as 15 separate nerve rootlets may be spread around the rostral half of the site where the main sensory cone enters the pons.[14] These rootlets are either motor or aberrant sensory rootlets. The aberrant sensory fibers are small rootlets that penetrate

the pons outside the main sensory root (Figures 8 and 9). The aberrant rootlets arise around the rostral two-thirds of the nerve and usually join the root a short distance from the brain stem. There may be as many as eight aberrant roots. Those arising rostral to the sensory root most frequently enter the first division and those arising more caudally enter the second or third division. No aberrant rootlets originate around the caudal third of the sensory root. Of 66 aberrant rootlets found in our study of 50 trigeminal nerves, 49 went into the first division, 10 into the second division, and 7 into the third division.[14] The findings that aberrant rootlets are most commonly related to the first division agree with Dandy's conclu-

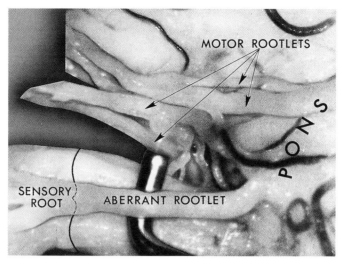

Figure 8. Lateral view of the left trigeminal nerve. A nerve hook is between the large aberrant sensory rootlet and the main sensory root. An aberrant rootlet arises from the pons directly lateral to the sensory root and joins the sensory root about 1 cm from the brain stem. Four motor rootlets are seen above the sensory root.[14]

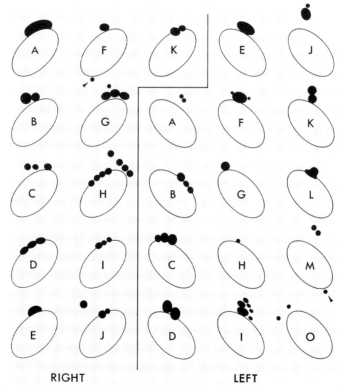

Figure 9. Origin of the aberrant sensory rootlets in relation to the main sensory root. The large, clear oval represents a cross section of the sensory root at the level of entry into the pons. Origin of aberrant rootlets is in solid black. All nerves to the left of the solid line are from the right side and are oriented the same as the nerves shown in Figure 5 (Upper). Those to the right of the line are from the left side and are oriented as shown in Figure 5 (Lower). The rootlet origin shown with the arrow below F (Right) goes with sensory root G, and the rootlet origin shown with the arrow below M (Left) goes with sensory root O. The rostral margin of the root is superior and the caudal margin is inferior on the diagrams. No aberrant sensory root originated caudal to the main sensory root.[14]

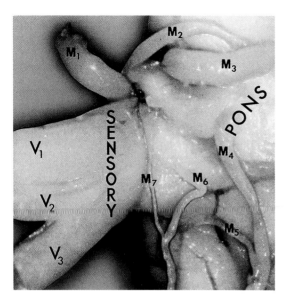

Figure 10. *Lateral view of the left trigeminal nerve at the level of entry into the pons. Seven different motor rootlets (M_{1-7}) joined to form the motor root and have been divided and reflected to show their separate sites of exit from the pons. M_{1-3} are rostral to the sensory root. M_{4-7} are lateral. The sensory root and fibers from each division are labeled appropriately. Most motor root fibers arise near the first division (V_1), but some arise in a more lateral or caudal location.*[14]

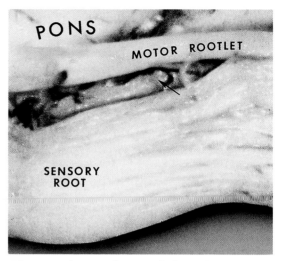

Figure 11A. *Lateral view of the right trigeminal nerve near its junction with the pons. The arrow points to the intermediate group of fibers between the motor rootlet and the sensory root.*

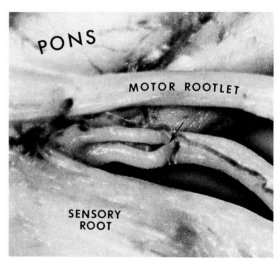

Figure 11B. *The same trigeminal nerve. The arrow points to intermediate fibers that proved to be a motor rootlet when traced distally. This illustrates the difficulty in telling whether an intermediate group of fibers is motor or sensory unless the nerve bundles can be separated and examined individually.*[14]

sion that when the accessory fibers are spared, sensation in the first division tends to be spared.[6] The aberrant rootlets appear to be nonspecific sensory fibers separated from the root by transverse pontine fibers.[14,58] Aberrant roots contribute mainly to the first division and probably do not convey a specific sensory modality from all three divisions.

Motor rootlets also arise around the rostral part of the nerve; however, they tend to arise further from the main sensory cone than do the accessory sensory rootlets. The motor root may be composed of 4-14 separate rootlets, each having a separate exit from the pons (Figures 5, 10, and 11).[14] The aberrant sensory fibers usually arise closer to the main sensory root than to the motor fibers. Some aberrant sensory fibers, however, will arise further from the main sensory root than does the origin of some motor filaments; for this reason, it is easy to confuse

aberrant sensory fibers and motor filaments at the nerve/pons junction.

Anastomoses between the motor and sensory roots are present in most nerves (Figure 12). Those sensory fibers associated with the motor root from the pons to just proximal to

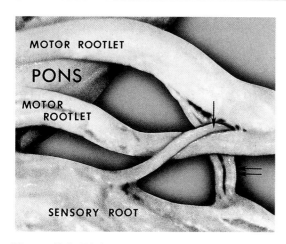

Figure 12A. Right sensory root below and motor rootlets above, showing anastomosis between the motor and sensory components. One rootlet (single arrow) actually leaves the sensory root and passes around the lower motor rootlet and back (double arrows) to the sensory root.

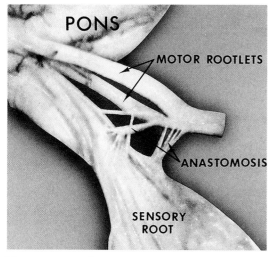

Figure 12B. Right trigeminal nerve showing complex anastomoses between the motor rootlet and the sensory root.[14]

the ganglion, where they anastomose with the sensory root, would be spared with a rhizotomy in the posterior fossa. Horsley et al[19] suspected that there were sensory fibers in the trigeminal motor root, and Adson implied this by suggesting that the motor root be sectioned if trigeminal neuralgia recurred after the complete section of the sensory root

(personal communication from Baker GS. 1969). Our studies offer two explanations for the accidental preservation of sensation after posterior rhizotomy: (1) sparing of the aberrant sensory rootlets and (2) sparing of the anastomotic sensory fibers that run with the motor root at the level of the rhizotomy.[14] Anastomosis is a more likely explanation for the accidental sensory preservation and recurrence of trigeminal neuralgia after the section of the posterior root because anastomotic rootlets are present throughout the interval from the pons to the ganglion. Aberrant sensory roots are present in only one-half of the nerves. They provide another explanation for the preservation of sensation following the section of the main sensory root.

Anatomy of Vascular Compression in the Upper Neurovascular Complex

In 1934, Dandy postulated that arterial compression and distortion of the trigeminal nerve might be the cause of trigeminal neuralgia.[7] He described the SCA as affecting the nerve in 30.7% of his 215 cases of trigeminal neuralgia. The vascular compression theory failed to gain acceptance at the time, but it awaited the better demonstration of these pathologic changes at surgery by Jannetta[23,25,26] using magnification provided by the operating microscope.

This author approaches the upper complex for a vascular decompression operation with the patient in the three-quarter prone position.[49] The surgeon should be positioned at the top of the head for approaching the upper neurovascular complex rather than behind the head as is common when approaching the middle and lower neurovascular complex (Figure 13). The vertical scalp incision crosses the asterion, which marks the junction of the transverse and sigmoid sinuses. The bone opening, which is approximately 3 cm in diameter, exposes the edge of the junction of the sigmoid and transverse sinuses in its superolateral margin. The cerebellum is relaxed by opening the arachnoid

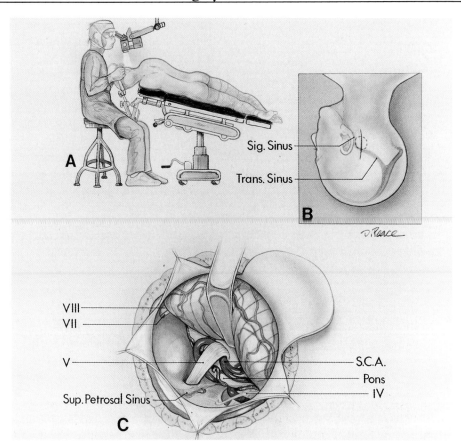

Figure 13. *Retrosigmoid approach to the trigeminal nerve for a microvascular decompression operation. (A) (Upper left) The patient is positioned in the three-quarter prone position. The surgeon is seated at the head of the table. The table is tilted so that the feet are lower than the heart. (B) The vertical paramedian incision crosses the asterion. The superolateral margin of the craniectomy is positioned at the junction of the transverse (Trans. Sinus) and sigmoid (Sig. Sinus) sinuses. (C) The superolateral margin of the cerebellum is gently elevated using a brain spatula tapered from 10 mm at the base to 3 or 5 mm at the tip to expose the site at which the trigeminal (V) nerve enters the pons. The brain spatula is advanced and aligned parallel to the superior petrosal sinus (Sup. Petrosal Sinus). The trochlear (IV) nerve is at the superior margin of the exposure and the facial (VII) and vestibulocochlear (VIII) nerves are at the lower margin. The dura is tacked up to the adjacent muscles to maximize the exposure along the superolateral margin of the cerebellum. The main trunk of the superior cerebellar artery (S.C.A.) loops down into the axilla of the trigeminal nerve.*[49]

and removing cerebrospinal fluid from the cisterns. A brain spatula, tapered from 10 mm at the base to 3 or 5 mm at the tip, is introduced parallel and just below the superior petrosal sinus to elevate the superolateral margin of the cerebellum (Figures 13 and 14). A bridging petrosal vein, which blocks access to the trigeminal nerve, is coagulated with gentle bipolar coagulation and divided

nearer its junction with the brain than to the superior petrosal sinus. Unexpected bleeding, encountered as the superolateral margin of the cerebellum is elevated, usually is related to stretching and tearing of the veins that pass from the superior surface of the cerebellum to the venous sinus in the tentorium or to tearing of the subarcuate branch of the AICA behind the internal auditory canal at

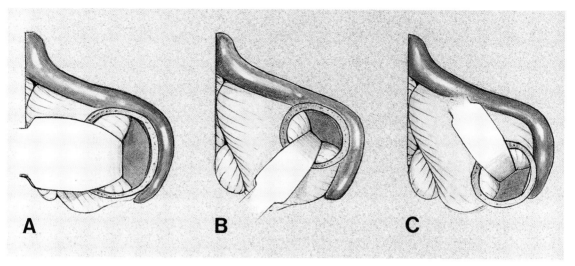

Figure 14. *Direction of the application of brain spatulas for surgery in the various compartments of the cerebellopontine angle (CPA). (A) Lateral exposure for a lesion in the midportion of the CPA such as an acoustic neuroma. The site of the craniectomy below the transverse sinus and medial to the sigmoid sinus is shown for removing an acoustic neuroma or other lesion involving multiple neurovascular complexes. The spatula protects the lateral surface of the cerebellum. A brain spatula tapered from 20 or 25 mm at the base to 15 or 20 mm at the tip is commonly used during acoustic neuroma removal. (B) Spatula application for exposing the upper neurovascular complex for a microvascular decompression operation for trigeminal neuralgia. A spatula tapered from 10 mm at the base to 3 or 5 mm at the tip is commonly selected. The spatula is placed parallel to the superior petrosal sinus. (C) Retractor application for the exposure of the lower neurovascular complex. This approach also is used in hemifacial spasm because the nerve root exit zone of the facial nerve is located only a few millimeters above the glossopharyngeal nerve and the PICA is commonly the compressing vessel. A brain spatula tapered from 10 mm at the base to 3 or 5 mm at the tip is commonly used for operations for hemifacial spasm.[51]*

its site of penetration of the dura covering the subarcuate fossa. The trochlear nerve is identified before opening the arachnoid behind the trigeminal nerve because it may be difficult to see the nerve after the arachnoid has been opened and shrinks into thick white clumps that may hide the nerve. Usually, the trochlear nerve is several millimeters above the trigeminal nerve; it may be carried downward, however, if it is adherent to a segment of the SCA that has looped into the axilla of the trigeminal nerve. The overhanging lip of the cerebellum must be retracted gently to expose the junction of the nerve with the pons. The identification and naming of the vessel compressing the nerve requires an understanding of the arterial and venous anatomy in the area. In the microvascular decompression operation, the offending vessel is displaced away from the trigeminal

nerve and the separation is maintained with a small prosthesis.

Arterial Relationships

The most common finding at a vascular decompression operation for trigeminal neuralgia is a segment of the SCA compressing the trigeminal nerve.[44,45,49] Normally, the SCA encircles the brain stem above the trigeminal nerve[16,17] (Figures 3 and 15). The SCA arises near the apex of the basilar artery. It passes below the oculomotor and trochlear nerves and above the trigeminal nerve. Its proximal portion courses medial to the free edge of the tentorium. Its distal segment passes below the tentorium to reach the tentorial surface of the cerebellum. After passing above the trigeminal nerve, it enters the cerebellomesencephalic fissure, the groove between the

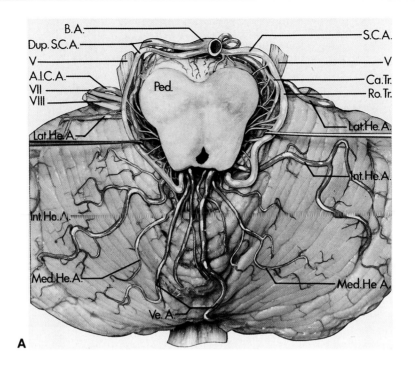

A

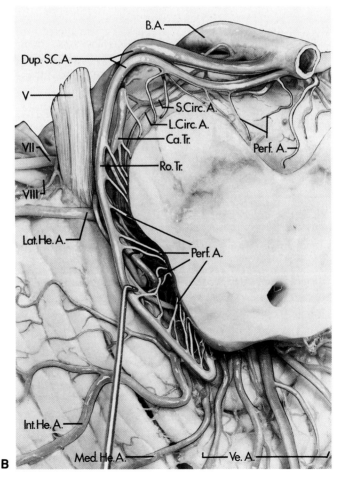

B

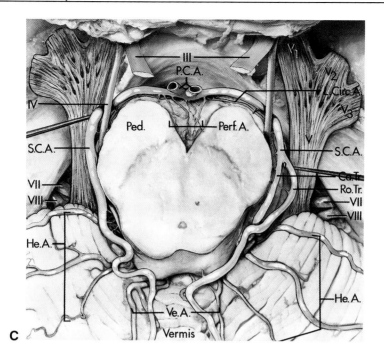

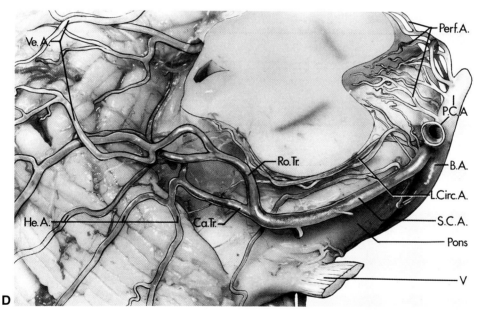

Figure 15. (A) Superior view. The left superior cerebellar artery (S.C.A.) arises from the basilar artery (B.A.) as a duplicate artery (Dup. S.C.A.). The right SCA bifurcates into rostral (Ro. Tr.) and caudal (Ca. Tr.) trunks medial to the trigeminal nerve (V). The cerebellum is supplied by the lateral (Lat. He. A.), intermediate (Int. He. A.), and medial (Med. He. A.) hemispheric, and vermian (Ve. A.) arteries. The SCAs give rise to multiple perforating arteries that enter the cerebral peduncles (Ped.) and the brain stem. The left anterior inferior cerebellar artery (A.I.C.A.) passes below the facial (VII) and vestibulocochlear (VIII) nerves. (B) Enlarged view of 15A shows the direct (Perf. A.), and long (L. Circ. A.), and short (S. Circ. A.) circumflex perforating arteries arising from the duplicate SCA. (C) Superior view. The SCAs pass below the oculomotor (III) and trochlear (IV) nerves and bifurcate above the trigeminal (V) nerves. Other structures include the posterior cerebral arteries (P.C.A.) and the ophthalmic (V_1), maxillary (V_2), and mandibular (V_3) divisions of the trigeminal nerve. (D) Superolateral view. Rostral and caudal trunks arise from the main trunk above the trigeminal (V) nerve.[17]

midbrain and the cerebellum (Figures 2 and 15). Its branches make several sharp turns to leave this fissure and are distributed to the tentorial surface of the cerebellum. The SCA gives off perforating arteries that penetrate the interpeduncular fossa, cerebral peduncle, and colliculi. The perforating vessels may limit the degree of repositioning of the artery achievable in a microvascular decompression operation.

The SCA commonly arises as a single main trunk at the basilar artery. The main trunk bifurcates on the side of the brain stem into a rostral trunk, which supplies the vermis, and a caudal trunk, which supplies the hemisphere. At times, the rostral and caudal trunks arise directly from the basilar artery, giving the SCA a duplicate origin (Figures 15A, B).

In adults, the SCA commonly makes a shallow, caudal loop and courses inferiorly for a variable distance on the lateral side of the pons (Figures 3, 13, and 15). In those cases with the most prominent caudally projecting loop, contact between the artery and the trigeminal nerve occurs. The point of contact with the SCA is usually on the superior or supermedial aspect of the nerve; and often a few fascicles of the nerve are distorted by an SCA that has looped down into the axilla between the medial side of the nerve and the pons (Figure 16). An arterial loop in the axilla may not be visible from the surgeon's view behind the trigeminal nerve if the SCA courses around the brain stem directly in front of the nerve. The loop of the SCA also may be difficult to see if the artery passes over the rostral aspect of the nerve very close to the brain stem, where it may be hidden by the overhanging lip of the cerebellum. The loop of the SCA may be seen dangling below the lower margin of the nerve, even though it is not visible above the nerve. These loops of the SCA, however, always pass rostrally along the medial and superior surfaces of the nerve to reach the fissure between the cerebellum and pons. The medial axilla of the nerve must be carefully explored with a teardrop dissector before concluding

that there is no arterial loop in the axilla of the nerve. It is important to remember that the trunks do not pass directly from the side of the brain stem to the superior surface of the cerebellum, but, rather, that they dip into the deep fissure between the cerebellum and midbrain at the posterior margin of the trigeminal nerve. The rostral and caudal trunks of the SCA loop deeply into this fissure and proceed to give branches to the superior cerebellar peduncle and dentate nucleus before reaching the tentorial surface of the cerebellum.

In the author's operative series, the most common site of compression of the trigeminal nerve on the SCA is at the junction of the main trunk with the origin of the rostral and caudal trunks (Figures 16, 17, and 18).[49] Other sites of compression are seen, however, depending on how far distal the artery bifurcates in relation to the trigeminal nerve. If the SCA bifurcates near the basilar artery or if there is a duplicate configuration in which the rostral and caudal trunks arise directly from the basilar artery, both trunks may loop down into the axilla and compress the nerve (Figure 16). Alternatively, if the artery bifurcates before reaching the nerve, the caudal trunk may compress the nerve and the rostral trunk may course well above the nerve. If the artery bifurcates distal to the nerve, only the main trunk will be involved in the compression. The point of bifurcation of the SCA does affect the caliber of the vessel that makes contact with the nerve. The contacting vessel will be of a smaller caliber if the SCA bifurcates before reaching the trigeminal nerve.

A less frequent source of compression of the trigeminal nerve is by the AICA (Figures 16-18). Jannetta, in 100 patients with trigeminal neuralgia, found 4 cases in which the AICA indented the inferior surface of the nerve root.[23,25,26] Normally, the AICA passes around the pons below the trigeminal nerve with the facial and vestibulocochlear nerves. The AICA, however, may have a high origin and loop upward to indent the medial or lower surface of the trigeminal nerve prior to passing downward to course with the facial and vestibulocochlear nerves. A serpentine

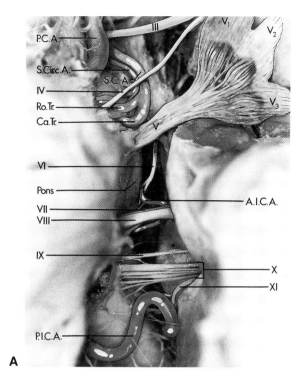

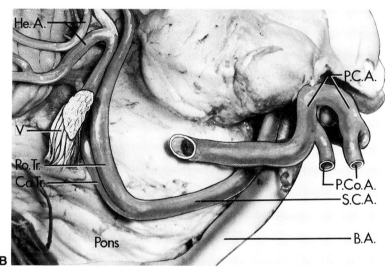

Figure 16A & B. *Relationship of the superior cerebellar artery to the trigeminal nerve. (A) Right posterior view. The rostral (Ro. Tr.) and caudal (Ca. Tr.) trunks and the short circumflex branch (S. Circ. A.) of the superior cerebellar artery (S.C.A.) pass above the trigeminal nerve (V). The oculomotor (III) and trochlear (IV) nerves pass between the SCA and the posterior cerebral artery (P.C.A.). Other structures include the abducens (VI), facial (VII), vestibulocochlear (VIII), glossopharyngeal (IX), vagus (X), and spinal accessory (XI) nerves; ophthalmic (V₁), maxillary (V₂), and mandibular (V₃) divisions; and anterior inferior cerebellar (A.I.C.A.) and posterior inferior cerebellar (P.I.C.A.) arteries. (B) Right lateral view. The SCA arises from the basilar artery (B.A.) and bifurcates into rostral and caudal trunks. The trunks loop caudally to reach the supermedial edge of the trigeminal root entry zone. Other structures include the posterior communicating (P. Co. A.) and hemispheric (He. A.) arteries.*

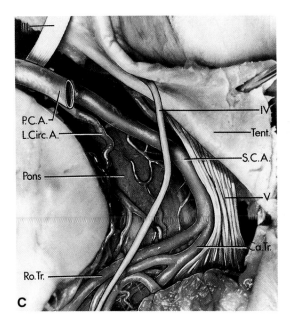
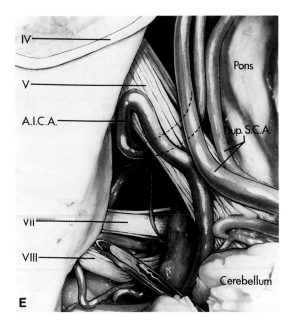

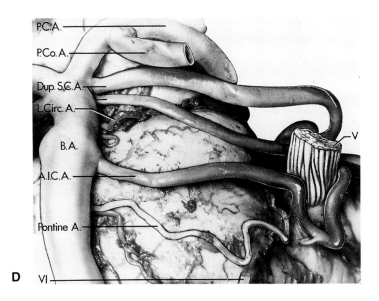

Figure 16C-E. *(C)* *The tentorium cerebelli (Tent.) has been divided to expose the trigeminal nerve. The junction of the main trunk with the rostral and caudal trunks indents the medial side of the nerve. A long circumflex artery (L. Circ. A.) encircles the brain stem. (D) Anterior view of a left trigeminal nerve that has points of contact on its superior surface with a duplicate SCA (Dup. S.C.A.) and on its inferior surface with the AICA. A pontine artery (Pontine A.) arises from the basilar artery. (E) Superior view of the trigeminal nerve shown in D surrounded by a duplicate SCA and an AICA (dotted line).[17]*

basilar artery also may wander laterally and compress the medial side of the trigeminal nerve.[57] This type of basilar artery often is elongated and has a fusiform configuration. More than one artery may compress the nerve. In a few cases, the SCA will compress the rostral surface of the nerve and the AICA will compress the caudal surface. Infrequently, the PICA may reach and groove the undersurface of the trigeminal nerve. The trigeminal nerve also may be compressed by a large pontine branch of the basilar artery

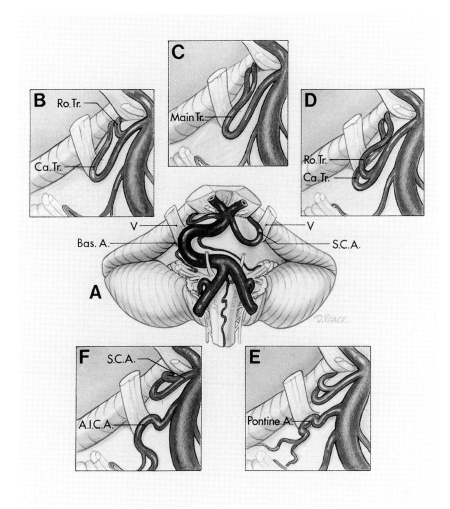

Figure 17. Sites of arterial compression of the trigeminal nerve. Orientation as shown in the central diagram. (A) Central diagram. The right trigeminal nerve (V) is compressed by a tortuous basilar artery (Bas. A.) and the left trigeminal nerve is compressed by the main trunk of the superior cerebellar artery (S.C.A.). (B) The SCA bifurcates into rostral (Ro. Tr.) and caudal (Ca. Tr.) trunks prior to reaching the trigeminal nerve. The nerve is compressed by the caudal trunk. (C) The SCA bifurcates distally to the nerve. The nerve is compressed by the main trunk (Main Tr.). (D) The SCA bifurcates prior to reaching the nerve. The nerve is compressed by both the rostral and caudal trunks. (E) The nerve is compressed by a large pontine artery (Pontine A.). (F) The nerve is compressed by an anterior inferior cerebellar artery (A.I.C.A.) that has a high origin and loops upward into the medial surface of the nerve. The SCA passes around the brain stem above the nerve.[49]

(Figures 17 and 18). Normally, these pontine branches pass around and penetrate the pons before reaching the trigeminal nerve. A large pontine artery, however, may indent the medial surface of the trigeminal nerve and then course rostral or caudal to the nerve

to supply the pons behind the nerve.

In a previous study of 50 cadaveric trigeminal nerves, we found that 26 had a point of contact with the SCA in the posterior cranial fossa.[16] In the 26 nerves having a point of contact with the SCA, the segment of the

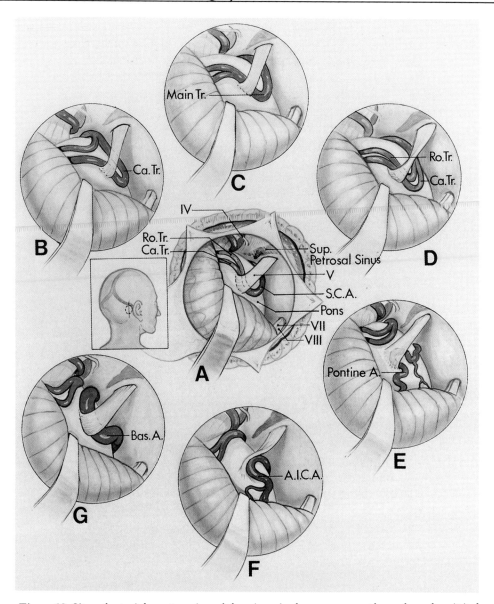

Figure 18. Sites of arterial compression of the trigeminal nerve as seen through a suboccipital craniectomy. *(A)* Central diagram. The site of the skin incision (solid line) and the craniectomy (interrupted line) are shown in the insert. The superolateral margin of the cerebellum is gently retracted to expose the trigeminal nerve (V) and the superior cerebellar artery (S.C.A.). The brain spatula is advanced parallel to the superior petrosal sinus (Sup. Petrosal Sinus). The trochlear nerve (IV) is at the superior margin of the exposure and the facial (VII) and vestibulocochlear (VIII) nerves are at the lower margin. The trigeminal nerve is compressed by a loop of the SCA that dangles down into the axilla of the nerve. The site of compression on the artery is at the junction of the main trunk with the rostral (Ro. Tr.) and caudal (Ca. Tr.) trunks. *(B)* The nerve is compressed by the caudal trunk. *(C)* The nerve is compressed by the main trunk (Main Tr.). *(D)* Compression by both the rostral and caudal trunks. *(E)* Compression by a pontine branch of the basilar artery. *(F)* Compression by the anterior inferior cerebellar artery (A.I.C.A.). *(G)* Compression by a tortuous basilar artery.[49]

SCA involved was the main trunk before its bifurcation in 8, the caudal trunk distal to the bifurcation in 11, the rostral trunk in 2, both the rostral and caudal trunk in 4, and a hemispheric branch of the caudal trunk in 1. In that study, the site of vascular contact was commonly a few millimeters peripheral to the point of entry of the nerve into the pons (average 3.7 mm) rather than at the root entry zone as is seen in most of our cases with trigeminal neuralgia. In 1 cadaveric specimen, the vascular contact was more than 1 cm from the pons. In 6 of the 50 cadaveric nerves, the contact occurred at the pontine root entry zone of the trigeminal nerve, usually by an arterial loop tucked into the axilla between the pons and the medial side of the nerve. Jannetta[23,25,26] stated that an association with trigeminal neuralgia occurs most frequently if the contact is at the root entry zone. The main trunk of the AICA also impinged on 4 of the 50 cadaveric trigeminal nerves that were examined, and in 3 of these, there was also a point of contact between the nerve and the SCA. One nerve also was contacted on its superior surface by the SCA and on its inferior surface by both trunks of a duplicated AICA.

Any study of cadaveric specimens must be of limited value in discussing the etiology of a pain-producing condition such as trigeminal neuralgia, but the fact that some degree of neurovascular contact occurs in at least one-half of the cadaveric specimens makes it possible that vascular compression and distortion of the trigeminal nerve may be important in its etiology. Not all of these neurovascular contacts seen in our anatomic studies produced distortion of the nerve or occurred at the sensory root entry zone, which Jannetta[23,25,26] postulated as a prerequisite for the production of trigeminal neuralgia. An equally reasonable conclusion to draw from the study, however, is that the high incidence of neurovascular contact in these specimens from a "nontic" population may mean that the findings of such neurovascular contacts at the operation is coincidental. In that case, the relief of pain that commonly follows the decompressive procedure must be achieved by some mechanism other than simple relief of the vascular compression.

Venous Relationships

Exposure of the trigeminal nerve through a suboccipital craniectomy commonly requires the sacrifice of one or more bridging veins, while exposure of the nerves entering the internal acoustic meatus infrequently requires sacrifice of a bridging vein (Figures 19 and 20).[33] The infrequent reports of adverse sequelae following intraoperative occlusion of veins in the posterior fossa probably is due to the diffuse anastomoses between the veins. However, we have seen two patients with transient cerebellar disturbance caused by venous infarction with hemorrhagic edema following the intraoperative occlusion of the veins above the trigeminal nerve.

Compression and distortion of the trigeminal nerve by the surrounding veins, although less frequent than arterial compression, also is found in trigeminal neuralgia[2,15,26] (Figures 21 and 22). The terminal end of the veins draining the brain stem and cerebellum form bridging veins that collect into three groups: (1) a galenic group that drains into the vein of Galen; (2) a petrosal group that drains into the petrosal sinuses; and (3) a tentorial group that drains into the tentorial sinuses converging on the torcula. The petrosal group is most frequently encountered in operative approaches to the trigeminal nerve in the posterior cranial fossa.[33] The petrosal veins drain the lateral part of the cerebellar hemisphere, much of the brain stem, and the walls of the fissures between the cerebellum and the brain stem. The petrosal veins also most commonly compress the trigeminal nerve.

The petrosal veins are divided into superior and inferior petrosal veins based on whether they enter the superior or inferior petrosal sinus. The superior petrosal veins are encountered in approaches to the trigeminal nerve and may compress the nerve. The superior petrosal veins are among the largest

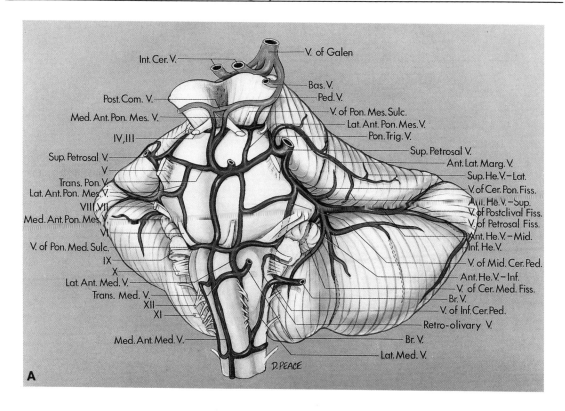

A

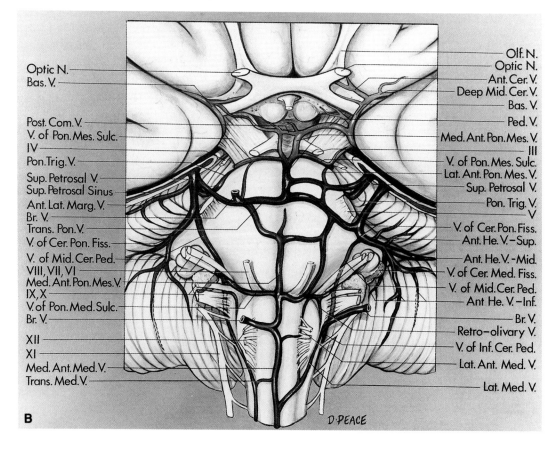

B

Figure 19. (Opposite page) Venous relationships of the trigeminal nerve. (A) Anterolateral view.(B) Anterior view. (A & B) The superior petrosal veins (Sup. Petrosal V.) converge on the superior petrosal sinus (Sup. Petrosal Sinus). The veins that commonly compress the trigeminal nerve (V) are tributaries of the superior petrosal veins. The most common veins to compress the nerve are the transverse pontine veins (Trans. Pon. V.) that course transversely on the anterior surface of the pons; the vein of the cerebellopontine fissure (V. of Cer. Pon. Fiss.) that drains the anterior surface of the cerebellum and ascends behind the trigeminal nerve; the vein of the middle cerebellar peduncle (V. of Mid. Cer. Ped.) that arises on the lower pons and ascends on the middle cerebellar peduncle; and the pontotrigeminal vein (Pon. Trig. V.) that exits the fissure between the midbrain and the cerebellum and passes above the trigeminal nerve. Other veins in the illustration include the internal cerebral (Int. Cer. V.), basal (Bas. V.), peduncular (Ped. V.), posterior communicating (Post. Com. V.), lateral anterior pontomesencephalic (Lat. Ant. Pon. Mes. V.), median anterior pontomesencephalic (Med. Ant. Pon. Mes. V.), anterior lateral marginal (Ant. Lat. Marg. V.), anterior hemispheric (Ant. He. V.), bridging (Br. V.), retro-olivary (Retro-olivary V), lateral medullary (Lat. Med. V.), lateral anterior medullary (Lat. Ant. Med. V.), median anterior medullary (Med. Ant. Med. V.), transverse medullary (Trans. Med. V.), anterior cerebral (Ant. Cer. V.), and deep middle cerebral (Deep Med. Cer. V.) veins and the veins of the postclival fissure (V. of Postclival Fiss.), petrosal fissure (V. of Petrosal Fiss), cerebellomedullary fissure (V. of Cer. Med. Fiss.), inferior cerebellar peduncle (V. of Inf. Cer. Ped.), pontomedullary sulcus (V. of Pon. Med. Sulc.), pontomesencephalic sulcus (V. of Pon. Mes. Sulc.), and the vein of Galen (V. of Galen). Other structures include the olfactory (Olf. N.), optic (Optic N.), oculomotor (III), trochlear (IV), abducens (VI), facial (VII), vestibulocochlear (VIII), glossopharyngeal (IX), vagus (X), spinal accessory (XI), and hypoglossal (XII) nerves.[33]

and most frequently encountered veins in the posterior fossa. The superior petrosal veins may be formed by the terminal segment of a single vein or by the common stem formed by the union of several veins. The most common tributaries of the superior petrosal veins are the transverse pontine and ponto-trigeminal veins, the veins of the cerebello-pontine fissure and the middle cerebellar peduncle, and the common stem of the veins draining the lateral part of the cerebellar hemisphere (Figures 19-22). The transverse pontine veins are the most frequent veins to compress the trigeminal nerve. They course transversely on the pons and pass above or below the trigeminal nerve to reach the bridging veins entering the superior petrosal sinus. They may course medially in the axilla of the nerve or they also may pass above, below, or lateral to the nerve and indent its upper, lower, or lateral surface. The vein of the middle cerebellar peduncle arises just above the facial nerve on the lower pons. It ascends on the pons and middle cerebellar peduncle and may compress the lateral or medial surface of the trigeminal nerve before joining the petrosal veins. The vein of the cerebellopontine fissure arises in the groove between the cerebellum and the pons and ascends posteriorly to the trigeminal nerve to join the vein of the middle cerebellar ped-

uncle and the transverse pontine veins prior to entering the superior petrosal sinus. The vein of the cerebellopontine fissure may indent the lateral margin of the trigeminal nerve as it ascends toward the superior petrosal sinus. The pontotrigeminal vein arises in the fissure between the cerebellum and the midbrain and passes above the trigeminal nerve to join the superior petrosal vein. The pontotrigeminal vein also may indent the upper margin of the nerve.

The junction of these veins, which converge and form a single trunk prior to entering the superior petrosal sinus, usually is lateral to the trigeminal nerve. This junction, however, may be located medial to the trigeminal nerve, in which case the common trunk must pass around the trigeminal nerve prior to reaching the superior petrosal sinus. These common trunks also may compress the trigeminal nerve.

Anatomy and Instrumentation

The anatomy of the area dictates the length and tip size of the instruments needed to complete a retrosigmoid operation on the trigeminal nerve while minimizing the damage to adjacent areas.[51] Exposing the trigeminal nerve requires the use of bayonet forceps

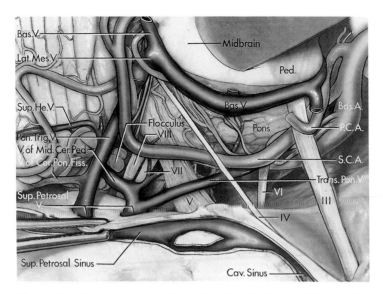

Figure 20A. *Venous relationships of the trigeminal nerve. (A) Superior view of the veins and arteries near the right trigeminal nerve. The superior cerebellar artery (S.C.A.) arises from the basilar artery (Bas. A.) and passes around the brain stem above the trigeminal nerve (V). The posterior cerebral artery (P.C.A.) and the basal vein (Bas. V.) course above the trochlear (IV) and oculomotor (III) nerves. Veins in the region of the trigeminal nerve include the transverse pontine (Trans. Pon. V.) and pontotrigeminal (Pon. Trig. V.) veins and the veins of the cerebellopontine fissure (V. of Cer. Pon. Fiss.) and middle cerebellar peduncle (V. of Mid. Cer. Ped.). The superior petrosal veins (Sup. Petrosal V.) empty into the superior petrosal sinus (Sup. Petrosal Sinus). Other structures in the exposure include the cavernous sinus (Cav. Sinus), cerebral peduncle (Ped.), superior hemispheric (Sup. He. V.) and lateral mesencephalic (Lat. Mes. V.) veins, and the abducens (VI), facial (VII), and vestibulocochlear (VIII) nerves.*

and scissors that have 9.5-cm shafts (Figure 23). A bipolar bayonet forceps with 9.5-cm shafts and 0.7-cm tips is used for coagulation of the petrosal veins and in the superficial intradural portion of the operation. The bipolar bayonet forceps with 9.5-cm shafts and 0.5-cm tips is used for gentle bipolar coagulation, if needed, along the brain stem or in the region around the trigeminal nerve. A small spatula dissector or a ball dissector with a 40° angle and a teardrop configuration at the tip is selected for separating the vessel and the nerve and for fitting the small prosthesis into the appropriate location. Avoid using a right-angle hook in the depths of the CPA because the hook may inadvertently catch and avulse a perforating vessel. Forty-

degree-angled dissectors are preferred for this area because they tend to slip off a perforating vessel without avulsing it. A series of tapered brain spatulas are used for elevating the cerebellum. The most commonly selected spatula for a microvascular decompression operation has a width of 10 mm at its base and tapers to 3 or 5 mm at the tip.

Middle Neurovascular Complex

The middle complex includes the AICA, pons, middle cerebellar peduncle, cerebellopontine fissure, petrosal surface of the cerebellum, and the abducens, facial, and vestibulocochlear nerves (Figure 1). The AICA arises

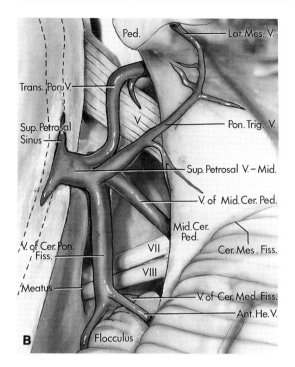
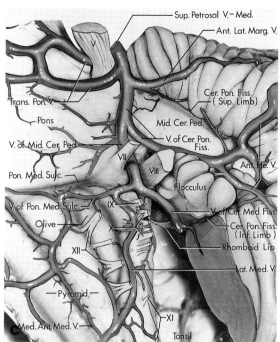

Figure 20B & C. Superior view. Left side. A large superior petrosal vein that empties into the midportion of the superior petrosal sinus is formed by the union of the transverse pontine and pontotrigeminal veins and the veins of the middle cerebellar peduncle and cerebellopontine fissure. Other structures in the exposure include the anterior hemispheric vein (Ant. He. V.) and the veins of the cerebellomedullary fissure (V. of Cer. Med. Fiss.) and middle cerebellar peduncle (V. of Mid. Cer. Ped.). (C) Anterolateral view of the left side of the brain stem and cerebellum. The transverse pontine (Trans. Pon. V.) and anterior lateral marginal (Ant. Lat. Marg. V.) veins and the veins of the cerebellopontine fissure and middle cerebellar peduncle converge on the region of the trigeminal nerve to form a superior petrosal vein that empties into the medial part of the superior petrosal sinus. Other structures in the exposure include the glossopharyngeal (IX), vagus (X), spinal accessory (XI), and hypoglossal (XII) nerves; the pontomedullary sulcus (Pon. Med. Sulc.); the cerebellopontine fissure (Cer. Pon. Fiss.); the median anterior medullary (Med. Ant. Med. V.) and lateral medullary (Lat. Med. V.) veins; and the vein of the pontomedullary sulcus (V. of Pon. Med. Sulc.). The cerebellopontine fissure (Cer. Pon. Fiss.) has superior (Sup. Limb) and inferior (Inf. Limb) limbs.[33]

at the pontine level, courses in relationship to the abducens, facial, and vestibulocochlear nerves to reach the surface of the middle cerebellar peduncle, where it courses along the cerebellopontine fissure and terminates by supplying the petrosal surface of the cerebellum (Figures 24 and 25).

The most common operations performed in the middle compartment are for the removal of acoustic neuromas and other tumors and for the relief of hemifacial spasm. The considerations related to acoustic neuromas will be dealt with first.

Anatomy of Acoustic Neuromas

Acoustic neuromas, as they expand, may involve a majority of the cranial nerves, cerebellar arteries, and parts of the brain stem. On the lateral side, in the meatus, they commonly expand by enlarging the meatus and infrequently may erode into the vestibule and cochlea. On the medial side, they compress the pons, medulla, and cerebellum. An understanding of microsurgical anatomy is especially important in preserving the facial and adjacent cranial nerves, which are the

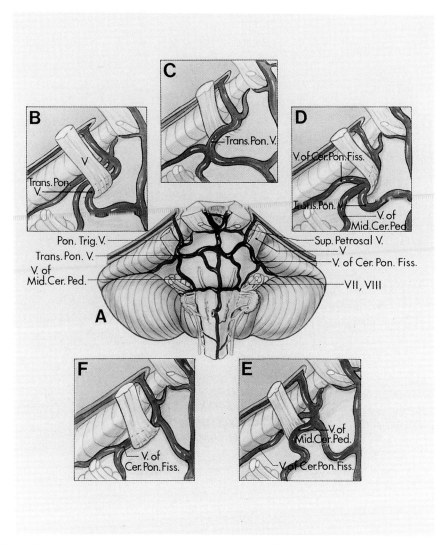

Figure 21. Sites of venous compression of the trigeminal nerve. (**A**) Central diagram. Anterior view. The veins that commonly compress the trigeminal nerve (V) are tributaries of the superior petrosal vein (Sup. Petrosal V.). The tributaries that converge on and may compress the nerve are the transverse pontine (Trans. Pon. V.) and pontotrigeminal (Pon. Trig. V.) veins and the veins of the cerebellopontine fissure (V. of Cer. Pon. Fiss.) and the middle cerebellar peduncle (V. of Mid. Cer. Ped.). The transverse pontine veins course transversely across the pons. The vein of the middle cerebellar peduncle arises in the region of the facial (VII) and vestibulocochlear (VIII) nerves and ascends on the pons. The vein of the cerebellopontine fissure arises along the cleft between the pons and the cerebellum and ascends behind the trigeminal nerve. The pontotrigeminal vein arises on the upper pons and passes above the trigeminal nerve. (**B**) A transverse pontine vein compresses the lateral side of the nerve and joins the vein of the middle cerebellar peduncle and the cerebellopontine fissure empties into a superior petrosal vein. (**C**) The medial side of the nerve is compressed by a tortuous transverse pontine vein. (**D**) The lateral side of the nerve is compressed by the junction of the transverse pontine vein with the veins of the middle cerebellar peduncle and the cerebellopontine fissure. (**E**) The nerve is compressed on the medial side by the vein of the middle cerebellar peduncle and on the lateral side by the vein of the cerebellopontine fissure. (**F**) The lateral side of the nerve is compressed by the vein of the cerebellopontine fissure.[49]

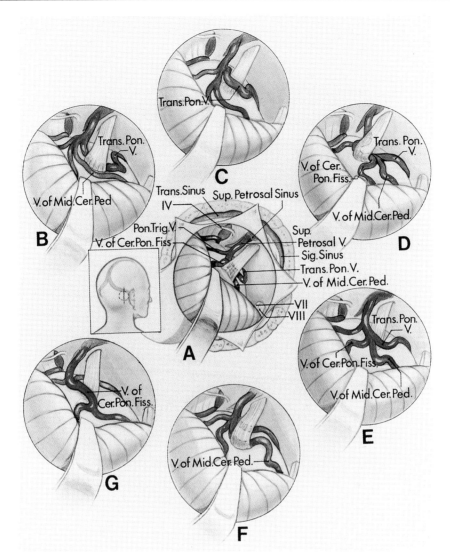

Figure 22. Sites of venous compression of the trigeminal nerve as seen through a retrosigmoid craniectomy. **(A)** The insert shows the site of the scalp incision (solid line) and the craniectomy (interrupted line). The cerebellum has been elevated to expose the junction of the trigeminal nerve with the pons. The superior petrosal veins (Sup. Petrosal V.) empty into the superior petrosal sinus (Sup. Petrosal Sinus). The trochlear nerve (IV) is at the superior margin and the facial (VII) and vestibulocochlear (VIII) nerves are at the lower margin of the exposure. The craniectomy exposes the junction of the sigmoid (Sig. Sinus) and transverse (Trans. Sinus) sinuses. The trigeminal nerve is compressed by the junction of a transverse pontine vein (Trans. Pon. V.) and the vein of the middle cerebellar peduncle (V. of Mid. Cer. Ped.) with the superior petrosal vein. The vein of the cerebellopontine fissure (V. of Cer. Pon. Fiss.) ascends behind the nerve and the pontotrigeminal vein (Pont. Trig. V.) passes above the nerve. **(B)** The trigeminal nerve is compressed on its medial side by a transverse pontine vein and on its lateral side by the vein of the middle cerebellar peduncle. **(C)** The lateral side of the nerve is compressed by a transverse pontine vein. **(D)** The medial side of the nerve is compressed by the junction of a transverse pontine vein with the veins of the middle cerebellar peduncle and the cerebellopontine fissure. **(E)** The lateral side of the nerve is compressed by the junction of the transverse pontine vein with the veins of the middle cerebellar peduncle and the cerebellopontine fissure. **(F)** The medial side of the nerve is compressed by the vein of the middle cerebellar peduncle. **(G)** The lateral side of the nerve is compressed by the vein of the cerebellopontine fissure.[49]

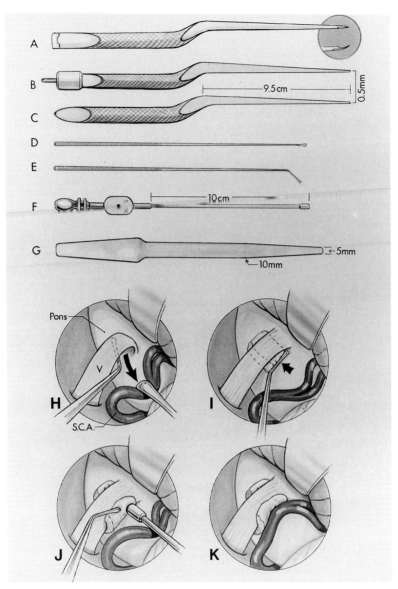

Figure 23. The size and type of instruments used for the microsurgical portion of a microvascular decompression operation are dictated by the anatomy of the area. *(A)* Bayonet scissors with 9.5-cm shafts and straight and curved blades are used for opening the arachnoid membrane and cutting in the depths of the exposure. *(B)* Bipolar bayonet forceps with 9.5-cm shafts and 0.5-mm tips are used for coagulation near the nerves or brain stem. A bipolar bayonet forceps with 0.7-mm tips may be used for coagulating large vessels in the superficial part of the exposure. *(C)* Fine dissection around the arteries and nerves is performed with plain bayonet forceps with 9.5-cm shafts and 0.5-mm tips. *(D-E)* The two dissectors most commonly used around the trigeminal nerve are the small spatula microdissector (D) and a 40°-angled ball dissector with a teardrop tip (E). *(F)* Suction around the nerve is performed with a blunt tip suction tube having a 10-cm shaft and a 5 French tip. *(G)* Retraction is maintained with a brain spatula tapered from 10 mm at the base to a 3- or 5-mm width at the tip. A self-retaining brain retractor system is used to hold the brain spatula in place. H to K are oriented as shown in Figure 13C. *(H)* The superior cerebellar artery (S.C.A.) is gently elevated away from the trigeminal nerve (V) with the spatula dissector and the area medial to the nerve is explored with a 40°-angled teardrop dissector. The tip of the brain spatula is 3 mm wide. *(I)* A small foam pad is fitted into the axilla of the nerve using a teardrop dissector. *(J)* The separation between the superior surface of the nerve and the artery is maintained with a small foam prosthesis. A blunt tip suction of 5 French size aids in positioning the small foam pad above the nerve. *(K)* The small foam pad protects the medial and superior surfaces of the nerve.[49]

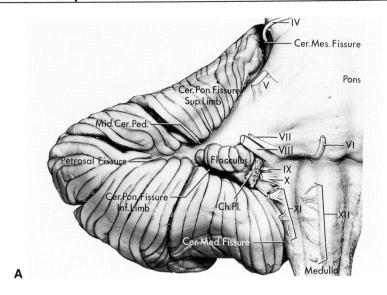

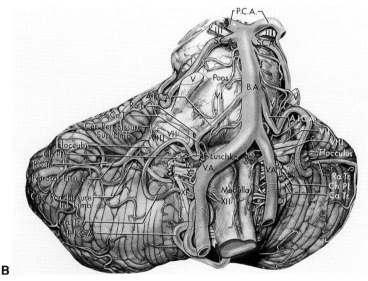

Figure 24. (*A*) *Anterior view of the petrosal surface of the cerebellum. The petrosal surface faces forward toward the petrous bone and is the surface that is elevated to expose the cerebellopontine angle. The petrosal (horizontal) fissure divides the petrosal surface into superior and inferior parts. The cerebellopontine fissure (Cer. Pon. Fissure) is a V-shaped fissure formed where the cerebellum wraps around the pons and the middle cerebellar peduncle (Mid. Cer. Ped.). The fissure has superior (Sup. Limb) and inferior (Inf. Limb) limbs, which meet at a lateral apex. The abducens nerve (VI) arises in the medial part of the pontomedullary sulcus (Pon. Med. Sulc.). The facial (VII) and vestibulocochlear (VIII) nerves arise near the flocculus at the lateral end of the pontomedullary sulcus. The glossopharyngeal (IX), vagus (X), spinal accessory (XI), and hypoglossal (XII) nerves arise from the medulla. The choroid plexus (Ch. Pl.) protrudes from the foramen of Luschka posterior to the glossopharyngeal and vagus nerves. The superior limb of the cerebellopontine fissure is continuous above with the cerebellomesencephalic fissure (Cer. Mes. Fissure), and the inferior limb is continuous below with the cerebellomedullary fissure (Cer. Med. Fissure). The trochlear nerve (VI) passes forward in the cerebellomesencephalic fissure.* (*B*) *Arterial relationships of the middle neurovascular complex. The basilar artery (B.A.) gives rise to the anterior inferior cerebellar arteries (A.I.C.A.). The right AICA bifurcates into rostral (Ro. Tr.) and caudal (Ca. Tr.) trunks. The rostral trunk passes above the flocculus and along the middle cerebellar peduncle to reach the petrosal surface. The caudal trunk loops below the flocculus. Other structures in the exposure include the vertebral (V.A.), posterior inferior cerebellar (P.I.C.A.), superior cerebellar (S.C.A.), and posterior cerebral (P.C.A.) arteries and the oculomotor nerves (III).*[34]

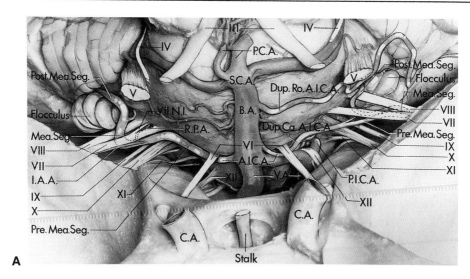

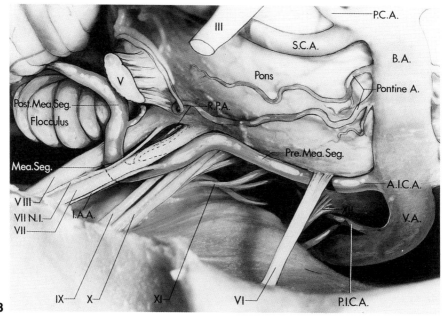

Figure 25. Anterosuperior view of the middle neurovascular complex. (A) The right anterior inferior cerebellar artery (A.I.C.A.) arises from the basilar artery (B.A.), courses below the abducens nerve (VI), and passes between the nervus intermedius (VII N.I.) and the facial motor root (VII) anteriorly and the vestibulocochlear nerve (VIII) posteriorly. The left AICA is a duplicate artery. The rostral duplicate AICA (Dup. Ro. A.I.C.A.) is not nerve related, but the caudal AICA (Dup. Ca. A.I.C.A.) is nerve related and passes between the facial and vestibulocochlear nerves. The premeatal segments (Pre. Mea. Seg.) approach the nerves, the meatal segments (Mea. Seg.) pass between the nerves, and the postmeatal segments (Post. Mea. Seg.) pass above the flocculus. Recurrent perforating (R.P.A.) and internal auditory (I.A.A.) arteries arise from the right AICA. The left posterior inferior cerebellar artery (P.I.C.A.) arises from the left vertebral artery (V.A.). The glossopharyngeal (IX), vagus (IX), spinal accessory (XI), and hypoglossal (XII) nerves are lateral to the vertebral arteries (V.A.). The carotid arteries (C.A.) and the pituitary stalk (Stalk) have been divided. The superior cerebellar (S.C.A.) and posterior cerebral (P.C.A.) arteries arise from the superior end of the basilar artery. The oculomotor (III) and trochlear (IV) nerves are above and the trigeminal (V) nerves are below the superior cerebellar arteries. (B) Enlarged view of the right CPA. The premeatal segment (Pre. Mea. Seg.) of the AICA passes below the abducens nerve. The meatal segment (Mea. Seg.) passes between the vestibulocochlear nerve and the nervus intermedius, and the postmeatal segment (Post. Mea. Seg.) passes above the flocculus. Pontine branches (Pontine A.) arise from the basilar artery.[32]

neural structures at greatest risk during acoustic neuroma removal. A widely accepted operative precept is that a nerve involved by a tumor should be identified proximally or distally to the tumor, where its displacement and distortion is the least, before the tumor is removed from the involved segment of the nerve. Considerable attention has been directed to the early identification of the facial nerve distal to the tumor at the lateral part of the internal acoustic canal, whether the operative route be through the middle fossa, labyrinth, or posterior meatal lip. Less attention has been directed to identification at the brain stem on the medial side of the tumor. These anatomic considerations are divided into sections dealing with the relationships at the lateral end of the tumor in the meatus and those on the medial end of the tumor at the brain stem.[46,47,50]

Meatal Relationships

The nerves in the lateral part of the internal acoustic meatus are the facial, cochlear, and inferior and superior vestibular nerves (Figures 26 and 27). The position of the nerves is most constant in the lateral portion of the meatus, which is divided into a superior and an inferior portion by a horizontal ridge, called either the transverse or falciform crest. The facial and the superior vestibular nerves are superior to the crest. The facial nerve is anterior to the superior vestibular nerve and is separated from it at the lateral end of the meatus by a vertical ridge of bone, called the vertical crest. The vertical crest is also called "Bill's bar" in recognition of William House's role in focusing on the importance of this crest in identifying the facial nerve in the lateral end of the canal.[20] The cochlear and inferior vestibular nerves run below the transverse crest with the cochlear nerve located anteriorly. Thus, the lateral meatus can be considered to be divided into four portions, with the facial nerve being anterior-superior, the cochlear nerve anterior-inferior, the superior vestibular nerve posterior-superior, and the inferior

vestibular nerve posterior-inferior.

The anatomy of the region offers the opportunity for three basic approaches to the tumor in the meatus and CPA. One is directed through the middle cranial fossa and the roof of the meatus. Another is directed through the labyrinth and posterior surface of the temporal bone. The third is directed through the posterior cranial fossa and pos-

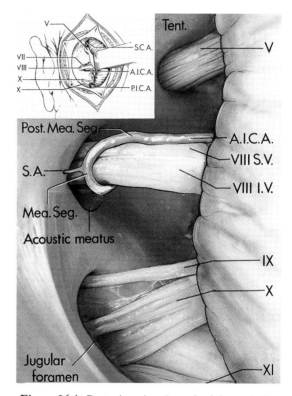

Figure 26A. Posterior view into the left cerebellopontine angle. The insert shows the orientation. The tentorium (Tent.) is above the trigeminal nerve (V). The facial (VII) and vestibulocochlear (VIII) nerves enter the internal acoustic meatus. The posterior surface of the vestibulocochlear nerve is formed by the inferior (VIII I.V.) and superior vestibular (VIII S.V.) nerves. The glossopharyngeal (IX), vagus (X), and spinal accessory (XI) nerves enter the jugular foramen. The premeatal segment of the anterior inferior cerebellar artery (A.I.C.A.) is not visible because it is anterior to the nerves. The meatal segment (Mea. Seg.) passes posterior to the nerves and gives rise to the subarcuate artery (S.A.). The postmeatal segment (Post. Mea. Seg.) passes above the nerves. The insert shows the superior cerebellar artery (S.C.A.) above the trigeminal nerve and the posterior inferior cerebellar artery (P.I.C.A.) below the glossopharyngeal nerve.

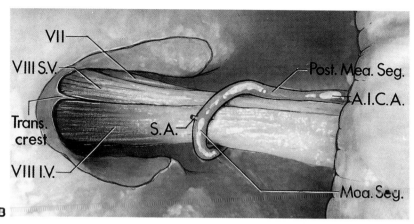

Figure 26B & C. (B) *The posterior wall of the internal acoustic canal has been removed. The facial nerve (VII) is anterior to the superior vestibular nerve. The subarcuate artery had to be divided to gain access to the posterior wall of the acoustic canal. The transverse crest (Trans. crest) separates the superior and inferior vestibular nerves at the lateral end of the canal.* **(C)** *The superior and inferior vestibular nerves have been divided to expose the facial and cochlear nerves (VIII Co.). The premeatal segment (Pre. Mea. Seg.) gives origin to the internal auditory (I.A.A.) and recurrent perforating (R.P.A.) arteries. The initial segment of the recurrent perforating artery loops toward the meatus before turning medially to reach the side of the brain stem.[32]*

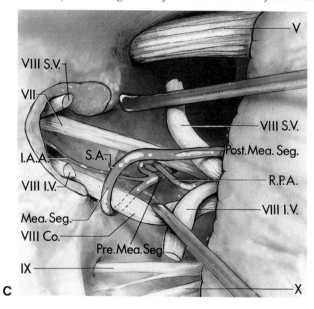

terior meatal tip. The anatomy presented by all three approaches will be reviewed.

Middle Fossa Approach

The middle fossa approach is suitable only for small tumors that are located predominantly within the internal acoustic meatus in which there is an opportunity to preserve hearing. With this approach, the meatus is approached from above, through a temporal craniotomy located anterior to the ear and above the zygoma (Figures 28-30).[4,37,50] The dura under the temporal lobe is elevated from the floor of the middle cranial fossa until the arcuate eminence and the greater petrosal nerve are identified. The distance from the inner table of the skull to the facial hiatus, through which the greater petrosal nerve passes, ranges from 1.3-2.3 cm (average 1.7 cm).[54] When separating the dura from the floor of the middle fossa, one

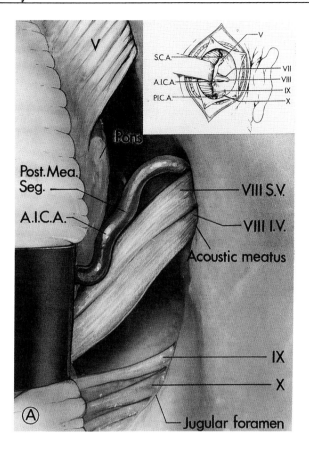

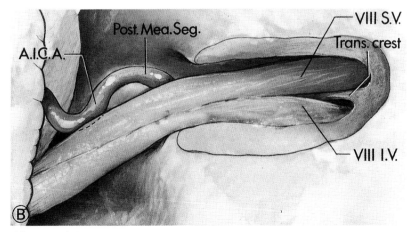

Figure 27 A & B. *Posterior view of the right cerebellopontine angle (CPA). (A) The insert shows the direction of view. The superior cerebellar artery (S.C.A.) is above the trigeminal nerve (V), and the posterior inferior cerebellar artery (P.I.C.A.) courses between the glossopharyngeal (IX) and vagus (X) nerves. The superior (VIII S.V.) and inferior (VIII I.V.) vestibular nerves enter the acoustic meatus, and the glossopharyngeal and vagus nerves pass through the dura over the jugular foramen. The postmeatal segment (Post. Mea. Seg.) of the anterior inferior cerebellar artery (A.I.C.A.) is above the vestibular nerves. (B) The posterior wall of the internal acoustic canal has been drilled away to expose the transverse crest (Trans. crest) and the division of the vestibular nerve into its superior and inferior parts.*

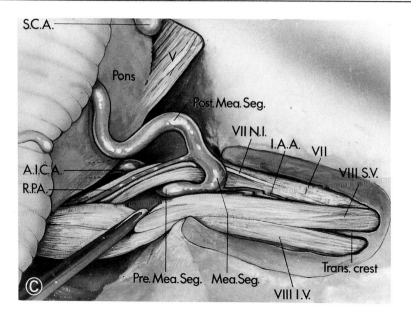

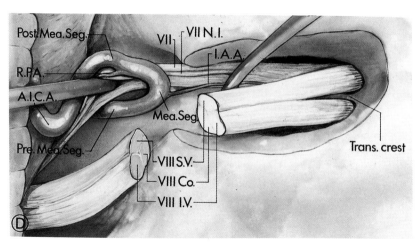

Figure 27C & D. (C) The vestibular nerves are displaced inferiorly to expose the premeatal (Pre. Mea. Seg.) and meatal (Mea. Seg.) segments of the AICA. The nervus intermedius (VII N.I.) is between the facial (VII) and vestibular nerves. The internal auditory (I.A.A.) and recurrent perforating (R.P.A.) arteries arise from the meatal segment. *(D)* The vestibulocochlear nerve has been divided near the meatus to show its superior and inferior vestibular and cochlear (VIII Co.) components in cross section.[32]

should remember that bone may be absent over all or part of the geniculate ganglion (Figure 29). In a previous study of 100 temporal bones, the author's group found that all or part of the geniculate ganglion and the genu of the facial nerve was exposed in the floor of the middle fossa in 15 bones (15%).[54] In 15 other specimens, the geniculate ganglion was completely covered but no bone

was extending over the greater petrosal nerve. The greatest length of greater petrosal nerve covered by bone was 6.0 mm. More than 50% of the specimens had less than 2.5 mm of greater petrosal nerve covered.

It also is important to remember that the petrous segment of the carotid artery may be exposed without a covering of bone in the floor of the middle fossa deep to the greater

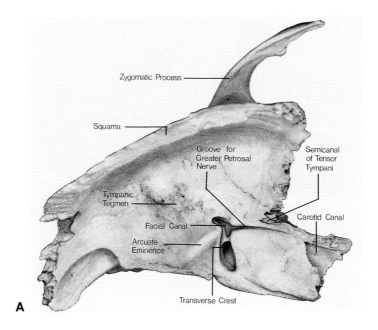

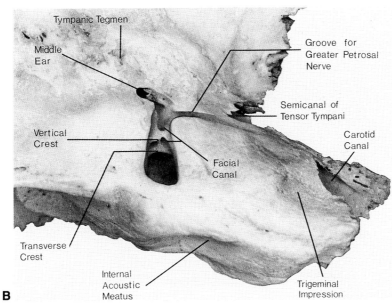

Figure 28A & B. Middle fossa approach to the internal acoustic meatus. (A) Superior view of the left temporal bone. The facial canal is exposed proximal and distal to its junction with the canal of the greater petrosal nerve. The internal auditory meatus is unroofed. (B) Enlarged view. The vertical and transverse crests are exposed at the lateral end of the internal auditory meatus.

petrosal nerve (Figure 29).[22,39] In a previous study, we found that a 7-mm length of petrous carotid artery may be exposed without a bony covering in the area below where the greater petrosal nerve passes below the lateral margin of the trigeminal ganglion.[18] The foramen spinosum and middle meningeal artery and the foramen ovale and third trigeminal division are situated at the anterior margin of the extradural exposure. The extra-

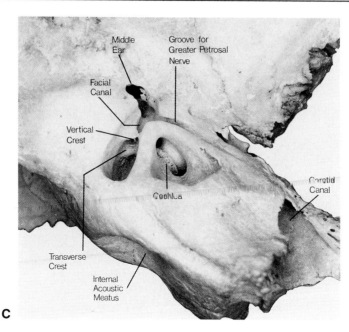

C

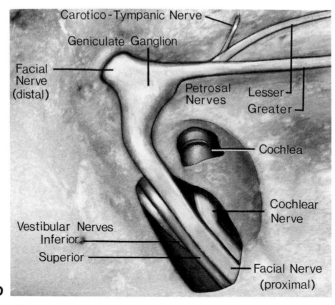

D

Figure 28C & D. (C) The cochlea is exposed in the angle between the groove for the greater petrosal nerve and the unroofed part of the internal acoustic meatus. (D) Specimen with nerves intact. The dura and bone above the facial canal and the internal acoustic meatus have been removed. The cochlea is exposed medial to the geniculate ganglion.

dural exposure usually can be completed without obliterating the middle meningeal artery at the foramen spinosum. The tensor tympani muscle and the eustachian tube, although not exposed in this approach, are located beneath the floor of the middle fossa roughly parallel to and in front of the horizontal portion of the petrous carotid (Figure 29).

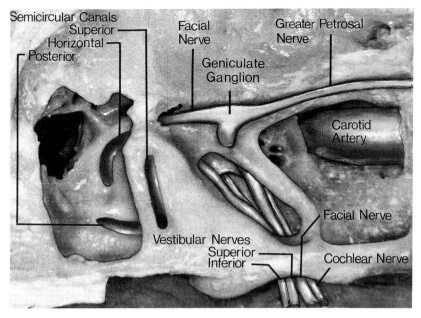

Figure 28E. All three semicircular canals, the nerves in the meatus, and the carotid artery are exposed.[37]

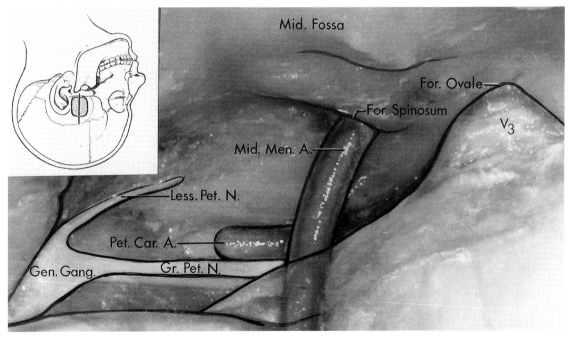

Figure 29A. Anatomy of the middle fossa approach to the internal acoustic meatus. The insert on the upper left shows the site of the scalp incision (straight line) and the craniectomy (stippled area). The dura has been elevated from the floor of the middle cranial fossa (Mid. Fossa). In this case, bone was absent over the geniculate ganglion (Gen. Gang.) and the petrous segment of the carotid artery (Pet. Car. A.) and both were exposed in the floor of the middle fossa. Elevation of the dura from the floor of the middle cranial fossa also exposes the middle meningeal artery (Mid. Men. A.) at the foramen spinosum (For. Spinosum), the mandibular division of the trigeminal nerve (V_3) at the foramen ovale (For. Ovale), and the lesser petrosal nerve (Less. Pet. N.). The geniculate ganglion is exposed by identifying the greater petrosal nerve and following it to the geniculate ganglion.

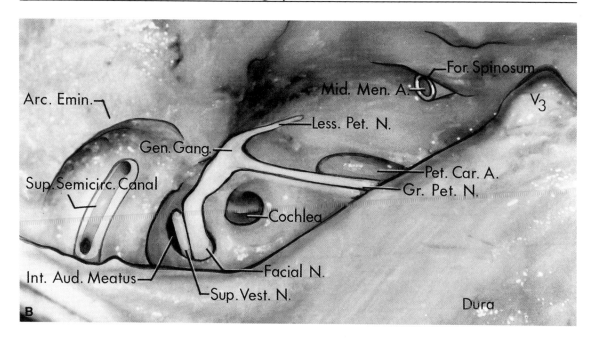

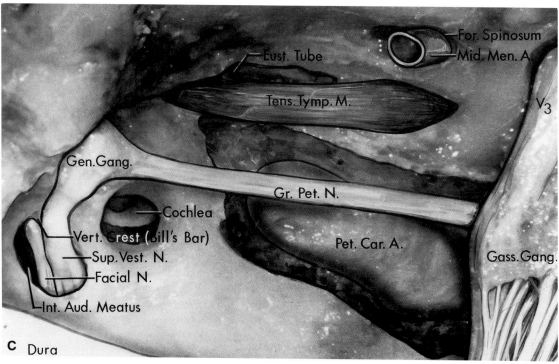

Figure 29B & C. (B) The middle meningeal artery has been divided at the foramen spinosum and bone removed over the internal auditory meatus (Int. Aud. Meatus) to expose the superior vestibular (Sup. Vest. N.) and facial (Facial N.) nerves. Bone has been removed to expose the cochlea in the angle between the greater petrosal nerve and the internal acoustic meatus. The superior semicircular canal (Sup. Semicirc. Canal) lies behind the superior vestibular nerve in the area deep to the arcuate eminence (Arc. Emin.). *(C)* The dura has been elevated to expose the gasserian ganglion (Gass. Gang.). The greater petrosal nerve courses above the petrous segment of the carotid artery. Bone has been removed in the floor of the middle fossa to expose the tensor tympani muscle (Tens. Tymp. M.) and the eustachian tube (Eust. Tube). The superior vestibular and facial nerves are separated at the lateral end of the meatus by the vertical crest (Vert. Crest—Bill's Bar).

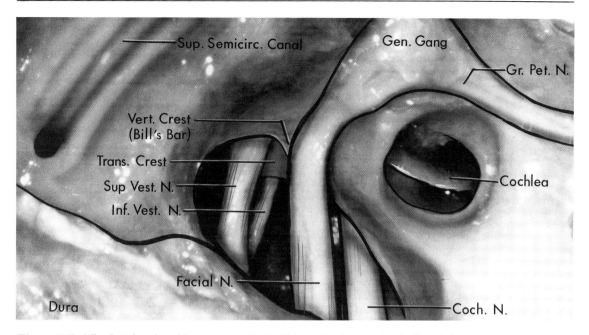

Figure 29D. The facial and cochlear nerves (Coch. N.) are in the anterior half and the superior and inferior vestibular nerves (Inf. Vest. N.) are in the posterior half of the meatus. The superior vestibular and facial nerves are separated from the inferior vestibular and cochlear nerves by the transverse crest (Trans. Crest). The cochlea lies in the angle between the facial and greater petrosal nerves.[50]

In completing the middle fossa approach, bone is removed over the greater petrosal nerve to expose the geniculate ganglion and the genu of the facial nerve. From here, the labyrinthine portion of the facial nerve is followed to the lateral end of the internal auditory canal by removing bone. During the middle fossa approach, care must be taken to avoid injury to the cochlea, which sits only a few millimeters anterior to the site of bone removal, and the semicircular canals, which are located a few millimeters behind the area of bone being removed. Entering either the cochlea or the semicircular canals will result in a loss of hearing.

The lateral part of the bone removal is limited posteriorly by the superior semicircular canal that is located a few millimeters behind and is oriented parallel to the labyrinthine segment of the facial nerve. The anterior edge of the exposure is limited by the cochlea, which sits only a few millimeters anterior to the site of bone removal in the angle between the labyrinthine portion of the facial nerve and the greater petrosal nerve.

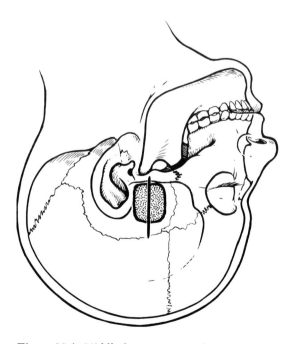

Figure 30A. Middle fossa approach for removing a small acoustic neuroma. The vertical skin incision is located anterior to the ear and the craniotomy is situated with its base on the floor of the middle cranial fossa (stippled area).

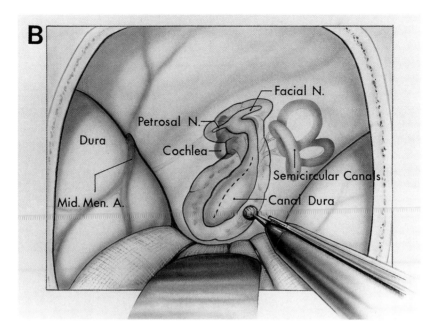

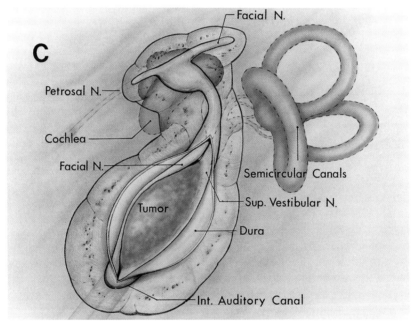

Figure 30B & C. *(B) The dura is elevated from the floor of the middle cranial fossa to identify the greater petrosal nerve (Petrosal N.). The middle meningeal artery (Mid. Men. A.) courses on the dura. Bone is removed over the greater petrosal nerve (Petrosal N.) to expose the facial nerve (Facial N.), which is followed proximally by removing bone to expose the superior wall of the internal auditory canal. Extreme care must be taken to avoid injuring the semicircular canals located in the bone at the posterior margin of the exposure and the cochlea situated in the bone between the greater petrosal nerve and the internal auditory canal. (C) Enlarged view of the area of bone removal. The dura has been opened to expose the tumor in the internal auditory canal (Int. Auditory Canal). The tumor arises in the superior vestibular nerve (Sup. Vestibular N.) and displaces the facial nerve anteriorly.*

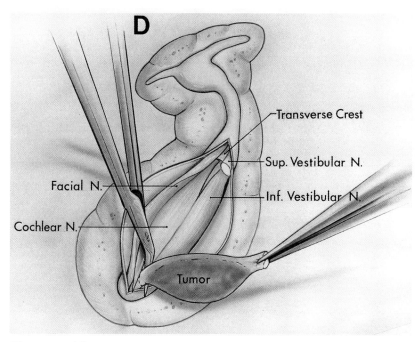

Figure 30D. The superior vestibular nerve has been divided above the transverse crest and elevated with the tumor. The superior vestibular nerve is being divided medial to the tumor. The facial, cochlear (Cochlear N.), and inferior vestibular (Inf. Vestibular N.) nerves are preserved.[50]

The cochlea and the semicircular canals must not be damaged in this approach if hearing is to be preserved. The vertical crest, which is identified at the upper edge of the lateral end of the internal acoustic canal, provides a valuable landmark for identifying the facial nerve. In the final stage of bone removal, the upper wall of the internal auditory canal is removed to expose the dura lining the entire superior surface of the internal auditory canal from the vertical crest to the porus.

The middle fossa approach is the least frequently performed operative approach to an acoustic neuroma. It is used for the removal of small tumors in which useful hearing may be preserved. The author prefers the retrosigmoid approach for these small tumors because this approach provides a wider exposure of the involved structures while allowing the preservation of hearing.

Translabyrinthine Approach

In the translabyrinthine approach, the meatus and CPA are approached through a mastoidectomy and labyrinthectomy (Figures 31-33).[20,37,50] This approach is suitable for the removal of small or medium-sized tumors in which there is no chance of preserving hearing because the labyrinthectomy, performed as a part of the approach, destroys hearing. Surgeons who operate by this route commonly combine the approach with a retrosigmoid craniectomy for the removal of large tumors. There are two goals of bone removal in this approach. The first is to remove enough bone to be able to identify the nerves lateral to the tumor as they course through the internal auditory canal and by the transverse and vertical crests. The second is to expose the dura on the posterior face of the temporal bone that faces the CPA. The triangular patch of dura facing the CPA, called Trautmann's triangle, extends from the sigmoid sinus laterally to the superior petrosal sinus above and to the jugular bulb below.

In the translabyrinthine exposure, the mastoid cortex is opened and the exposure is

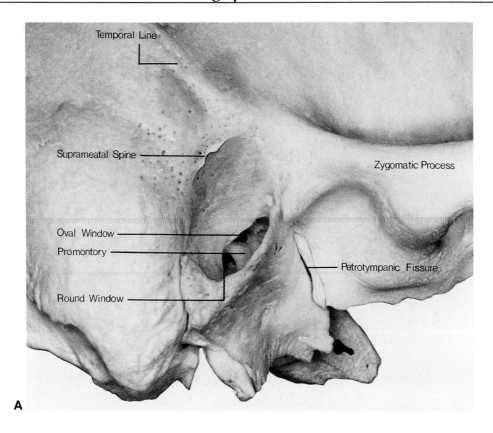

A

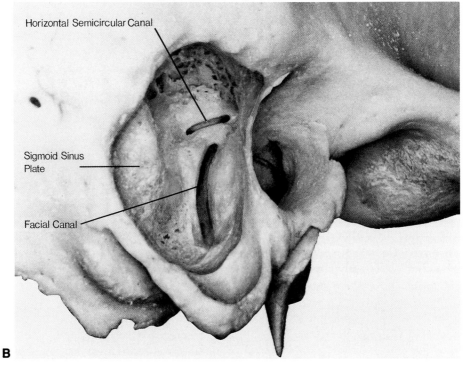

B

Figure 31 A-D. Translabyrinthine approach to the internal acoustic meatus. Lateral view of the right temporal bone showing the external acoustic meatus, the oval and round windows, and the promontory. (B) The sigmoid

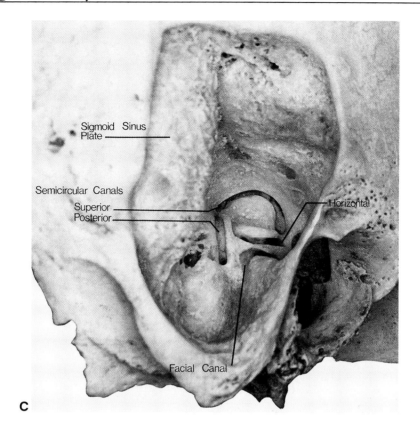

Sigmoid Sinus Plate

Semicircular Canals
Superior
Posterior

Horizontal

Facial Canal

C

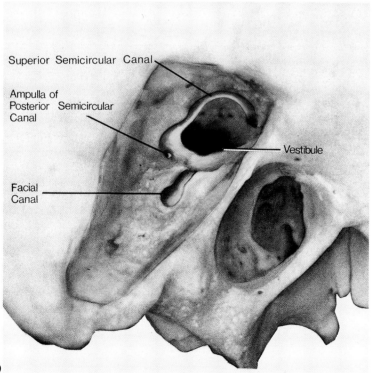

Superior Semicircular Canal

Ampulla of Posterior Semicircular Canal

Facial Canal

Vestibule

D

sinus plate, facial canal, and horizontal semicircular canal are exposed. (C) The three semicircular canals and the facial canal are exposed. (D) The canals have been removed to open into the vestibule.

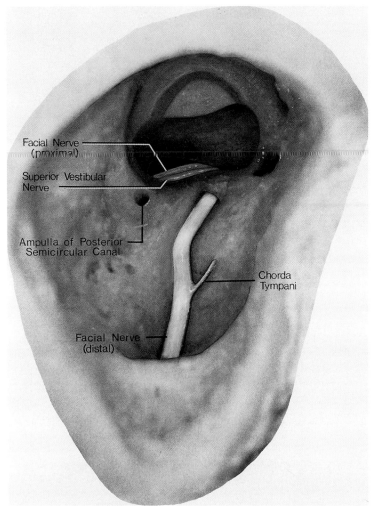

Facial Nerve
(proximal)

Superior Vestibular
Nerve

Ampulla of Posterior
Semicircular Canal

Chorda
Tympani

Facial Nerve
(distal)

Figure 31E. Specimen with nerves intact. The upper part of the internal acoustic meatus has been exposed by drilling through the vestibule and the ampulla of the posterior canal.[37]

directed through the triangular gateway between the facial nerve anteriorly, the sigmoid sinus posteriorly, and the floor of the middle fossa above. Bone is removed to skeletonize the dura covering the sigmoid sinus, middle fossa, facial nerve, the angle between the sigmoid sinus and middle fossa dura, called the sinodural angle, and the upper surface of the jugular bulb. The mastoidectomy is carried down to the horizontal semicircular canal, which provides the landmark for identifying the other canals and the facial nerve.

The labyrinthectomy portion of the procedure involves removing the semicircular canals

and the vestibule to expose the dura lining the internal auditory canal. In the process of removing the semicircular canals, the dura of the middle fossa above the internal acoustic meatus is skeletonized and the dura on the posterior fossa plate behind the canal is exposed. After opening and removing the canals, the vestibule is opened and removed, and the dura lining the posterior half of the internal auditory canal is exposed. Care is required to avoid injury to the facial nerve as it courses below the horizontal canal and the ampullae of the posterior canal and around the superolateral margin of the vestibule.

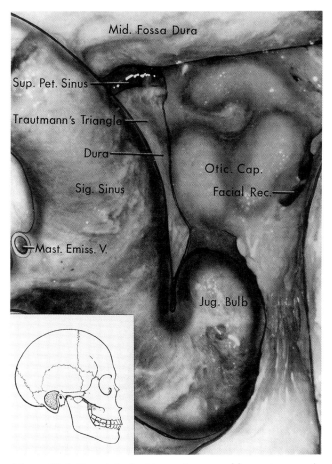

Figure 32A. Translabyrinthine and transcochlear exposure. A mastoidectomy has been completed to expose the otic capsule (Otic Cap.), sigmoid sinus (Sig. Sinus), jugular bulb (Jug. Bulb), and dura lining the floor of the middle cranial fossa (Mid. Fossa Dura). Trautmann's triangle is the triangular portion of the dura that faces the cerebellopontine angle (CPA). This triangle is located between the superior petrosal sinus (Sup. Pet. Sinus) above, the sigmoid sinus laterally, and the jugular bulb below. Mastoid emissary veins (Mast. Emiss. V.) join the sigmoid sinus. The facial recess (Facial Rec.) is located in front of the facial canal.

Further bone removal at the lateral end of the meatus exposes the transverse and vertical crests and the covering of the superior and inferior vestibular and facial nerves. In removing bone behind the internal acoustic meatus, it is important to remember that the jugular bulb may bulge upward behind the posterior semicircular canal or internal auditory meatus. The vestibular aqueduct and the endolymphatic sac will be opened and removed as bone is removed between the meatus and the jugular bulb. The cochlear canali-

culus will be seen deep to the vestibular aqueduct as bone is removed in the area between the meatus and the jugular bulb. The lower end of the cochlear canaliculus is situated just above the area where the glossopharyngeal nerve enters the medial side of the jugular foramen.

The subarcuate artery, or the AICA, may be encountered in the dura of Trautmann's triangle. Usually, the subarcuate artery arises from the AICA and passes through the dura on the upper posterior wall of the meatus as a fine stem.

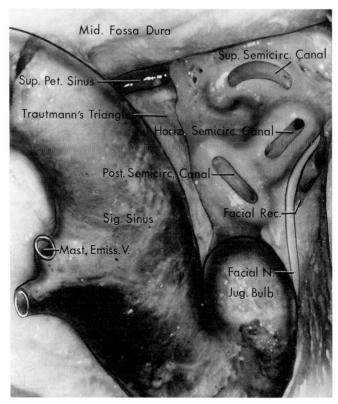

Figure 32B. Additional bone has been removed to expose the horizontal (Horiz. Semicirc. Canal), posterior (Post. Semicirc. Canal), and superior semicircular (Sup. Semicirc. Canal) canals. The facial nerve (Facial N.) passes below the horizontal canal.

Occasionally, however, the subarcuate artery along with its origin from the AICA may be incorporated into the dura on the posterior face of the temporal bone.

Retrosigmoid Approach

The retrosigmoid approach to the meatus is directed through a vertical scalp incision and cranial opening situated just behind the sigmoid sinus and down the plane between the posterior face of the temporal bone and the petrosal surface of the cerebellum (Figures 26, 27, 34, and 35).[41,42,46-48] The cerebellum, which commonly bulges outward upon opening the dura, usually relaxes after the arachnoid membrane over the cisterna magna is opened and cerebrospinal fluid is allowed to escape. A tapered brain spatula 20-25 mm

wide at its base and 15-20 mm at its tip is commonly used to support the lateral margin of the cerebellum. When removing the posterior meatal wall, it often is necessary to sacrifice the subarcuate artery because it passes through the dura on the posterior meatal wall to reach the subarcuate fossa.[32] This artery usually has a sufficiently long stem so that its obliteration does not risk damage to the AICA from which it arises. In a few cases, however, the subarcuate artery and the segment of the AICA from which it arises will be incorporated into the dura covering the subarcuate fossa. In this case, the dura and the artery will have to be separated together from the posterior meatal lip in preparation for opening the meatus.

The posterior wall of the internal auditory canal may be removed prior to opening the arachnoid membrane around the tumor. The

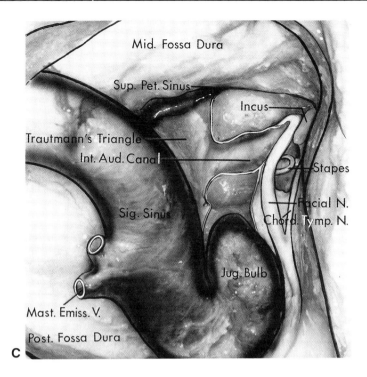

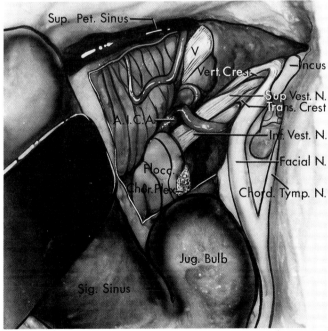

Figure 32C & D. (C) *The semicircular canals and the vestibule have been removed to expose the dura lining the internal auditory canal (Int. Aud. Canal). The chorda tympani (Chord. Tymp. N.) arises from the facial nerve. The posterior fossa dura (Post. Fossa Dura) is behind the sigmoid sinus. (**D**) The dura lining the internal auditory canal and facing the cerebellopontine angle (CPA) has been removed to expose the trigeminal (V), facial, and vestibulocochlear nerves. The transverse crest (Trans. Crest) separates the superior (Sup. Vest. N.) and inferior vestibular (Inf. Vest. N.) nerves. The vertical crest (Vert. Crest) separates the facial and superior vestibular nerves. The flocculus (Flocc.) is behind the vestibulocochlear nerve. The choroid plexus (Chor. Plex.) protrudes from the foramen of Luschka. The anterior inferior cerebellar artery (A.I.C.A.) courses around the facial and vestibulocochlear nerves.*

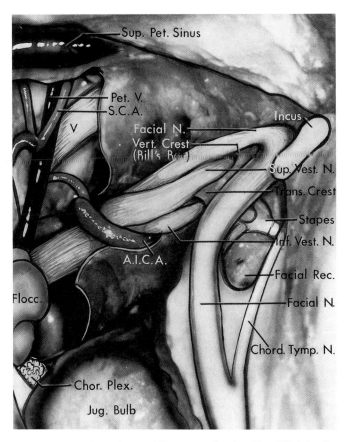

Figure 32E. Enlarged view. The petrosal veins (Pet. V.) join the superior petrosal sinus. The superior cerebellar artery (S.C.A.) courses above the trigeminal nerve.

preservation of the arachnoid membrane (which lies posterior to an acoustic neuroma) during the drilling of the posterior meatal wall prevents bone dust from entering the subarachnoid space. The posterior semicircular canal and its common crus with the superior canal, both of which are situated just lateral to the posterior meatal lip, should be preserved when exposing the meatal contents if there is the possibility of preserving hearing, since hearing will be lost if damage occurs. Care also is required to avoid injury to the vestibular aqueduct, which is situated inferolateral to the meatal lip, and the endolymphatic sac, which expands under the dura on the posterior surface of the temporal bone inferolateral to the posterior meatal lip. The endolymphatic sac may be entered in removing the dura from the posterior meatal lip. There

is little danger of encountering the cochlear canaliculus, which has a more anterior course below the internal auditory canal. An unusually high projection of the jugular bulb presents an anomaly that may block access to the posterior meatal lip. Mastoid air cells commonly are encountered in the posterior meatal lip.

After removing the posterior wall of the meatus, the dura lining the meatus is opened to expose its contents. The facial nerve is identified near the origin of the facial canal at the anterior-superior quadrant of the meatus rather than in a more medial location where the direction of displacement is variable. If the tumor extends into the vestibule, the latter can easily be exposed by drilling along the posterior and superior semicircular canals. The strokes of the fine dissecting

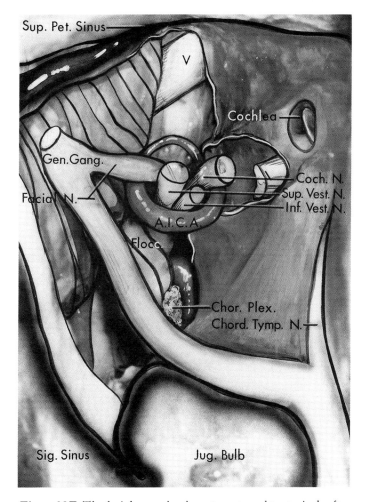

Figure 32F. The facial nerve has been transposed posteriorly after dividing the greater petrosal nerve distal to the geniculate ganglion (Gen. Gang.). The superior and inferior vestibular and cochlear nerves (Coch. N.) have been divided. Additional bone has been removed to expose the cochlea. The distal segment of the cochlear nerve penetrates the lateral end of the meatus to enter the cochlea.

instruments along the vestibulocochlear nerve should be directed from medial to lateral rather than from lateral to medial, because traction medially may tear the tiny filaments of the cochlear nerve at the site where these filaments penetrate the lateral end of the meatus to enter the cochlea.

The retrosigmoid approach is used by this author because it is suitable for the removal of both small and large tumors. Unlike the translabyrinthine approach, which is directed through the vestibule and semicircular canals, the retrosigmoid approach is not necessarily

associated with hearing loss. The retrosigmoid approach provides a broader exposure of the small tumor than does the middle fossa approach. Also, once the nerves are identified lateral to the tumor, there are advantages to being able to separate the tumor capsule off the nerves beginning medially for this more often results in preservation of hearing than dissection starting laterally.

Brain Stem Relationships

A consistent set of neural, arterial, and

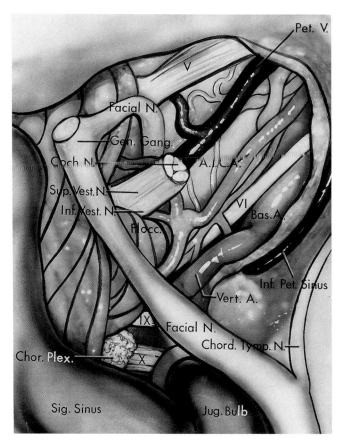

Figure 32G. The bone surrounding the cochlea has been removed to complete the transcochlear exposure. The bone removal extends to the lateral margin of the clivus and the inferior petrosal sinus (Inf. Pet. Sinus). The abducens nerve (VI) ascends beside the basilar artery (Bas.A.). The glossopharyngeal (IX) and vagus (X) nerves are in the lower margin of the exposure behind the vertebral artery (Vert. A.).

venous relationships at the brain stem facilitates the identification of the nerves on the medial side of the tumor.[47]

Neural Relationships

The neural structures most intimately related to the medial side of an acoustic neuroma are the pons, medulla, and cerebellum (Figures 24, 36, and 37). The landmarks on these structures that are helpful in guiding the surgeon to the junction of the facial nerve with the brain stem are the pontomedullary sulcus; the junction of the glossopharyngeal, vagus, and spinal accessory nerves

with the medulla; the foramen of Luschka and its choroid plexus; and the flocculus.

Pontomedullary Sulcus

The facial nerve arises from the brain stem near the lateral end of the pontomedullary sulcus. This sulcus extends along the junction of the pons and the medulla and ends immediately in front of the foramen of Luschka and the lateral recess of the fourth ventricle (Figures 36 and 37). The facial nerve arises in the pontomedullary sulcus 1-2 mm anterior to the point at which the vestibulocochlear nerve joins the brain stem at

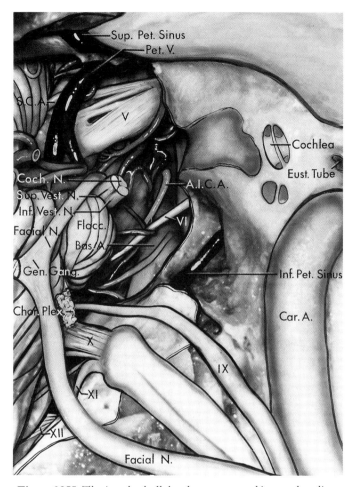

Figure 32H. *The jugular bulb has been removed in another dissection to expose the glossopharyngeal, vagus, and spinal accessory (XI) nerves as they course through the medial side of the jugular foramen. The internal carotid artery (Car. A.) and the eustachian tube (Eust. Tube) are in the anterior part of the exposure.*[50]

the lateral end of the sulcus. The interval between the vestibulocochlear and facial nerves is greatest at the level of the pontomedullary sulcus and decreases as these nerves approach the meatus.

Glossopharyngeal, Vagus, and
Spinal Accessory Nerves

The facial nerve enjoys a consistent relationship to the junction of the glossopharyngeal, vagus, and spinal accessory nerves with the lateral side of the medulla (See Figures 36 and 37). The facial nerve arises 2-3 mm

above the most rostral rootlet contributing to these nerves. A helpful way of visualizing the point where the facial nerve will exit from the brain stem, even when displaced by a tumor, is to project an imaginary line along the medullary junction of the rootlets forming the glossopharyngeal, vagus, and spinal accessory nerves upward through the pontomedullary junction. This line, at a point 2-3 mm above the junction of the glossopharyngeal nerve with the medulla, will pass through the pontomedullary junction at the site where the facial nerve exits from the brain stem. The glossopharyngeal and vagus nerves are seen and should be carefully protected below the lower margin of the tumor in both the translabyrinthine and retrosigmoid approaches.

Nervus Intermedius

The filaments of the nervus intermedius also are stretched around an acoustic neuroma (Figure 38). The nervus intermedius usually is described as a component of the facial nerve. Relatively little note has been taken of the fact that it may be closely bound to the vestibulocochlear nerve for a variable distance before it enters the brain stem, and that in the CPA, it may consist of as many as four rootlets. In previous studies, the nervus intermedius was found divisible into three parts: a proximal segment that adheres closely to the acoustic nerve, an intermediate segment that lies freely between the acoustic nerve and the motor root of the facial nerve, and a distal segment that joins the motor root to form the facial nerve.[53] Twenty-two percent of the nerves were adherent to the acoustic nerve for 14 mm or more (the entire course of the nerve in the posterior cranial fossa) and could be found as a separate structure only after opening the internal acoustic meatus (Figure 38). In most instances, the nerve was a single trunk, but in some cases, it was composed of as many as four rootlets. A single large root most frequently arose at the brain stem anterior to the superior vestibular nerve and, in the meatus, lay anterior to the superior vestibular nerve. When multiple rootlets are present, they may arise along the whole anterior surface of the acoustic nerve; however, they usually converge immediately proximal to the junction with the facial motor root to form a single bundle that lies anterior to the superior vestibular nerve.

Cerebellar-Brain Stem Fissures

Acoustic neuromas are closely related to the cerebellopontine and cerebellomedullary fissures, the clefts formed by the folding of the cerebellum around the pons and medulla

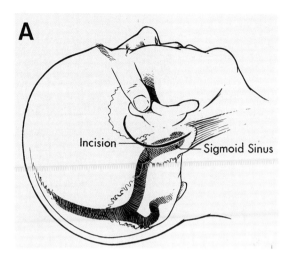

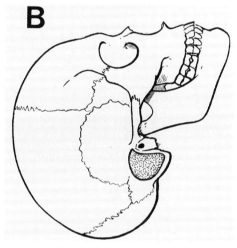

Figure 33A, B. Translabyrinthine approach to the removal of acoustic neuromas.(A) The operation is performed with the patient in the supine position with the face turned toward the side opposite the tumor. The retromastoid skin incision is located about 2 cm behind the ear. (B) The stippled area shows the site of the bony opening through the mastoid.

(Figures 1, 24, 36, and 37).[34] The cerebellopontine fissure is a V-shaped fissure formed by the folding of the petrosal surface of the cerebellum around the lateral side of the pons and the middle cerebellar peduncle. The petrosal surface is the cerebellar surface that faces the posterior surface of the petrous bone, and is the cerebellar surface compressed by an acoustic neuroma. The cerebellopontine fissure has a superior limb situated between the rostral half of the pons and the superior

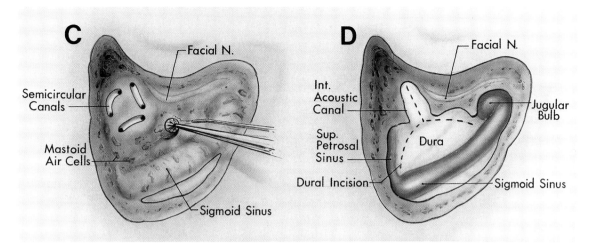

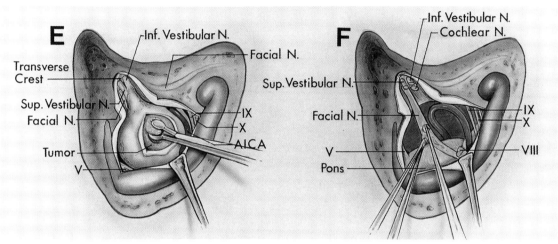

Figure 33C-F. (C) The mastoidectomy has been completed to expose the semicircular canals. The bone removal will be carried medially through the semicircular canals and the vestibule. The sigmoid sinus and the facial nerve (Facial N.) have been skeletonized. (D) The labyrinthectomy has been completed to expose the dura lining the internal auditory canal. The dura between the superior petrosal (Sup. Petrosal Sinus) and the sigmoid sinuses and the jugular bulb has been exposed. The interrupted lines show the site of the dural opening. (E) The intracapsular contents of the tumor are being removed. The superior (Sup. Vestibular N.) and inferior vestibular (Inf. Vestibular N.) nerves are seen lateral to the tumor where they are separated by the transverse crest. The anterior inferior cerebellar artery (A.I.C.A.) courses around the lower margin of the tumor. The facial nerve is anterior to the tumor. The trigeminal nerve (V) is above and the glossopharyngeal (IX) and vagus (X) nerves are below the tumor. (F) The final fragments of the tumor are being removed from the surface of the facial nerve. The superior and inferior vestibular and cochlear nerve (Cochlear N.) have been removed along with the tumor. The central stump of the vestibulocochlear nerve (VIII) is exposed at the brain stem.[50]

part of the petrosal surface, and an inferior limb located between the caudal half of the pons and the inferior part of the petrosal surface. The apex of the fissure is located laterally where the superior and inferior limbs meet. The V-shaped area between the superior and inferior limbs, which has the middle cerebellar peduncle in its floor, corresponds to the area that is called the CPA. The facial and vestibulocochlear nerves arise just anterior to the inferior limb of the fissure and just below the middle cerebellar peduncle. The trigeminal nerve arises near the superior limb of the fissure.

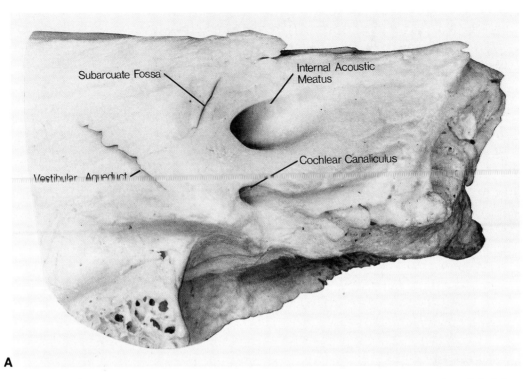

A

Figure 34A, B. Retrosigmoid approach to internal acoustic meatus. (*A*) Posterior view of the left temporal bone showing the subarcuate fossa, the vestibular aqueduct, and the cochlear canaliculus. (*B*) The bone has been removed to expose the transverse crest, the vestibular aqueduct, and the posterior semicircular canal.

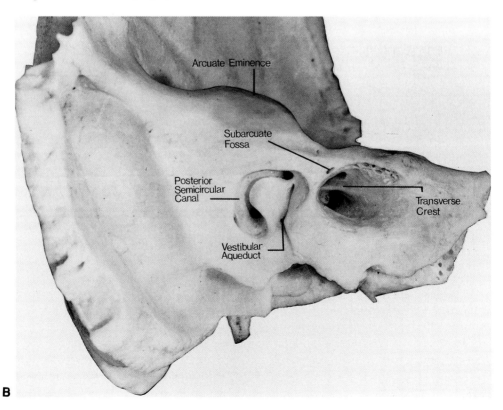

B

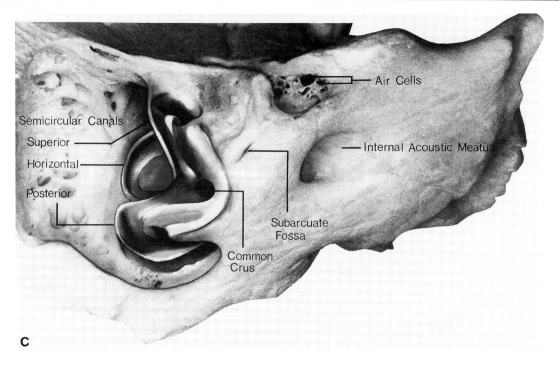

C

Figure 34C, D. (C) Relationship of the three semicircular canals to the internal acoustic meatus. The horizontal canal was exposed by removing bone anterior to the posterior canal and lateral to the superior canal. (D) Bone removed to show the lateral end of the internal acoustic meatus. The transverse crest separates the facial canal and the superior vestibular area from the cochlear and inferior vestibular areas. The vertical crest, also called Bill's Bar, separates the facial canal and the superior vestibular area.

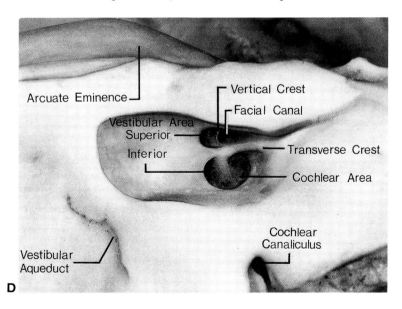

D

The cerebellomedullary fissure, the cleft between the cerebellum and the medulla that extends upward between the cerebellar tonsil and the medulla, communicates with the inferior limb of the cerebellopontine fissure near the lateral recess of the fourth ventri-

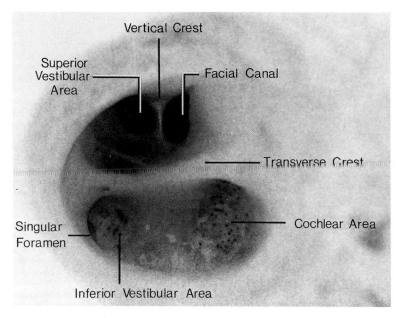

Figure 34E. *Enlarged view of the lateral end of the canal.*

cle.[34] Several structures related to the lateral recess and the foramen of Luschka project into the CPA near the facial and the vestibulocochlear nerves.

Foramen of Luschka, Choroid Plexus and Flocculus

The structures related to the lateral recess of the fourth ventricle that have a consistent relationship to the facial and vestibulocochlear nerves are the foramen of Luschka and its choroid plexus, and the flocculus (Figures 36 and 37).[12,34] The foramen of Luschka is situated at the lateral margin of the pontmedullary sulcus, just behind the junction of the glossopharyngeal nerve with the brain stem, and immediately posteroinferior to the junction of the facial and vestibulocochlear nerves with the brain stem. The foramen of Luschka is infrequently well visualized. A consistently identifiable tuft of choroid plexus, however, hangs out of the foramen of Luschka and sits on the posterior surface of the glossopharyngeal and vagus nerves just inferior to the junction of the facial and vestibulocochlear nerves with the brain stem.

Another structure related to the lateral recess is the flocculus. It is a fan-shaped cerebellar lobule projecting from the margin of the lateral recess into the CPA. The flocculus, together with the nodule of the vermis, forms the primitive flocculonodular lobe of the cerebellum. The flocculus is attached to the rostral margin of the lateral recess and foramen of Luschka. The flocculus is continuous medially with the inferior medullary velum, a butterfly-shaped sheet of neural tissue that forms on the surface of the nodule and sweeps laterally above the tonsil to form part of the lower half of the roof of the fourth ventricle. The lateral part of the inferior medullary velum narrows to a smaller bundle, the peduncle of the flocculus, which fuses to the rostral margin of the lateral recess and the foramen of Luschka. The flocculus projects from the peduncle of the flocculus into the CPA just posterior to where the facial and vestibulocochlear nerves join the pontomedullary sulcus.

Arterial Relationships

The arteries crossing the CPA, especially the AICA, enjoy a consistent relationship to the facial and vestibulocochlear nerves, the

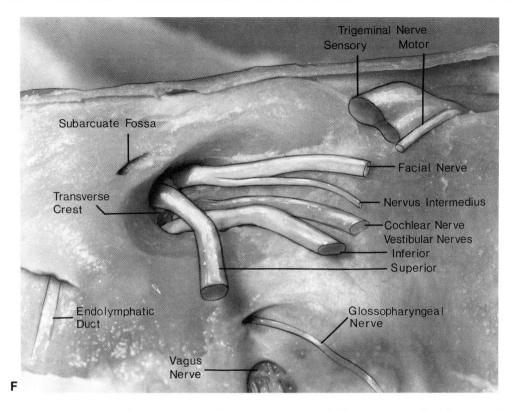

Figure 34F, G. (F) Temporal bone with the nerves preserved. The posterior wall of the internal auditory meatus has been removed to expose the nerves. (G) The bone lateral to the internal auditory canal has been removed to expose the posterior and superior semicircular canals.[37]

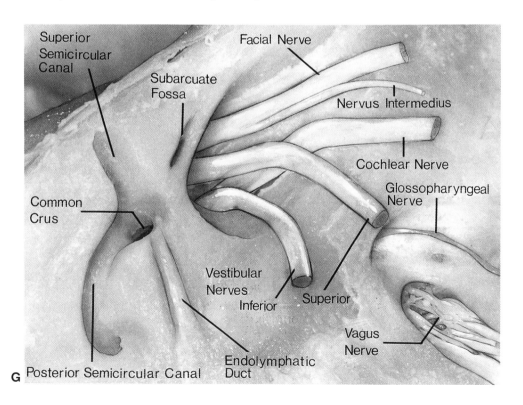

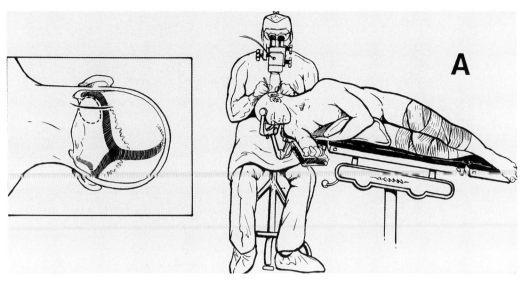

Figure 35A. *Retrosigmoid approach for the removal of acoustic neuromas. The patient is positioned in the three-quarter prone position with the surgeon behind the head. The insert shows the site of the scalp incision (continuous line) and the bony opening (interrupted line).*

foramen of Luschka, and the flocculus (Figures 25 to 27 and 37 to 40).[3,17,31,32] The AICA originates from the basilar artery and encircles the pons near the pontomedullary sulcus. After coursing near and sending branches to the nerves entering the acoustic meatus and the choroid plexus protruding from the foramen of Luschka, it passes around the flocculus to reach the surface of the middle cerebellar peduncle and terminates by supplying the lips of the cerebellopontine fissures and the petrosal surface of the cerebellum. The AICA usually bifurcates near the facial and vestibulocochlear nerves to form a rostral and a caudal trunk. The rostral trunk courses along the middle cerebellar peduncle to supply the upper part of the petrosal surface, and the caudal trunk passes near the lateral recess and supplies the lower part of the petrosal surface.

The trunk of the AICA is divided into three segments based on its relationship to the nerves and the meatus: the premeatal, the meatal, and the postmeatal segments (Figures 24, 39, and 40). The premeatal segment begins at the basilar artery and courses around the brain stem to reach the region of the meatus. The meatal segment is located in the vicinity of the internal acoustic meatus. The postmeatal segment begins distal to the nerves and courses medially to supply the brain stem and the cerebellum. This meatal segment often forms a laterally convex loop, the meatal loop, directed toward or into the meatus. In a prior study, the author's group found that the meatal segment was located medial to the porus in 46% of 50 cases and formed a loop that reached the porus or protruded into the canal in 54% of the cases.[32] When opening the meatus by the middle fossa, translabyrinthine, or posterior approaches, care is required to avoid injury to the meatal segment if it is located at or protrudes through the porus.

In most cases, the AICA passes below the facial and vestibulocochlear nerves as it encircles the brain stem, but it also may pass above or between these nerves in its course around the brain stem (Figures 25 and 39). In the most common case, in which the artery passes below the nerves, the tumor would displace the artery inferiorly (Figure 16). If the artery courses between the facial and vestibulocochlear nerves, a tumor arising in the latter nerve will displace the artery forward. Tumor growth would displace the

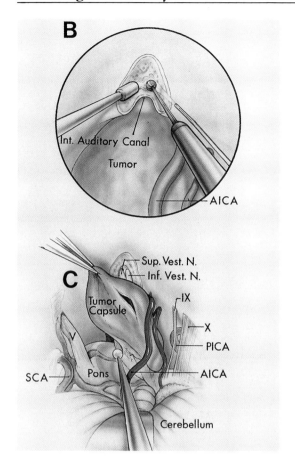
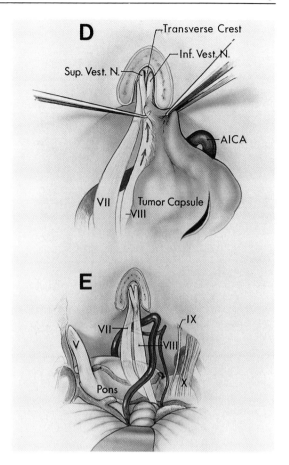

Figure 35B-E. *(B)* *The posterior wall of the internal auditory canal is being removed. The anterior inferior cerebellar artery (A.I.C.A.) courses around the lower margin of the tumor. (C) The intracapsular contents of the tumor have been removed. The capsule of the tumor is being separated from the pons and the posterior surface of the superior (Sup. Vest. N.) and inferior vestibular (Inf. Vest. N.) nerves. The trigeminal nerve (V) and the superior cerebellar artery (S.C.A.) are above the tumor and the glossopharyngeal (IX) and vagus (X) nerves and the posterior inferior cerebellar artery (P.I.C.A.) are below the tumor. (D) The dissection along the vestibulo-cochlear nerve (VIII) is performed in a medial to lateral direction (arrows) to avoid tearing the tiny filaments of the cochlear nerve in the lateral end of the canal where they pass through the lamina cribosa. The transverse crest separates the superior and inferior vestibular nerves in the lateral end of the canal. The facial nerve (VII) is anterior to the superior vestibular nerve. (E) The cerebellopontine angle (CPA) and the internal auditory canal after tumor removal with the facial and cochlear nerves preserved.[50]*

artery superiorly if it passes above the nerves.

The branches of the AICA that arise near the facial and vestibulocochlear nerves are the labyrinthine (internal auditory) arteries, which supply the facial and vestibulocochlear nerves and adjacent structures; the recurrent perforating arteries, which initially may pass toward the meatus but subsequently may turn medially and supply the brain stem; and the subarcuate artery, which enters the subarcu-

ate fossa (Figures 25, 26, and 40). The subarcuate artery usually ends in the bone below the superior canal, but it infrequently may supply the distal territory of the labyrinthine arteries.

The SCA, which is separated from the tumor by the trigeminal nerve, is displaced rostrally by the tumor, and the PICA is displaced caudally with the glossopharyngeal and vagus nerves by the tumor.

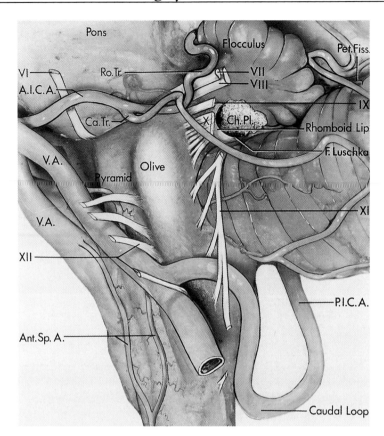

Figure 36. *Anterolateral view of the brain stem. A line drawn along the origin of the glossopharyngeal (IX), vagus (X), and spinal accessory (XI) nerves from the posterior margin of the olive will pass through the site at which the facial nerve (VII) exits the brain stem. The facial nerve usually exits the brain stem 2-3 mm rostral to where the glosso-pharyngeal nerve enters the brain stem. The rootlets of the hypoglossal nerves (XII) arise along the anterior margin of the olive. The glosso-pharyngeal and vagus nerves course anterior to the choroid plexus (Ch. Pl.) protruding from the foramen of Luschka (F. Luschka). The facial and vestibulocochlear (VIII) nerves arise in front of the flocculus. The anterior inferior cerebellar artery (A.I.C.A.) courses below the abducens nerve (VI) and gives rise to the rostral (Ro. Tr.) and caudal (Ca.Tr.) trunks. The rostral trunk courses above the flocculus to reach the petrosal fissure (Pet. Fiss.). The caudal trunk passes inferiorly. The posterior inferior cerebellar artery (P.I.C.A.) courses between the spinal accessory (XI) rootlets. The anterior spinal arteries (Ant. Sp. A.) arise from the vertebral arteries (V.A.).[31]*

Venous Relationships

The veins on the side of the brain stem that have a predictable relationship to the facial and vestibulocochlear nerves are those draining the petrosal surface of the cerebellum, the pons and the medulla, and the cerebellopontine and cerebellomedullary fissures (Figures 19, 20, and 37).[33,34,47] The identification of any of these veins during the removal of the tumor makes it easier to identify the site of the junction of the facial and vestibulocochlear nerves with the brain stem. These veins on the medial side of the tumor are the vein of the pontomedullary sulcus, which courses transversely in the pontomedullary sulcus; the lateral medullary vein, which courses longitudinally along the line of origin of the rootlets of the glossopharyngeal, vagus, and spinal accessory nerves; the vein of the

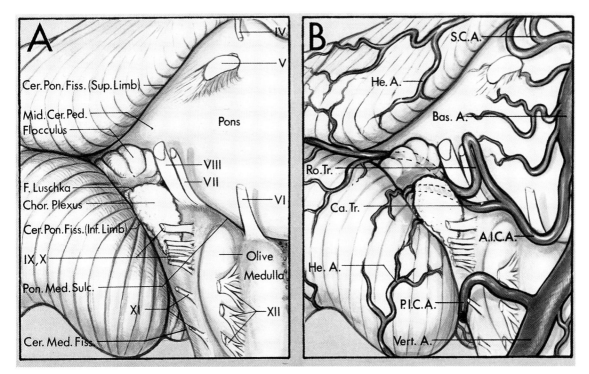

Figure 37 A, B. *Neurovascular relationships on the brain stem side of an acoustic neuroma. Anterolateral view of the right cerebellopontine angle (CPA). (A) Neural relationships. The facial (VII) and vestibulocochlear (VIII) nerves arise from the brain stem near the lateral end of the pontomedullary sulcus (Pon. Med. Sulc.); anterior-superior to the choroid plexus (Chor. Plexus) protruding from the foramen of Luschka (F. Luschka); anterior to the flocculus; rostral to a line drawn along the junction of the rootlets of the glossopharyngeal (IX), vagus (X), and spinal accessory (XI) nerves with the brain stem; and slightly posterior to the rostral pole of the inferior olive. The abducens nerve (VI) arises in the medial part of the pontomedullary sulcus. The hypoglossal rootlets (XII) arise anterior to the olive. The cerebellopontine fissure (Cer. Pon. Fiss) formed by the cerebellum wrapping around the lateral side of the pons and the middle cerebellar peduncle (Mid. Cer. Ped.) has a superior limb (Sup. Limb) that passes above the trigeminal nerve (V) and an inferior limb (Inf. Limb) that extends below the foramen of Luschka. The cerebellomedullary fissure (Cer. Med. Fiss.), which extends superiorly between the medulla and the cerebellum, communicates in the region of the foramen of Luschka with the cerebellopontine fissure. The trochlear nerve (IV) is above the trigeminal nerve. (B) Arterial relationships. The anterior inferior cerebellar artery (A.I.C.A.) arises from the basilar artery (Bas. A.) and divides into the rostral (Ro. Tr.) and caudal (Ca. Tr.) trunks. The rostral trunk, which is usually the larger of the two trunks, courses below the facial and vestibulocochlear nerves and then above the flocculus to reach the surface of the middle cerebellar peduncle. The posterior inferior cerebellar artery (P.I.C.A.) arises from the vertebral artery (Vert. A.) and passes first between the hypoglossal rootlets and then between the vagus and spinal accessory nerves on its way to the cerebellar hemisphere. The superior cerebellar artery (S.C.A.) passes above the trigeminal nerve. The cerebellar arteries give rise to the hemispheric branches (He. A.).*

cerebellomedullary fissure, which passes dorsal or ventral to the flocculus before joining the other veins in the CPA; the vein of the middle cerebellar peduncle, which is formed by the union of the lateral medullary vein and the vein of the pontomedullary sulcus and ascends on the middle cerebellar peduncle to join the vein of the cerebellopontine fissure; and the vein of the cerebellopon-

tine fissure, which is formed by the union of the veins that arise on the petrosal surface of the cerebellum and converge on the apex of the cerebellopontine fissure. All of these veins course near the lateral recess and the junction of the facial and vestibulocochlear nerves with the brain stem (Figure 37).

The veins surrounding an acoustic neuroma terminate by forming bridging veins,

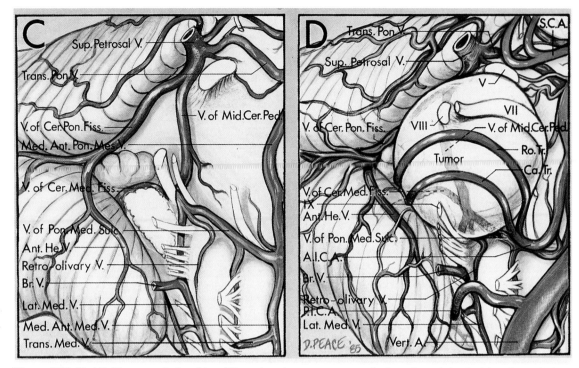

***Figure* 37C, D. (C)** *Venous relationships. The veins that converge on the junction of the facial and vestibulo-cochlear nerves with the brain stem are the veins of the pontomedullary sulcus (V. of Pon. Med. Sulc.), cerebellomedullary fissure (V. of Cer. Med. Fiss), middle cerebellar peduncle (V. of Mid. Cer. Ped.), and the retro-olivary (Retro-olivary V.) and lateral medullary veins (Lat. Med. V.). The vein of the cerebellopontine fissure (V. of Cer. Pon. Fiss.) that passes above the flocculus on the middle cerebellar peduncle is formed by the anterior hemispheric veins (Ant. He. V.) that arise on the cerebellum. Transverse pontine (Trans. Pon. V.) and transverse medullary (Trans. Med. V.) veins cross the pons and the medulla. The median anterior medullary (Med. Ant. Med. V.) and median anterior pontomesencephalic veins (Med. Ant. Pon. Mes. V.) ascend on the anterior surface of the medulla and the pons. The veins of the middle cerebellar peduncle and the cerebellopon-tine fissure and a transverse pontine vein join to form a superior petrosal vein (Sup. Petrosal V.) that empties into the superior petrosal sinus. A bridging vein (Br. V.) passes below the vagal rootlets toward the jugular foramen. **(D)** Neurovascular relationships of an acoustic neuroma. The tumor arises from the vestibulocochlear nerve and displaces the facial nerve anteriorly, the trigeminal nerve superiorly, and the vagus and glossopharyn-geal nerves inferiorly. The facial nerve, even though displaced by the tumor, exits the brain stem along the lateral margin of the pontomedullary sulcus, rostral to the glossopharyngeal and vagus nerves, anterior to the flocculus, and rostral to the choroid plexus protruding from the foramen of Luschka. The rostral trunk of the anterior inferior cerebellar artery, after passing below the tumor, returns to the surface of the middle cerebellar peduncle above the flocculus. The veins displaced around the medial side of the tumor are the veins of the middle cerebellar peduncle, cerebellomedullary fissure, cerebellopontine fissure, and pontomedullary sulcus, and the retro-olivary and lateral medullary veins.*[47]

called petrosal veins, that empty into the superior petrosal sinus (Figures 19, 20, and 37). These veins, which cross the CPA to reach the superior petrosal sinus, are the ones most frequently occluded in the course of operations in the CPA. Bridging veins are exposed more frequently and sacrificed in the rostral part of the CPA during operations

near the trigeminal nerve than during opera-tions near the nerves entering the internal acoustic meatus. The exposure of an acoustic neuroma in the central part of the CPA near the lateral recess usually can be completed without sacrificing a bridging vein. If a vein is obliterated during acoustic tumor removal, it is usually one of the superior petrosal

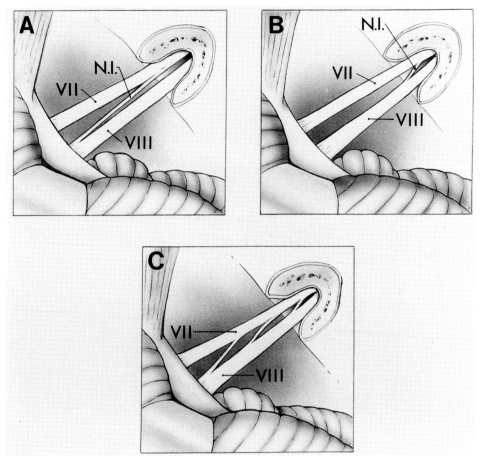

Figure 38. *View of the cerebellopontine angle (CPA) from above to show the relationship of the nervus intermedius to the facial (VII) and vestibulocochlear (VIII) nerves. (A) Most common relationship. The nervus intermedius (N.I.) is joined to the ventral surface of the vestibulocochlear nerve for a few millimeters adjacent to the brain stem, then has a free segment in the CPA as it courses to join the facial motor root. (B) Pattern present in 20% of the nerves studied. The free segment is entirely in the meatus. (C) The nervus intermedius consists of three free segments. Two are in the CPA and one is in the meatus. The nervus intermedius in A could be exposed in the CPA without drilling off the posterior lip of the meatus. In B, the free segment could not be found in the angle but only in the meatus.[50]*

veins, which is sacrificed near the superior pole of the tumor during the later stages of the removal of a large tumor. Small acoustic neuromas usually are removed without sacrificing a petrosal vein. The largest vein encountered around the superior pole of an acoustic neuroma is the vein of the cerebellopontine fissure, which passes from the petrosal surface of the cerebellum above the facial and vestibulocochlear nerves to join tributaries of the superior petrosal sinus.

Summary: Anatomy of Acoustic Neuromas

Because acoustic neuromas most frequently arise in the posteriorly placed vestibular nerves, they usually displace the facial and cochlear nerves anteriorly (Figures 30, 33, and 35). The facial nerve is stretched around the anterior half of the tumor capsule. Variability in the direction of the growth of the tumor arising from the vestibular nerves may result in

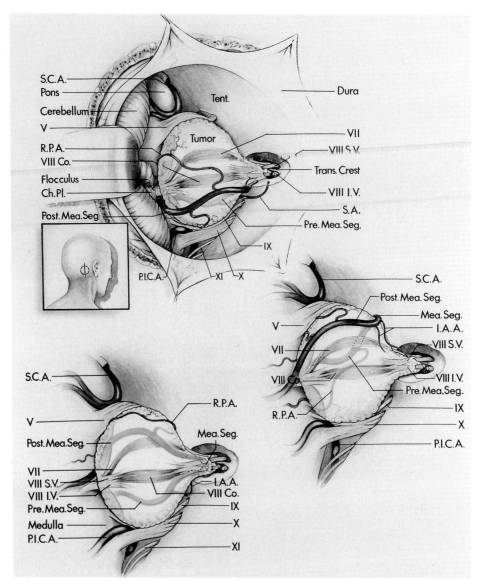

Figure 39. Posterior views of the direction of displacement of the anterior inferior cerebellar artery around an acoustic neuroma. Top left. The insert shows the direction of view. Both the premeatal (Pre. Mea. Seg.) and the postmeatal (Post. Mea. Seg.) segments are in their most common locations around the lower margin of the tumor. The premeatal segment approaches the meatus from anteroinferior, and the postmeatal segment passes posteroinferior to the tumor. The superior cerebellar artery (S.C.A.) and the trigeminal nerve (V) are above the tumor, and the posterior inferior cerebellar artery (P.I.C.A.) and the glossopharyngeal (IX), vagus (X), and spinal accessory (XI) nerves are below the tumor. The choroid plexus (Ch. Pl.) protrudes into the cerebellopontine angle (CPA) medial to the tumor. The posterior wall of the internal acoustic canal has been removed to expose the transverse crest (Trans. Crest) and the superior vestibular (VIII S.V.) and inferior vestibular (VIII I.V.) nerves. The vestibular nerves disappear into the tumor; however, the cochlear (VIII Co.) and facial (VII) nerves are displaced around the anterior margin of the tumor. A subarcuate artery (S.A.) arises from the premeatal segment, and a recurrent perforating artery (R.P.A.) arises from the postmeatal segment. Center right. In a less common pattern of displacement of the AICA, the premeatal and postmeatal segments are above the tumor. The internal auditory arteries (I.A.A.) arise from the meatal segment (Mea. Seg.). Bottom left. Both the premeatal and the postmeatal segments are displaced anteriorly to the tumor. This occurs if the AICA courses between the vestibulocochlear and facial nerves. The tumor arises in the vestibular nerves, and tumor growth displaces both the premeatal and the postmeatal segments anteriorly.[32]

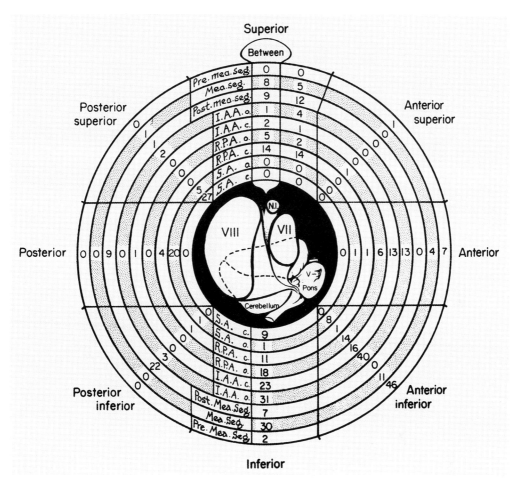

Figure 40. *Diagram showing the relationship of nerve-related arteries to the nerves in the cerebellopontine angle (CPA). The nerves are oriented as shown in the central diagram of the right side of the brain stem. The trigeminal nerve (V) arises from the pons. The facial (VII) and vestibulocochlear (VIII) nerves and the nervus intermedius (N.I.) are oriented as shown. The terms* superior, anterosuperior, *etc., refer to the relationship of the arteries to the nerves. The number of arteries and arterial segments found in 50 CPAs are listed according to their location in relationship to the nerves. The most common locations were as follows: premeatal segment (Pre. Mea. Seg.), anteroinferior; meatal segment (Mea. Seg.), inferior; postmeatal segment (Post. Mea. Seg.), posteroinferior; internal auditory artery origin (I.A.A.o.) and course (I.A.A.c.), inferior and anteroinferior; recurrent perforating artery origin (R.P.A.o.), inferior and anteroinferior, and course (R.P.A.C.), superior and between; and subarcuate artery origin (S.A.o.), posterior, and course (S.A.c.), posterosuperior.*[32]

the facial nerve being displaced, not only directly anteriorly, but also anterior-superiorly or anterior-inferiorly. The nerve infrequently is found on the posterior surface of the tumor. Because the facial nerve always enters the facial canal at the anterior-superior quadrant of the lateral margin of the meatus, it usually is easiest to locate it here, rather than at a more medial location where the degree

of displacement of the nerve is more variable. The cochlear nerve also lies anterior to the vestibular nerve and is stretched most frequently around the anterior half of the tumor. The strokes of the fine dissecting instruments used in removing the tumor should be directed along the vestibulocochlear nerve from medial to lateral rather than from lateral to medial, because traction

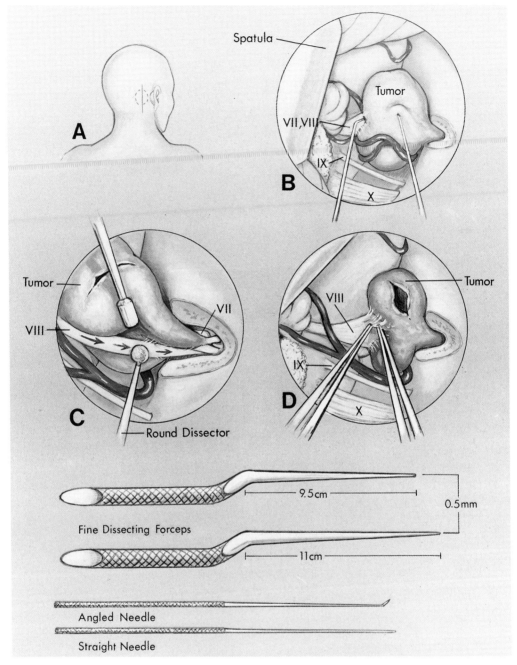

Figure 41. *Three methods for separating the capsule of an acoustic neuroma from the involved nerves using fine dissecting instruments. (A) Site of the skin incision (solid line) and the craniectomy (interrupted line). (B) A small acoustic neuroma is being separated from the vestibulocochlear nerve (VIII) using angled and straight needles (shown below). The straight needle is used to retract the tumor capsule and the angled needle separates the tumor capsule and the nerve. A brain spatula protects the cerebellum. The glossopharyngeal (IX) and vagus (X) nerves are below the tumor. (C) The nerve and the tumor capsule are separated with a round dissector. The strokes of the dissectors should be directed from medial to lateral if there is a chance of preserving hearing. The facial nerve (VII) is exposed at the lateral end of the meatus. (D) The residual capsule of a large tumor is being separated from the vestibulocochlear nerve using fine dissecting bayonet forceps having 0.5-mm tips. Bayonet dissecting forceps with 9.5-cm shafts are used in deep sites such as the cerebellopontine angle (CPA). Bayonet forceps with 11-mm shafts are used at extra deep sites such as in front of the brain stem.[51]*

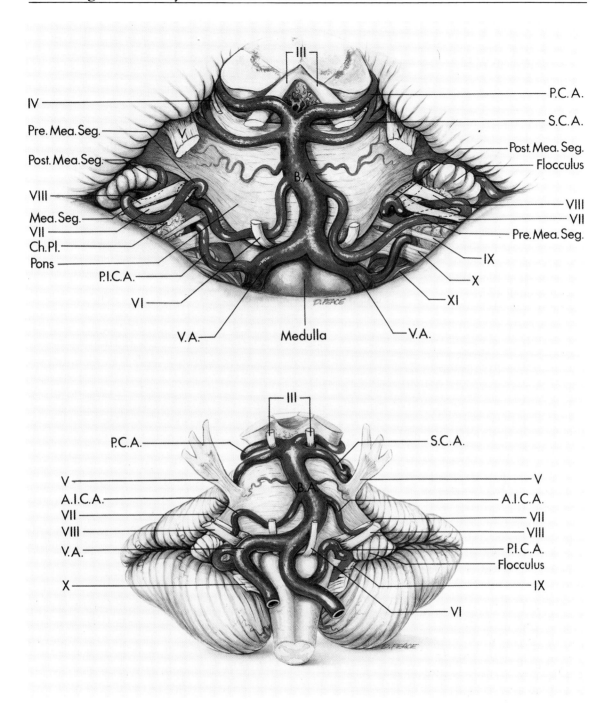

Figure 42. Sites of arterial compression of the facial nerve in hemifacial spasm. **(A)** Anterosuperior view. The facial (VII) and vestibulocochlear (VIII) nerves are distorted at their junction with the brain stem by the right premeatal (Pre. Mea. Seg.) and the left postmeatal (Post. Mea. Seg.) segments of the anterior inferior cerebellar arteries. Other structures exposed include the oculomotor (III), trochlear (IV), trigeminal (V), abducens (VI), glossopharyngeal (IX), vagus (X), and spinal accessory (XI) nerves; the posterior cerebral (P.C.A.), superior cerebellar (S.C.A.), basilar (B.A.), posterior inferior cerebellar (P.I.C.A.), and vertebral (V.A.) arteries; the choroid plexus (Ch. Pl.) protruding from the foramen of Luschka; and the meatal segments (Mea. Seg.) of the AICAs. **(B)** Anterior view. The junction of the right facial and vestibulocochlear nerves with the brain stem is compressed by a tortuous vertebral artery. The nerves on the left side are compressed by the PICA.[32]

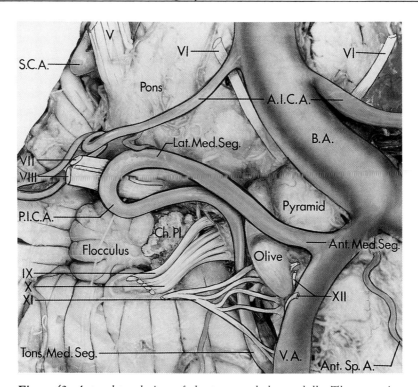

Figure 43. Anterolateral view of the pons and the medulla. The posterior inferior cerebellar artery (P.I.C.A.) arises from the vertebral artery (V.A.) and loops upward against the facial (VII) and vestibulocochlear (VIII) nerves before descending in front of the choroid plexus (Ch. Pl.) protruding from the foramen of Luschka and the glossopharyngeal (IX) and vagus (X) nerves. The PICA reaches the posterior medullary surface by passing between the rootlets of the vagus and spinal accessory nerves (XI). This portion of the PICA is divided into the anterior medullary (Ant. Med. Seg.), lateral medullary (Lat. Med. Seg.), and tonsillomedullary (Tons. Med. Seg.) segments. Other structures in the exposure include the basilar (B.A.), anterior inferior cerebellar (A.I.C.A.), superior cerebellar (S.C.A.), and anterior spinal (Ant. Sp. A.) arteries and the trigeminal (V), abducens (VI), and hypoglossal (XII) nerves.[31]

medially may tear the tiny filaments of the cochlear nerve at the site where these filaments penetrate the lateral end of the meatus to enter the cochlea (Figures 34E and 35D). The motor responses of the facial nerve are monitored using electromyographic techniques. Auditory-evoked potentials also are monitored if a goal is to preserve hearing.

The operation for a CPA tumor should be planned so that the tumor surface is allowed to settle away from the neural tissue rather than the neural structures being retracted away from the tumor.[48] No attempt is made to see the whole tumor upon initial exposure. The surface of the tumor then is opened and

the intracapsular contents are removed. As the intracapsular contents are evacuated, the tumor shifts laterally, allowing more of the tumor to be removed through the small exposure. The most common reason for the tumor appearing to be tightly adherent to the neural structures is not adhesions between the capsule and surrounding tissue but, rather, the residual tumor within the capsule wedging the tumor into position. As the intracapsular contents are removed, the tumor capsule folds laterally, revealing the structures on the brain stem side of the tumor.

The landmarks that are helpful in identifying the facial and vestibulocochlear nerves at the brain stem on the medial side of the tumor have been reviewed (Figures 36 and 37).[47] These nerves, although distorted by the tumor, usually can be identified on the brain stem side of the tumor at the lateral end of the pontomedullary sulcus just rostral to the glossopharyngeal nerve and just anterior-superior to the foramen of Luschka, the flocculus, and the choroid plexus protruding from the foramen of Luschka. After the facial and vestibulocochlear nerves are identified on the medial and lateral sides of the tumor, the final remnants of the tumor are separated from the intervening segment of the nerves using fine dissecting instruments (Figure 41).

It is especially important to preserve the segment of the cerebellar arteries adherent to the tumor capsule because a major cause of operative mortality and morbidity is the loss of perforating arteries and branches of the cerebellar arteries that may be adherent to and displaced by the tumor (Figures 37 and 39). Any vessel that stands above or is stretched around the tumor capsule should be dealt with initially as if it were an artery that runs over the tumor surface to supply the brain. After the tumor has been removed from within the capsule, an attempt should be made to displace the vessel off the tumor capsule using a small dissector. When dissected free of the capsule, vessels that initially appeared to be adherent to the capsule often prove to be neural vessels.

The number of veins sacrificed should be kept to a minimum because of the undesirable consequences of their loss. Obliteration of the petrosal veins, which pass from the surface of the cerebellum and the brain stem to the superior petrosal sinus, is inescapable when reaching and removing some CPA tumors (Figures 19 and 20). Occlusion of these veins, which drain much of the cerebellum and the brain stem, infrequently may cause hemorrhagic edema of the cerebellum and the brain stem. Some of these veins may need to be sacrificed if the tumor extends into the area above the internal acoustic meatus. Small acoustic neuromas and other tumors in the lower part of the CPA, however, frequently may be removed without

sacrificing a petrosal vein.

In the three approaches to the meatus and CPA (retrosigmoid, translabyrinthine, and middle fossa), a communication may be established between the subarachnoid space and the mastoid air cells that will require careful closure to prevent a cerebrospinal fluid leak.

Anatomy of Vascular Compression in the Middle Neurovascular Complex

Compression of the facial and vestibulocochlear nerves by tortuous arteries is postulated to cause dysfunction of these nerves, and cases in which surgical liberation of the vessels from these nerves has relieved the symptoms provide strong support for a vascular compressive etiology of these cranial nerve dysfunction syndromes[13,27,43] (Figures 42-44). Ectasia and elongation of the arteries are important in forcing the arteries into the nerves.

Gardner was the first to treat hemifacial spasm by removing a compressive arterial loop from the facial nerve.[13] Jannetta et al, using the suboccipital approach to the CPA, found mechanical compression and distortion of the root exit zone of the facial nerve in all of 47 patients with hemifacial spasm.[27] The distorting vessel not only was the AICA and its branches, but in some cases was found to be the PICA, the vertebral or basilar artery, veins, or an arteriovenous malformation (Figures 42-44).[27] It is expected that the AICA would be the compressing vessel in most cases because the facial nerve is located in the middle neurovascular complex. A tortuous PICA, a member of the lower neurovascular complex, however, is the most frequent offending vessel in hemifacial spasm, followed in order by the AICA, vertebral artery, basilar artery, veins, and combination of these vessels. The proximal part of the PICA usually passes around the brain stem below the facial and vestibulocochlear nerves. In some

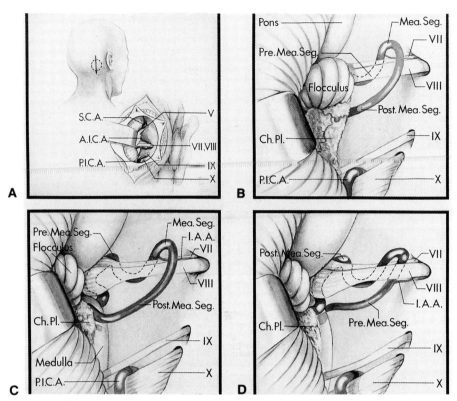

Figure 44A, B, C, D. Arterial compression of the facial nerve in hemifacial spasm as viewed posteriorly through a retrosigmoid craniectomy performed with the patient in the three-quarter prone position. *(A)* The upper drawing shows the site of the incision (straight line) and the location of the bone opening (broken line). The lower drawing shows the surgical exposure obtained with this approach. The anterior inferior cerebellar artery (A.I.C.A.) and the facial (VII) and vestibulocochlear (VIII) nerves are in the midportion of the exposure. The vertebral artery (Vert. A) and the posterior inferior cerebellar artery (P.I.C.A.) and the glossopharyngeal (IX), vagus (X), and spinal accessory (XI) nerves are below. *(B)* The cerebellum is elevated to expose the facial and vestibulocochlear nerves and the premeatal (Pre. Mea. Seg.), meatal (Mea. Seg.), and postmeatal (Post. Mea. Seg.) segments of the AICA. The flocculus and the choroid plexus (Ch. Pl.) block the view of the junction of the facial and vestibulocochlear nerves with the brain stem. *(C)* The flocculus and the choroid plexus have been elevated to expose the root entry/exit zone of the facial and vestibulocochlear nerves. The premeatal segment compresses the nerves at the junction with the pons and the medulla. *(D)* The nerve root entry/exit zone is compressed by the postmeatal segment.[32]

CPAs, however, the proximal part of the PICA, after coursing posteriorly to the level of the hypoglossal rootlets, will loop superiorly toward the facial and vestibulocochlear nerves before descending to pass between the glossopharyngeal, vagus, and spinal accessory nerves (Figures 42-44).

The offending arterial loop may be located on either the superior or the inferior aspect of the facial nerve at its exit from the brain stem. In the most common type of hemifa-

cial spasm, that beginning in the orbicularis oculi muscle and gradually spreading downward to involve the lower face, the anterior-inferior aspect of the nerve root exit zone will commonly be compressed. Atypical hemifacial spasm, beginning in the midface and spreading upward to involve the frontalis muscle, will be caused by the compression of the posterosuperior aspect of the facial nerve at the brain stem. Jannetta and others thought that the arteries frequently seen coursing

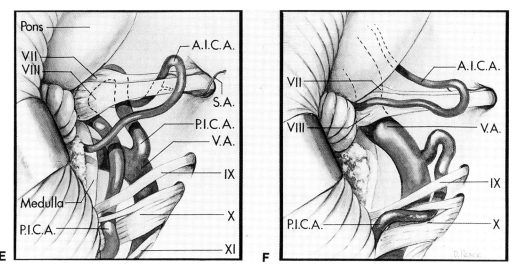

Figure 44E, F. *(E) A tortuous PICA loops upward to compress the nerves at their junction with the brain stem before turning inferiorly to pass between the glossopharyngeal and vagus nerves. (F) A tortuous vertebral artery compresses the nerve root entry/exit zone.*[32]

around or between the facial and vestibulocochlear nerves in the interval between the brain stem and the porus acusticus, as found by Gardner,[13] were not the cause of hemifacial spasm, but that cross compression of the facial nerve by the same arteries coursing at right angles to the nerve at the root exit zone was the essential element.[27]

This author performs the operation for hemifacial spasm with the patient in the three-quarter prone position with the anterior-posterior axis of the head parallel to the floor. The surgeon, for operations in the middle compartment, is positioned behind the head of the patient rather than at the head of the table as shown for operations in the upper complex (Figures 13A and 35A). It is helpful for the top of the head to be tilted slightly downward toward the floor to keep the inferolateral exposure away from the patient's upper shoulder, which may block the exposure. One should avoid placing tape on the upper shoulder to pull it downward to keep it from blocking access to the operative site because this may injure the brachial plexus. It is best to let the patient and the upper shoulder roll slightly forward to position the shoulder out of the route of passage of the instruments for the inferolateral exposure. Care should be taken to avoid injuring

the vertebral artery as it courses along the upper margin of the atlas. It is not necessary to extend the bone opening downward to the foramen magnum or upward to the transverse sinus. The opening has its lateral edge along the medial edge of the lower half of the sigmoid sinus. When the dura is opened, the arachnoid covering the cisterna magna is opened for aspiration of cerebrospinal fluid, which will increase the extracerebellar space. The inferolateral margin of the cerebellum behind the glossopharyngeal and vagus nerves is elevated with a small brain spatula that is tapered from 10 mm at the base to 3 mm at the tip. The arachnoid behind the glossopharyngeal and vagus nerves is opened. This will expose the tuft of choroid plexus protruding from the foramen of Luschka, which sits on the posterior surface of the glossopharyngeal and vagus nerves. The arachnoid then is opened posterior to the facial and vestibulocochlear nerves. Commonly, the flocculus is seen protruding behind the nerves and blocks their visualization at the junction with the brain stem. It also may be difficult to see the facial nerve that is hidden in front of the vestibulocochlear nerve. At this time, it is important to recall that the facial nerve root exits the brain stem 2-3 mm rostral to the point at which the glossopharyngeal nerve enters the brain stem. To expose the nerve root exit zone of the facial nerve, it may be necessary to gently separate the choroid plexus from the posterior margin of the glossopharyngeal and upper vagal rootlets so that their junction with the brain stem can be seen. The brain spatula is advanced upward to elevate the choroid plexus away from the posterior margin of the glossopharyngeal nerve. The exposure then is directed several millimeters above the glossopharyngeal nerve to where the facial nerve will be seen joining the brain stem in front of the vestibulocochlear nerve. The spatula often needs to be positioned so that it elevates the lower margin of the flocculus. Care must be taken to avoid damage to the vestibulocochlear nerve, which may be adherent to the posterior margin of the flocculus. The most common offending arterial loop is a PICA that loops upward prior to passing between the glossopharyngeal, vagus, and spinal accessory nerves (Figure 43). After looping into the facial nerve exit zone, the PICA then passes distally between the rootlets of the lower cranial nerves. The compressing artery also may be the premeatal or postmeatal segments of the AICA or a tortuous vertebral or basilar artery (Figures 42 to 44). Care is taken to explore the interval between the facial and vestibulocochlear nerves because it would be easy to miss a vessel compressing the facial nerve in this location.

Venous compression is less commonly encountered. The most common venous compression is by the vein of the pontomedullary sulcus, the retro-olivary vein, or the vein of the middle cerebellar peduncle (Figures 19, 20, and 37C).[33] The vein of the pontomedullary sulcus courses in the groove between the pons and the medulla and joins the retro-olivary vein that courses along the origin of the rootlets of the glossopharyngeal and vagus nerves from the retro-olivary sulcus. These two veins join in the region of the facial nerve to form the vein of the middle cerebellar peduncle, which ascends on the middle cerebellar peduncle toward the superior petrosal sinus. The vein of the middle cerebellar peduncle commonly passes between the facial

and vestibulocochlear nerves. It is not uncommon to encounter a bridging vein that passes from the lateral side of the medulla to the jugular bulb. At the time of elevating the cerebellum, it is best to obliterate this vein with gentle bipolar coagulation.

The same dissecting instruments described for trigeminal neuralgia are useful in operations for hemifacial spasm.[51] Scissors and bayonet forceps with 9.5-cm shafts are needed to work comfortably at this depth. Bayonet and bipolar forceps with tips no larger than 0.5 mm are used for gentle bipolar coagulation in this area. The 40°-angled teardrop dissectors are especially helpful in exploring the area around the junction of the nerves with the brain stem.

Cochlear and Vestibular Nerve Compression Syndromes

Vascular compression has been reported as a cause of cochlear and vestibular nerve dysfunction manifested by tinnitus, hearing loss, dysequilibrium, and disabling positional vertigo.[24,29,35,36] The site of the compressive lesion with vestibulocochlear nerve dysfunction, however, may be more peripheral along the nerve rather than at the junction with the brain stem, as commonly seen in trigeminal neuralgia and hemifacial spasm. Jannetta and others have restricted the use of the operation for vestibulocochlear nerve symptoms to those patients who are disabled and have documented unilateral disease on neuro-otologic testing.[29] Jannetta et al[29] and Gardner[13] have postulated that vascular compression of a cranial nerve is more likely to be symptomatic when it is located on the nerve proximal to the Obersteiner-Redlich zone where the axons are insulated by central myelin produced by oligodendroglia. It is proximal to this glial-neurilemmal junction that the compression causes transaxonal excitement between the afferent and efferent fibers. This glial-neurilemmal junction on the facial and trigeminal nerves is situated at the nerve root junction with the brain stem, but the entire intracranial portion of the vestibulocochlear nerve is sensitive to compression because the glial-neurilemmal junction is located at or in the internal acoustic meatus. Cochlear nerve dysfunction has been related to compression at any site between the brain stem and the meatus, but vestibular nerve dysfunction has been found to be related to compression at or near the junction of the nerve with the brain stem.[29]

Compression by veins is less common around the facial and vestibulocochlear nerves than in the region of the trigeminal nerve because the veins around the facial and vestibulocochlear nerves tend to be smaller. Because no large bridging veins cross the subarachnoid space around the facial and vestibulocochlear nerves, as are seen frequently around the trigeminal nerve, any vascular cross compression of the facial and vestibulocochlear nerves peripheral to the brain stem is likely to be caused by arteries that loop through the CPA and even into the meatus. The veins at the level of the junction of the facial and vestibulocochlear nerves with the brain stem tightly hug the pontomedullary junction where they adhere to the pial membrane as described in the section on hemifacial spasm. The same operative approach as described for hemifacial spasm is used for vestibulocochlear nerve dysfunction.

Geniculate Neuralgia

When sectioning the nervus intermedius for geniculate neuralgia, it is important to recall that the nervus intermedius may be composed of as many as four rootlets[53] (see Figure 38). It also is important to recall that these rootlets are composed of a medial segment that adheres to the vestibulocochlear nerve at the brain stem, an intermediate segment between where it leaves the vestibulocochlear nerve and joins the facial motor root, and a distal segment joined to the facial motor root. It is the intermediate segment that would be divided in geniculate neuralgia. This segment, where the nervus intermedius is free of both the facial and vestibulocochlear nerves, may be located in the CPA or in the meatus if the nervus intermedius is composed of a single rootlet. If the nervus

intermedius is composed of more than one rootlet, however, there may be free segments both in the CPA and in the meatus. Geniculate neuralgia with or without vestibulocochlear dysfunction also has been postulated to be caused by vascular compression of the nervus intermedius or the vestibulocochlear nerve.[24,37]

Lower Neurovascular Complex

The lower complex, which is related to the PICA, includes the medulla, inferior cerebellar peduncle, cerebellomedullary fissure, suboccipital surface of the cerebellum, and the glossopharyngeal, vagus, spinal accessory, and hypoglossal nerves (Figures 1, 45, and 46). The PICA arises at the medullary level, encircles the medulla, passing in relationship to the glossopharyngeal, vagus, spinal accessory, and hypoglossal nerves to reach the surface of the inferior cerebellar peduncle, where it dips into the cerebellomedullary fissure and terminates by supplying the suboccipital surface of the cerebellum. The more common surgically treatable conditions involving the lower complex include glossopharyngeal neuralgia and tumors of the lower clivus and jugular foramen.

Jugular Foramen

Three of the four nerves in the lower complex exit the skull through the jugular foramen (Figure 47). The anterolateral bony wall of the jugular foramen is formed by the temporal bone and the posteromedial wall by the occipital bone. The bony foramen is subdivided into a larger posterolateral compartment called the pars venosa and a smaller anteromedial compartment called the pars nervosa.[8,52] The pars venosa contains the jugular bulb, the vagus and spinal accessory nerves, and a posterior meningeal artery. The pars nervosa contains the inferior petrosal sinus and the glossopharyngeal nerve (Figures 47 and 48). These two parts usually are separated by a fibrous bridge connecting the jugular spine of the petrous temporal bone to the jugular process of the occipital bone. This

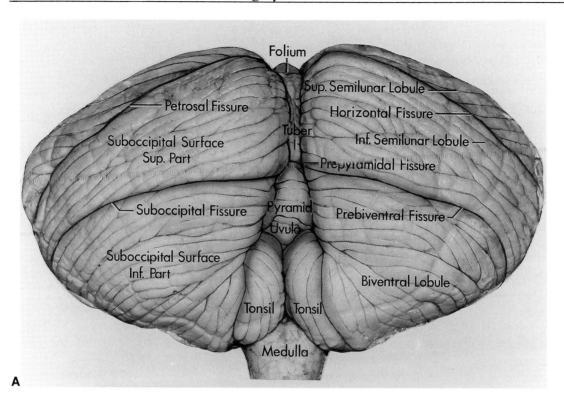

A

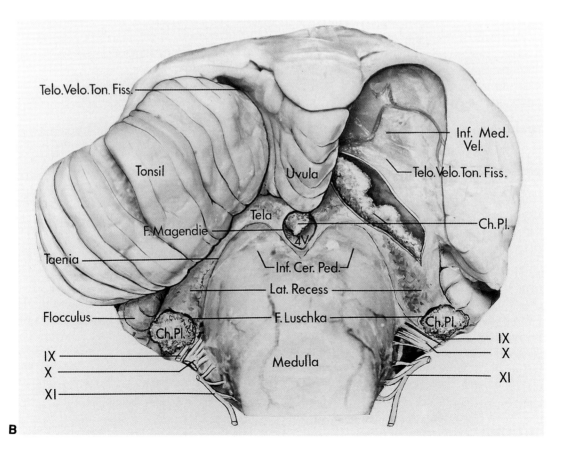

B

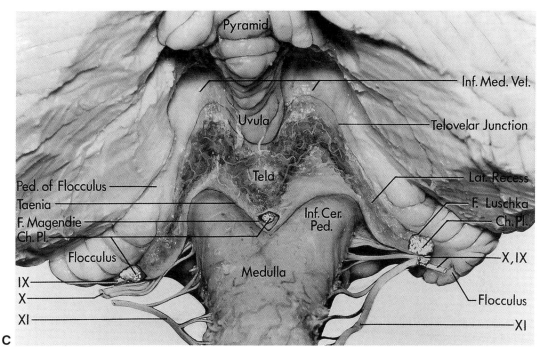

Figure 45A, B, C. Relationships in the lower neurovascular complex. **(A)** Suboccipital surface of the cerebellum. This is the surface exposed in a wide suboccipital craniectomy. It extends from the transverse sinuses above to the foramen magnum below and to the sigmoid sinuses laterally. The corresponding vermian and hemispheric portions of the suboccipital surface are the folium and the superior (Sup.) semilunar lobule, the tuber and the inferior (Inf.) semilunar lobule, the pyramid and the biventral lobule, and the uvula and the tonsil. There are two significant fissures on this surface. The most important, the suboccipital fissure, divides the suboccipital surface into superior (Sup. Part) and inferior (Inf. Part) parts. This fissure divides the hemispheres between the biventral and the inferior semilunar lobules and the vermis between the tuber and the pyramid. The hemispheric component of this fissure is called the prebiventral fissure, and the vermian part is called the prepyramidal fissure. The petrosal fissure, which also is called the horizontal fissure, begins on the petrosal surface of the cerebellum and divides the superior half of the suboccipital surface into the superior and inferior semilunar lobules. **(B)** The right tonsil has been removed. The upper pole of the left tonsil has been reflected inferiorly to show the telovelotonsillar fissure (Telo. Velo. Ton. Fiss.), which is situated between the tonsil below and the inferior medullary velum (Inf. Med. Vel.) and the tela choroidea (Tela) above. The tela choroidea is attached to the caudal margin of the inferior medullary velum and extends inferiorly over the lower part of the roof of the fourth ventricle (4 V). The tela choroidea is attached to the edge of the floor of the fourth ventricle along small ridges called the taenia. The choroid plexus (Ch. Pl.) protrudes from the foramen of Luschka (F. Luschka) at the lateral end of the lateral recess (Lat. Recess.) and from the foramen of Magendie (F. Magendie) in the midline. On the right side, the tela has been opened to expose the choroid plexus in the lateral recess. The choroid plexus is attached to the inner surface of the tela choroidea. The glossopharyngeal (IX) and vagus (X) nerves arise anterior to the foramen of Luschka. The spinal accessory nerves (XI) arise caudal to the vagus nerves. **(C)** Both tonsils and the adjacent part of the cerebellum have been removed to show the inferior medullary velum and the tela choroidea covering the lower one-half of the roof of the fourth ventricle. The peduncle of the flocculus (Ped. of Flocculus) is anterosuperior to the lateral recess. The inferior cerebellar peduncle (Inf. Cer. Ped.) passes anterior and then superior to the lateral recess to reach the cerebellum.

bridge separating the pars venosa and the pars nervosa will be ossified in about one-quarter of foramina. The right foramen usually is larger than the left.[61] In a previous

study, the right foramen was larger than the left in 68%, equal in 12%, and smaller than the left in 20% of the cases.[52] The cranial nerves course along the anteromedial wall of

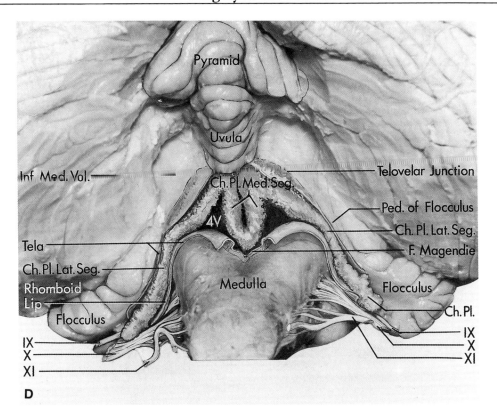

D

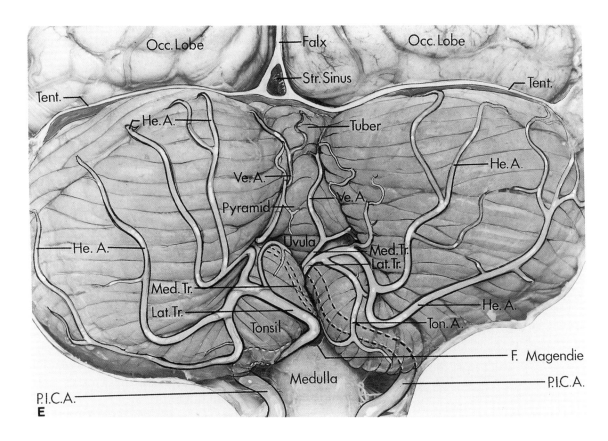

E

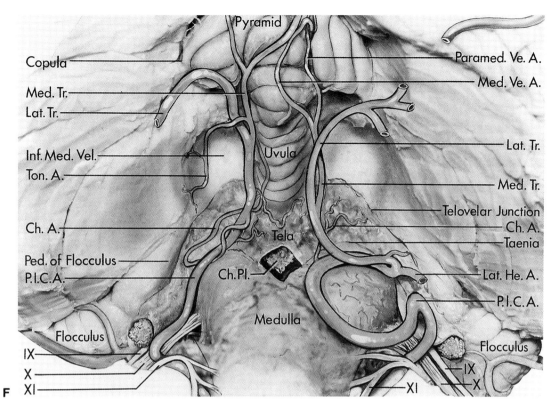

Figure 45D, E, F. (D) The tela choroidea has been opened at its junction with the inferior medullary velum to show the choroid plexus in the fourth ventricle. Each half of the choroid plexus has a medial (Ch. Pl. Med. Seg.) and a lateral (Ch. Pl. Lat. Seg.) segment. The medial segment protrudes from the foramen of Luschka. *(E)* The posterior inferior cerebellar arteries (P.I.C.A.) pass around the medulla (dashed lines) to supply the suboccipital surface. The PICAs bifurcate into lateral (Lat. Tr.) and medial (Med. Tr.) trunks. The medial trunk gives rise to the vermian arteries (Ve. A.) and the lateral trunk gives rise to the tonsillar (Ton. A.) and hemispheric (He. A.) arteries. Other structures in the exposure include the tentorium cerebelli (Tent.), occipital lobe (Occ. Lobe), and straight sinus (Str. Sinus). *(F)* The tonsils and part of the biventral lobules have been removed to show the relationship of the trunks of the PICA to the tela choroidea, inferior medullary velum, and flocculus. The PICAs give rise to choroidal (Ch. A.), lateral hemispheric (Lat. He. A.), and median (Med. Ve. A.) and paramedian vermian (Paramed. Ve. A.) arteries.

the jugular foramen and the jugular bulb (Figure 49). The vagus and spinal accessory nerves pass through the part of the pars venosa adjacent to the pars nervosa through which the glossopharyngeal nerve passes. In a few cases, the glossopharyngeal nerve exits the skull through a separate bony canal anterior to, rather than through, the pars nervosa.

The dura mater over the anteromedial part of the jugular foramen has two characteristic perforations forming a glossopharyngeal meatus, through which the glossopharyngeal nerve passes to enter the pars nervosa, and a vagal meatus, through which the vagus and spinal accessory nerves reach the ante-

romedial part of the pars venosa and the jugular bulb (Figures 47, 50-52).[52] The glossopharyngeal and vagal meati are consistently separated by a dural septum ranging from 0.5-4.9 mm. The only site at which the glossopharyngeal nerve is consistently distinguishable from the vagus is just proximal to this dural septum. The glossopharyngeal meatus is funnel shaped, becoming narrower as the nerve passes distally. The vagal meatus is a shallow, sievelike dural depression, approximately twice the width of the glossopharyngeal meatus; it lies over the anteromedial part of the pars venosa and varies in shape from elliptical to round or even rectangular.

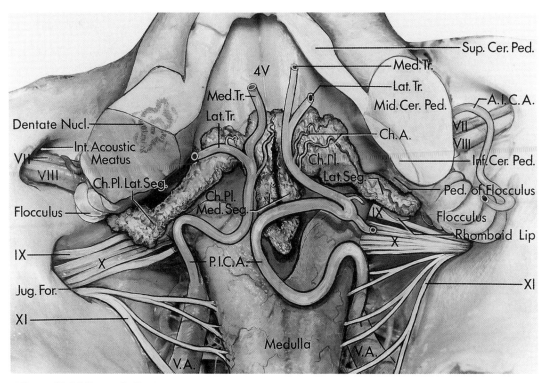

Figure 45G. *The cerebellar hemispheres and the tela choroidea have been removed to expose the floor of the fourth ventricle and the choroid plexus. The glossopharyngeal, vagus, and spinal accessory nerves enter the jugular foramen (Jug. For.), and the facial (VII) and vestibulocochlear (VIII) nerves enter the internal acoustic meatus (Int. Acoustic Meatus). The level of removal of the cerebellum on the left side extends through the dentate nucleus (Dentate Nucl.), and on the right side it extends through the superior (Sup. Cer. Ped.), middle (Mid. Cer. Ped.) and inferior cerebellar peduncles. The anterior inferior cerebellar artery (A.I.C.A.) passes above the facial and glossopharyngeal nerves.*[31]

The anterior and lateral margins of the glossopharyngeal and vagal meati frequently form a roof or lip that projects posteromedially over the respective dural exits of the nerves (Figures 47, 50-52). This lip projects most prominently over the glossopharyngeal meatus and is comparable to, but smaller than, the posterior lip of the acoustic meatus. It is either predominantly bony or fibrous and may project a maximum of 2.5 mm over the margin of the glossopharyngeal meatus.[52] The vagal lip is present infrequently and projects a maximum of 1 mm over the margin of the meatus.

Neural Relationships

The glossopharyngeal, vagus, spinal accessory, and hypoglossal nerves arise from the medulla along the margin of the infe-

rior olive. The glossopharyngeal, vagus, and spinal accessory nerves arise as a line of rootlets that exit the brain stem along the posterior edge of the olive in the postolivary sulcus, a shallow groove between the olive and posterolateral surface of the medulla (Figures 46, 47, and 53-55). The hypoglossal nerve arises as a line of rootlets that exit the brain stem along the anterior margin of the lower two-thirds of the olive in the preolivary sulcus, a groove between the olive and the medullary pyramid. The glossopharyngeal and vagus nerves arise at the level of the superior one-third of the olive. The spinal accessory rootlets arise along the posterior margin of the inferior two-thirds of the olive and from the lower medulla and the upper segments of the cervical spinal cord. The glossopharyngeal and vagus nerves arise rostral to the level of origin of the hypoglossal rootlets.

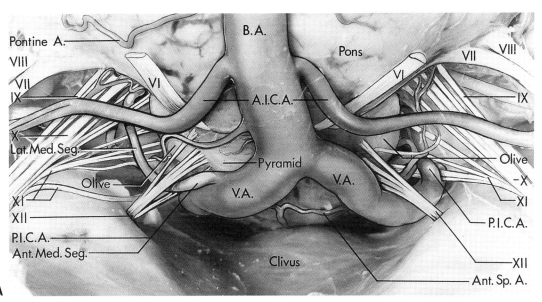

Figure 46. Anterior-superior views of the lower neurovascular complex. *(A)* The posterior inferior cerebellar arteries (P.I.C.A.) arise from the vertebral arteries (V.A.). The right PICA passes posteriorly between the rootlets of the hypoglossal (XII) and vagus (X) nerves. The anterior medullary segment (Ant. Med. Seg.) of the right PICA is anterior to the inferior olive, and the lateral medullary segment (Lat. Med. Seg.) extends from the level of the most prominent part of the inferior olive to the level of the rootlets of the glossopharyngeal (IX), vagus, and spinal accessory nerves. The left PICA arises caudal to the rootlets of the hypoglossal nerve and passes posteriorly between the rootlets of the spinal accessory nerve. The vertebral arteries always pass anterior to the rootlets of the glossopharyngeal, vagus, spinal accessory, and hypoglossal nerves. The anterior inferior cerebellar arteries (A.I.C.A.) arise from the basilar artery (B.A.) and course in front of the abducens nerves (VI) to reach the facial (VII) and vestibulocochlear (VIII) nerves. The anterior spinal arteries (Ant. Sp. A.) arise from the vertebral arteries, and the pontine arteries (Pontine A.) arise from the basilar artery. *(B)* Enlarged view showing the complex relationships of rootlets of the lower cranial nerves to the right PICA. The hypoglossal rootlets arise along the preolivary sulcus, the groove between the medullary pyramid and the olive. The glossopharyngeal, vagal, and spinal accessory rootlets arise near the postolivary sulcus, the groove between the olive and the posterolateral medulla. The tonsillomedullary segment (Tons. Med. Seg.) of the PICA begins at the level of the glossopharyngeal, vagal, and spinal accessory rootlets.[31]

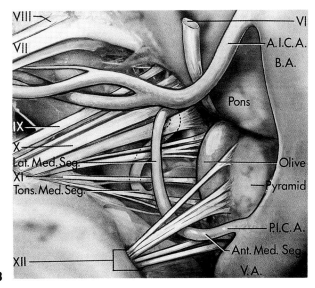

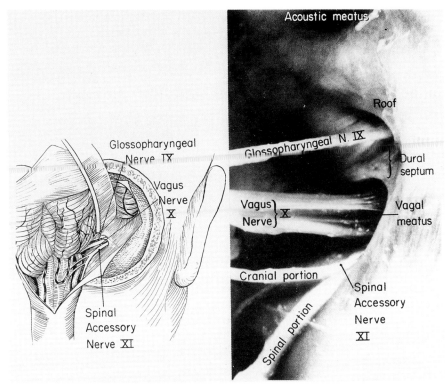

Figure 47. (A) Orientation of specimen in photograph. *(B)* The glossopharyngeal and vagus nerves are separated by a dural septum as they pass through their dural meati. The vagus and spinal accessory nerves have a separate entrance into the vagal meatus. The glossopharyngeal meatus is covered by a lip or roof arising laterally and projecting medially over the nerves' passage through the dura.[52]

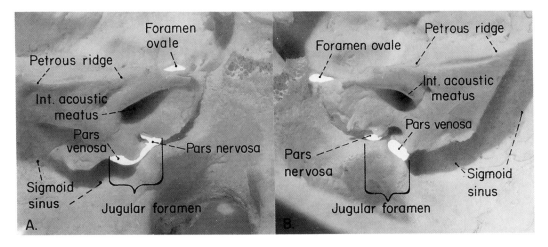

Figure 48. Posterior view of the skull and the jugular foramen. *(A)* Left. *(B)* Right. A bony strut separates the pars nervosa and pars venosa on the right but not on the left. *(C)* Posterior view of the skull, the brain stem, and the jugular foramen with the same orientation as A and B. The glossopharyngeal nerve (IX) on the left leaves the skull through a bony canal separate from the jugular foramen. On the right, this nerve leaves through a pars nervosa separated by a bony bridge from the pars venosa. The vagus (X) and spinal accessory (XI) nerves leave the skull through the medial part of the pars venosa.[52]

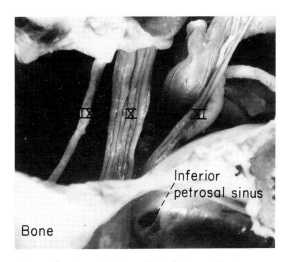

Figure 49. Lateral view of the left jugular foramen and the glossopharyngeal (IX), vagus (X), and spinal accessory (XI) nerves. The vagus nerve enters the anteromedial wall of the jugular bulb just anterior to where the inferior petrosal sinus joins the bulb.[52]

The spinal accessory rootlets arise at both the level of, and inferior to, the origin of the hypoglossal rootlets.

The glossopharyngeal nerve arises as one or rarely two rootlets from the upper medulla, posterior to the upper one-third of the olive, just caudal to the origin of the facial nerve. It courses ventral to the choroid plexus protruding from the foramen of Luschka on its way to the jugular foramen (Figures 54 and 55). Its length from the brain stem to the dura ranges from 15-21 mm (average 17.6 mm). Frequently, a larger dorsal and a smaller ventral component can be seen at the junction with the brain stem.[9,52] Tarlov[58] demonstrated that the smaller ventral rootlets are motor and the larger main bundle is sensory. The larger dorsal component usually arises from the medulla as one root except in a few cases in which it will originate as two rootlets. The two rootlets may remain separate throughout their course to the meatus (Figure 54).

The vagus nerve arises inferior to the glossopharyngeal nerve as a line of tightly packed rootlets along a line 2-5.5 mm in length posterior to the superior one-third of the olive (Figures 46, 53-55). The most rostral vagal fibers arise adjacent to the glossopharyngeal origin, from which they are sometimes separated by as much as 2 mm. The vagal rootlet diameter varies from 0.1-1.5 mm. The vagus is composed of multiple combinations of large and small rootlets that pass ventral to the choroid plexus protruding from the foramen of Luschka on its way to the anteromedial part of the pars venosa. Occasionally, several small rootlets are found originating ventral to the majority of the vagal rootlets (Figures 53 and 55). These small ventral rootlets are considered to be motor.[9]

The spinal accessory nerve arises as a widely separated series of rootlets that originate from the medulla at the level of the lower two-thirds of the olive and from the upper cervical cord. The cranial rootlets of the spinal accessory nerve arise as a line of rootlets ranging in diameter from 0.1-1 mm just caudal to the vagal fibers (Figures 46, 53, and 56). The cranial rootlets of the spinal accessory nerve are more properly regarded as inferior vagal rootlets because they arise from vagal nuclei.[38] It may be difficult to separate the lower vagal fibers from the upper spinal accessory rootlets because the vagal and cranial accessory fibers usually enter the vagal meatus as a single bundle.

The upper rootlets of the spinal portion of the accessory nerve originate several millimeters caudal to the lowest cranial accessory fibers and either course to join the cranial accessory bundle or enter the lower border of the vagal meatus separate from the cranial accessory rootlets. The spinal accessory fibers pass superolaterally from their origin to reach the jugular foramen. Although the cranial and spinal portions of the accessory nerve most frequently enter the vagal meatus together, they infrequently may be separated by a dural septum.

Anatomy of Glossopharyngeal Neuralgia

Dandy[5] described endocranial sectioning of the glossopharyngeal nerve for neuralgia, but because this alone did not adequately control

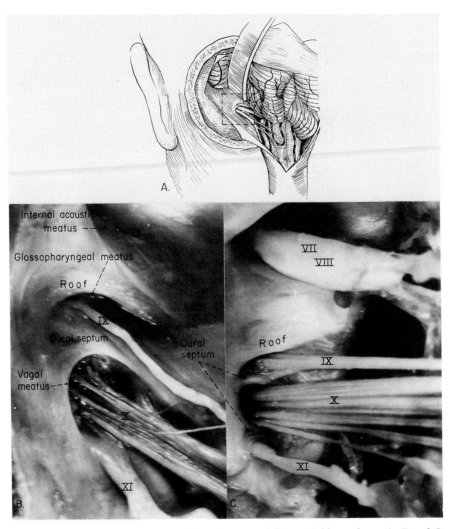

Figure 50. (A) The broken line outlines the area of the cranial base shown in B and C. (B) A wide dural septum (4 mm) separates the glossopharyngeal (IX) and vagus (X) nerves at the glossopharyngeal and vagal meati. The vagal fibers diverge as they enter the vagal meatus. (C) A small dural septum (0.5 mm) separates the glossopharyngeal (IX) and vagus (X) nerves and their meati. The vagal fibers converge as they enter the foramen. A narrow dural septum separates the vagus (X) and spinal accessory (XI) nerves.[52]

the neuralgia, he later advocated the additional sectioning of "perhaps 1/8 to 1/6 of the vagus." Tarlov[58,59] sectioned the cephalic third of the vagal-spinal accessory group and produced analgesia of the epiglottis but only hypalgesia over the mucosa of the lower pharynx and larynx. In his second case, he sectioned the cephalic half of the vagal-spinal accessory complex; this caused both analgesia and transient paralysis of the ipsilateral soft palate, pharynx, and larynx. In our study, the structure of the vagus nerve was variable, being composed of all large or all small rootlets or any combination of the two. This author suggests that fewer of the rostral rootlets be cut if the diameters of the upper rootlets are large rather than small; the diameter of the largest rootlet was 1.5 mm and the smallest was 0.1 mm.

A large glossopharyngeal nerve diameter might be associated with a small diameter of the upper rootlets of the vagus nerve or a

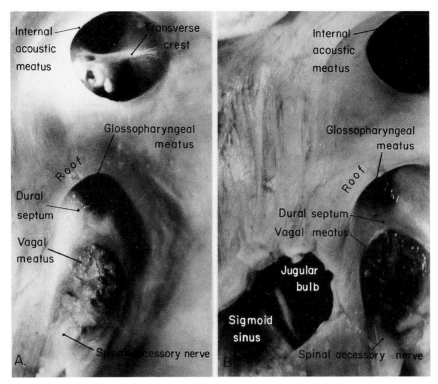

Figure 51. (A) Superior view of the left jugular foramen showing the dural roof over the glossopharyngeal meatus. A dural septum separates the glossopharyngeal and vagal meati. The transverse crest is at the lateral end of the internal acoustic meatus. (B) Same specimen with the dural roof removed to show the relation of the nerves to the sigmoid sinus and the jugular bulb. The nerves are medial to the jugular bulb.[52]

large vagus nerve might be associated with a small glossopharyngeal nerve because the two nerves arise from the same nuclei and have a similar function.[9] This idea that more fibers might be distributed to one nerve, leaving the other smaller, was not confirmed in our studies.[32] When the diameter of the dorsal root of the glossopharyngeal nerve is compared to the mean of the upper rootlets of the vagus nerve, no significant correlation is found.[52] A smaller diameter of the glossopharyngeal nerve is not commonly associated with a large mean diameter of the upper rootlets of the vagus, nor is a large glossopharyngeal nerve diameter associated with a small diameter of the vagal rootlets.

The only location where the glossopharyngeal nerve can consistently be distinguished from the vagus is just proximal to the dural meati where a dural septum separates the glossopharyngeal and vagus nerves.[52] This septum varies in width from 0.5-4.9 mm and serves to differentiate the glossopharyngeal nerve from the vagus nerve. The close medullary origin of the glossopharyngeal and vagus nerves and the frequent arachnoid adhesions between the two makes separation difficult in their course through the subarachnoid space or adjacent to the brain stem except in the few cases in which there will be a 1-2-mm separation between their origin at the medulla.

The superior glossopharyngeal and vagal ganglia may be visible intracranially. In glossopharyngeal neuralgia, Adson[1] noted the need to section the glossopharyngeal nerve proximal to the superior ganglion. The superior ganglion was intracranial in 32% of 50 jugular foramina that were examined and within or extracranial to the foramen in 68%.[52] The superior ganglion of the vagus

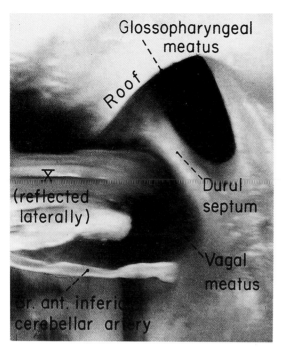

Figure 52. *Left jugular foramen. Same view as Figure 50. The dural septum separates the glossopharyngeal and vagal meati. The dural and bony lip projects medially, partially covering the meati. The meningeal branch of the posterior inferior cerebellar artery passes into the jugular foramen. The vagus nerve (X) is reflected laterally.*[52]

Figure 53. (Opposite page) *The broken line on the drawing of the lateral surface of the brain stem outlines the area shown in each diagram, demonstrating the brain stem origin and variations of the rootlet size of the glossopharyngeal (IX), vagus (X), and spinal accessory (XI) nerves. The large ovoid structure is the inferior olive. The broken-line circles outline the origin of the facial (VII) and vestibulocochlear (VIII) nerves. The most cephalad-shaded circles indicate glossopharyngeal rootlet origins, intermediate open circles indicate vagal rootlet origins, and caudal-black circles outline spinal accessory rootlet origins. The glossopharyngeal nerve usually originates as one large rootlet, the vagus as a series of large and small rootlets, and the spinal accessory as a series of small rootlets. (Top) Note the small ventral rootlets of the glossopharyngeal nerve in A, B, and C and the small ventral rootlet between the glossopharyngeal and vagus nerves in A. The glossopharyngeal rootlet is larger than the rostral rootlet of the vagus nerve in all except D, in which the rostral vagal rootlet is larger than the glossopharyngeal nerve. (Bottom) Note the wide separation of the origin of the glossopharyngeal and vagus nerves in C, the small ventral rootlet of the glossopharyngeal nerve in C, and the small ventral rootlets of the glossopharyngeal and vagus nerves in A. The glossopharyngeal nerve is smaller than the upper vagal rootlet in A and D.*[52]

could be seen intracranially in only 14% of the cases.

The dura mater surrounding the jugular foramen contains the sigmoid and inferior petrosal sinuses. The sigmoid sinus passes through the pars venosa and becomes the jugular bulb. The inferior petrosal sinus drains from the clival area and consists of one or more channels that course rostrally or caudally to or between the three nerves entering the jugular foramen (Figures 49 and 57). The sinus terminates anterior to the point where the cranial nerves descend in the anteromedial wall of the jugular bulb in 48 of 50 foramina and posterior to the nerves in 2 foramina (Figure 57). The inferior petrosal sinus may pass through either the pars nervosa or the pars venosa before joining the medial wall of the jugular bulb. A posterior meningeal artery that passed through the subarachnoid space to enter the jugular foramen, as described by Hovelacque,[21] was

noted in only 4 of the 50 foramina that were examined; in each case, the artery was a branch of the AICA (Figure 52).

Vascular Relationships

The vertebral artery courses anterior to all the nerves in the lower neurovascular complex. The PICA has a much more complex relationship to these nerves (Figures 45, 46, 56, and 58).[31] The proximal part of the PICA passes around or between and often stretches or distorts the rootlets of the nerves in the lower complex.

The PICA arises from the vertebral artery at the anterolateral aspect of the brain stem near the inferior olive and passes posteriorly around the medulla. At the anterolateral margin of the medulla, it passes around or between the rootlets of the hypoglossal nerve. At the posterolateral margin of the medulla, it passes between the fila of the glossopharyngeal, vagus, and spinal accessory nerves.

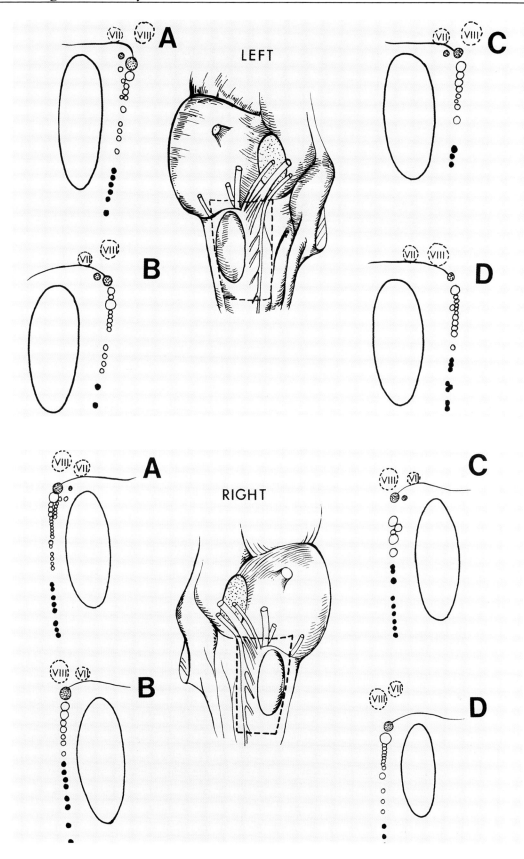

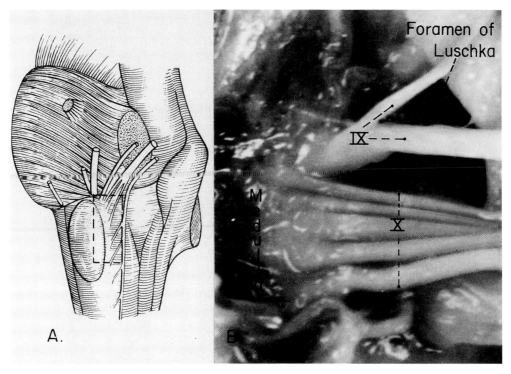

Figure 54. (A) The broken line outlines the area of the left side of the brain stem shown in B. (B) The glossopharyngeal (IX) and vagus (X) nerves arise just ventral to the foramen of Luschka. The vagal rootlets originate immediately adjacent to the glossopharyngeal nerve. (C) Anterior view. The glossopharyngeal nerve consists of two rootlets with a separate brain stem origin. The glossopharyngeal (IX) and vagus (X) nerves course ventral to the choroid plexus protruding from the foramen of Luschka to exit at the glossopharyngeal and vagal meati. The facial (VII) and vestibulocochlear (VIII) nerves are in the upper part of the exposure.[52]

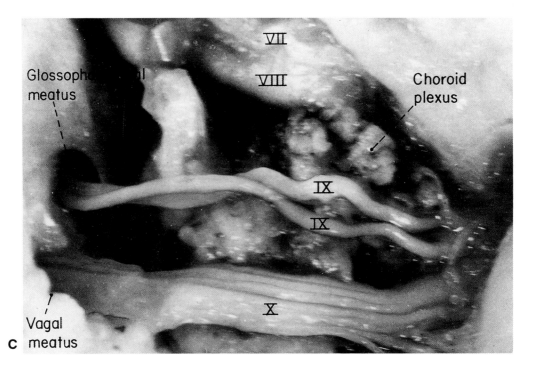

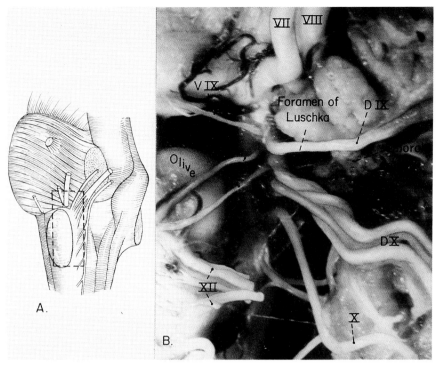

Figure 55. *(A) Lateral view of the left side of the brain stem as outlined by the broken line. (B) Note the ventral (V IX, V X) and dorsal (D IX, D X) rootlets of the glossopharyngeal and vagus nerves. One ventral glossopharyngeal and two ventral vagal rootlets are seen.*[52]

After passing the latter nerves, it courses around the cerebellar tonsil and passes posteriorly to the lower half of the roof of the fourth ventricle, which is formed by the inferior medullary velum and the tela choroidea. Both of the latter structures have important relationships in the CPA as described in the section on the middle neurovascular complex. After turning away from the roof of the fourth ventricle, the PICA enters the fissures between the tonsil, vermis, and hemisphere. Upon exiting these fissures, its branches are distributed to the suboccipital surface of the cerebellum.

The PICA most commonly courses from the lateral to the posterior aspect of the medulla by passing between the rootlets of the glossopharyngeal, vagus, and spinal accessory nerves. The most common site of passage is between the rootlets of the vagus or spinal accessory nerve or between the two nerves. The PICA may be ascending, descending, or passing laterally or medially or

may be involved in a complex loop that stretches and distorts these nerves as it passes between them (Figures 45, 46, 56, and 58). Of the 42 PICAs found in 50 cerebellar hemispheres in our studies,[31] 16 passed between the rootlets of the spinal accessory nerve, 10 passed between the rootlets of the vagus nerve, 13 passed between the vagus and spinal accessory nerves, 2 passed above the glossopharyngeal nerve between the latter nerve and the vestibulocochlear nerve, and 1 passed between the glossopharyngeal and the vagus nerves (Figure 58).

The hypoglossal rootlets also are intimately involved with the vertebral artery and the PICA. These rootlets, in their course from the preolivary sulcus to the hypoglossal canal, always pass posterior to the vertebral artery. If the vertebral artery is elongated or tortuous and courses laterally to the olive, it will stretch the hypoglossal rootlets over its posterior surface (Figures 46, 56, and 58). Some tortuous vertebral arteries will stretch the

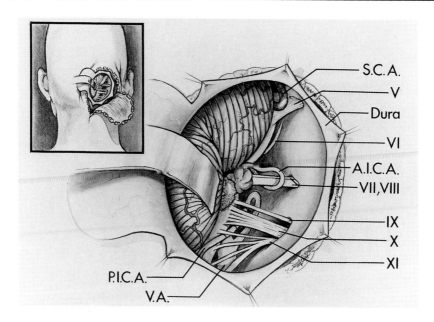

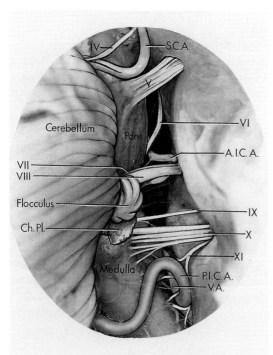

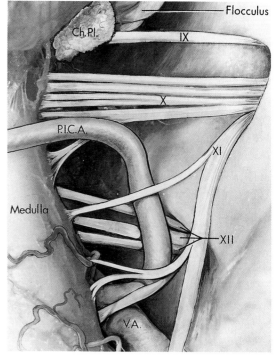

Figure 56A, B, C. Posterior views of the cerebellopontine angle (CPA). (A) Orientation of the posterior view shown in B through G. B, C, and D are from the right side, and E, F, and G are from the left side. The superior cerebellar artery (S.C.A.) is above the trigeminal nerve (V). The anterior inferior cerebellar artery (A.I.C.A.) courses near the abducens (VI), facial (VII), and vestibulocochlear (VIII) nerves. The posterior inferior cerebellar artery (P.I.C.A.) arises from the vertebral artery (V.A.) and passes near the glossopharyngeal (IX), vagus (X), and spinal accessory (XI) nerves. (B) In the superior third of the right CPA, the SCA passes between the trochlear (IV) and the trigeminal nerves. In the middle third of the posterior fossa, the AICA passes below the abducens, facial, and vestibulocochlear nerves. In the inferior third, the PICA passes between the rootlets of the spinal accessory nerve. The choroid plexus (Ch. Pl.) protrudes from the foramen of Luschka. (C) The PICA arises from the posterior surface of the vertebral artery and ascends between the rootlets of the hypoglossal (XII) and spinal accessory nerves to reach the posterior surface of the medulla.

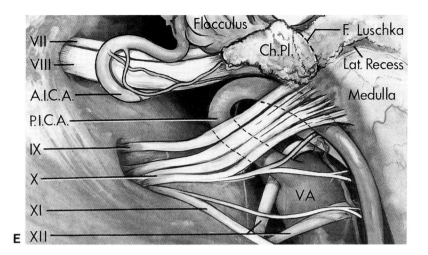

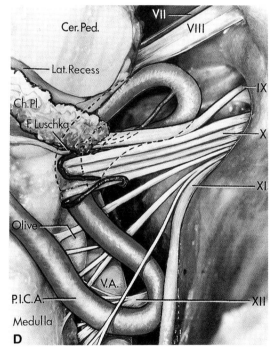

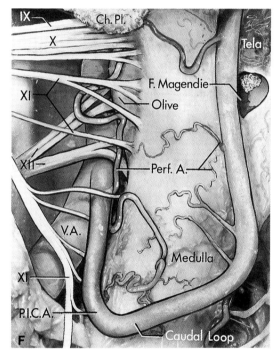

Figure 56D, E, F. (D) *A tortuous PICA arises from the vertebral artery and passes rostrally toward the vestibulocochlear and facial nerves. At the level of the vestibulocochlear nerve, it loops inferiorly and descends anterior to the glossopharyngeal and vagus nerves, and passes between the vagus and spinal accessory nerves. The PICA compresses the medulla anterior to the origin of the glossopharyngeal and vagus nerves. The choroid plexus protrudes from the foramen of Luschka (F. Luschka) posterior to the glossopharyngeal nerve. The cerebellar peduncles (Cer. Ped.) are above the lateral recess (Lat. Recess) of the fourth ventricle. (E) The PICA arises from the vertebral artery, passes between the rootlets of the hypoglossal nerve, and loops superiorly under the glossopharyngeal and vagus nerves before passing posteroinferiorly between the rootlets of the vagus and spinal accessory nerves. The vertebral artery stretches the rootlets of the hypoglossal nerve posteriorly. The AICA loops posterior to the facial and vestibulocochlear nerves. (F) The vertebral artery displaces and stretches the hypoglossal rootlets so far posteriorly that they intermingle with the rootlets of the spinal accessory nerve. The PICA descends between the rootlets of the spinal accessory nerve. This PICA forms a well-defined caudal loop posterior to the medulla before ascending beside the foramen of Magendie (F. Magendie) and the tela choroidea (Tela.) in the roof of the fourth ventricle. The PICA and the vertebral artery give rise to several perforating arteries (Perf. A.).*

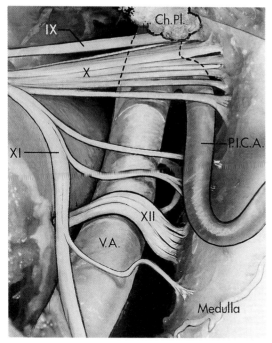

Figure 56G. The hypoglossal rootlets are displaced posteriorly over the vertebral artery. The PICA descends between the rootlets of the vagus and spinal accessory nerves.[31]

hypoglossal rootlets so far posterior that they intermingle with the glossopharyngeal, vagus, and spinal accessory nerves.

The relation of the origin of the PICA to the hypoglossal rootlets varies markedly. The PICA arises either rostral or caudal to, or at the level of, the hypoglossal rootlets. The hypoglossal rootlets frequently are stretched around the origin and initial segment of the PICA that arise at the level of the lower two-thirds of the olive in addition to being stretched posteriorly by the vertebral artery (Figures 46 and 56). In reaching the lateral medulla, the PICA may pass above, below, or between the hypoglossal rootlets. However, some PICAs will loop upward, downward, or laterally in front of the hypoglossal rootlets before passing posteriorly between or around them.

Vascular Compression in the Lower Neurovascular Complex

The close relationship of the PICA and

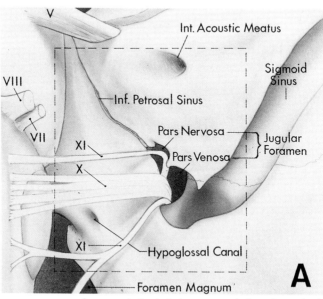

Figure 57A. Most frequent patterns of entry of the inferior petrosal sinus into the jugular bulb. Orienting diagram. Right side. The inferior petrosal sinus empties into the jugular bulb or the jugular vein at the jugular foramen. The glossopharyngeal nerve (IX) passes through the pars nervosa, and the vagus (X) and spinal accessory (XI) nerves pass through the pars venosa of the jugular foramen. The internal acoustic meatus is located above and the hypoglossal canal inferomedial to the jugular foramen. The trigeminal (V), facial (VII), and vestibulocochlear (VIII) nerves also are shown. The inferior petrosal sinus is shown as a single- or multipronged dark arrow in B to E.

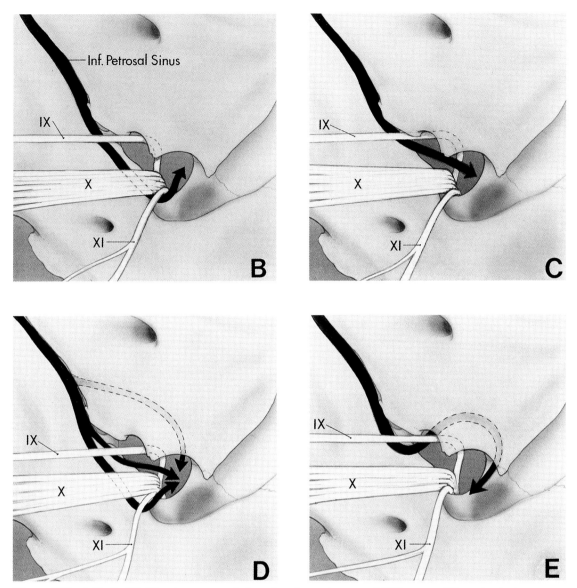

Figure 57B, C, D, E. (B) The sinus passes below the glossopharyngeal (IX), vagus (X), and spinal accessory (XI) nerves before entering the pars venosa. *(C)* The inferior petrosal sinus passes between the glossopharyngeal (IX) and vagus (X) nerves. *(D)* Different branches of the sinus pass around the nerves as shown. *(E)* The sinus passes rostral to the glossopharyngeal (IX) nerve, enters the pars nervosa, and passes extracranially to join the anterior medial part of the jugular bulb.

the vertebral artery to the glossopharyngeal and vagus nerves makes it logical to explore these relationships in glossopharyngeal neuralgia.[30,60] During operations on six patients with glossopharyngeal neuralgia, Laha and Jannetta found that the glossopharyngeal and vagus nerves were compressed at their junction with the brain stem by the PICA in three cases and by the vertebral artery in two.[30] In the sixth case, the junction of the nerves and the brain stem could not be visualized because of scarring from a prior operation. Three of the six patients were treated by separating the artery and the nerves, and the remaining three had rhizotomies because the patients' anatomies or scarring from prior operations prevented mobilization of the arterial loops. Two of the three who had the

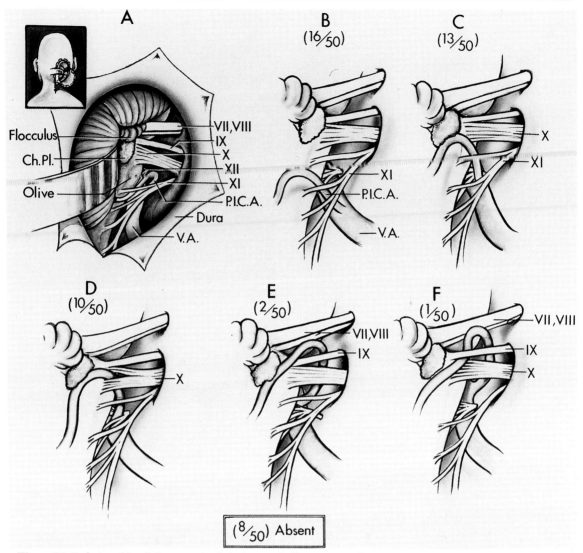

Figure 58. *Relationship of the posterior inferior cerebellar artery to the rootlets of the glossopharyngeal, vagus, and spinal accessory nerves. (A) Orientation of illustrations B through F. The cerebellum has been retracted to show the facial (VII), vestibulocochlear (VIII), glossopharyngeal (IX), vagus (X), spinal accessory (XI), and hypoglossal (XII) nerves. The choroid plexus (Ch. Pl.) and the flocculus project into the cerebellopontine angle (CPA) behind the glossopharyngeal and vagus nerves. The posterior inferior cerebellar artery (P.I.C.A.) arises from the vertebral artery (V.A.) and passes inferiorly (B, C), superiorly (E, F), or between (D) the rootlets of the hypoglossal nerve. Of the 42 PICAs found in 50 cerebellar hemispheres, 16 passed between the rootlets of the spinal accessory nerve (B), 13 passed between the vagus and accessory nerves (C), 10 passed between the rootlets of the vagus nerve (X) (D), 2 passed between the glossopharyngeal and vestibulocochlear nerves (E), and 1 passed between the glossopharyngeal and vagus nerves (F). A tortuous PICA may ascend anterior to the glossopharyngeal and vagus nerves and compress and distort the facial and vestibulocochlear nerves before passing posteriorly between the glossopharyngeal, vagus, and spinal accessory nerves (E, F).[31]*

arteries and nerves separated achieved complete pain relief.

The junction of the nerves with the medulla is exposed through a small retromastoid craniectomy using superior and medial retraction of the inferolateral margin of the cerebellum as described for hemifacial spasm. The glossopharyngeal and vagus nerves enter the brain stem anterior to the choroid plexus protruding from the foramen of Luschka.

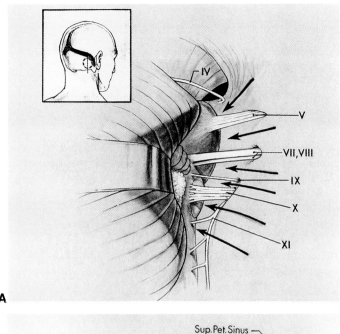

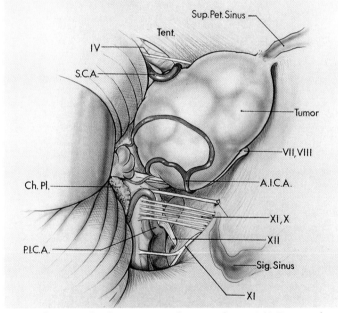

Figure 59A, B. Tumors involving multiple neurovascular complexes. *(A)* Routes that can be taken between the cranial nerves to expose and remove a tumor situated medial to and involving multiple neurovascular complexes. The insert (upper left) shows the site of the vertical scalp incision and the craniectomy. The approach to pathology located medial to the nerves can be directed (arrows) between the trochlear nerve (IV) above and the trigeminal nerve (V) below; between the trigeminal above and the facial (VII) and vestibulocochlear (VIII) nerves below; between the facial and vestibulocochlear nerves above and the glossopharyngeal nerve (IX) below; between the glossopharyngeal and vagus (X) nerves; between the vagus nerve and spinal accessory rootlets (XI) and between the widely separated rootlets of the spinal accessory nerve. Tumor located medial to the nerves often will widen the intervals between the nerves depending on the type and the site of origin of the tumor. *(B)* Meningioma involving the upper and middle complex that has its attachment lateral to the trigeminal nerve in the region of the superior petrosal sinus (Sup. Pet. Sinus). The trochlear nerve is elevated, the trigeminal nerve is pushed medially, and the facial and vestibulocochlear nerves are stretched below the tumor. Other structures exposed include the superior cerebellar (S.C.A.), anterior inferior cerebellar (A.I.C.A.), and posterior inferior cerebellar (P.I.C.A.) arteries; the sigmoid sinus (Sig. Sinus); the hypoglossal nerve (XII), and the choroid plexus (Ch. Pl.) protruding from the foramen of Luschka.

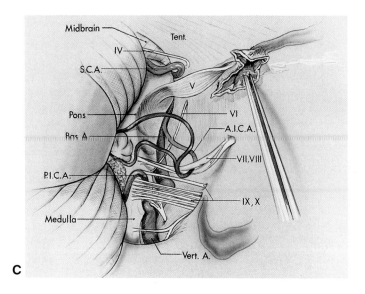

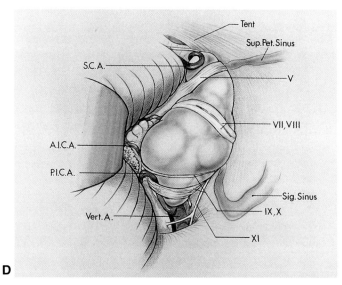

Figure 59C, D. (C) The tumor has been removed. The thin distorted nerves have been preserved and the remaining dural attachment is removed or cauterized with bipolar coagulation. The vertebral (Vert. A.) and basilar (Bas. A.) arteries and the abducens nerve (VI) are exposed. **(D)** Large meningioma arising from the clivus in the region of the inferior petrosal sinus with involvement of cranial nerves IV-X. The nerves are displaced laterally around the tumor. The tumor is removed by working through the intervals between the nerves.

The tortuous or ectatic artery and the nerves are separated at the nerve root entry zone, and the interval between them is maintained with a foam prosthesis. Compression, by the PICA, of the facial and vestibulocochlear nerves also has been found in hemifacial spasm, geniculate neuralgia, and vestibulo-cochlear dysfunction producing symptoms such as Meniere's disease.[24,27,28,29,36]

Jannetta and Gendell have proposed that compression of the lateral side of the medulla by the PICA or the vertebral artery may be a cause of hypertension.[28] The fact that hypertension is a component of the Cushing re-

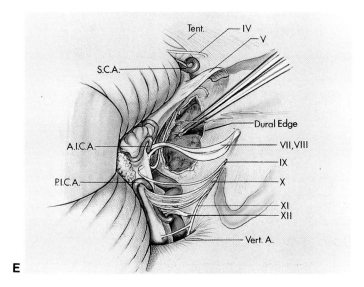

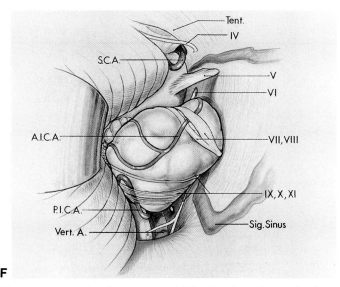

Figure 59E, F. *(E) The meningioma has been removed. The dural attachment has been partially removed and the base is being cauterized. (F) Meningioma arising medial to the jugular bulb in the region of the jugular tubercle. The tumor involves the middle and lower neurovascular complexes.*

sponse to medullary compression has been well established.[11,56] Jannetta and Gendell reported their observations on 16 hypertensive patients who were undergoing exploration of the left CPA for trigeminal or glossopharyngeal neuralgia or hemifacial spasm.[28] All were found to have compression of the left side of the medulla in the area between the glossopharyngeal and the vagus nerves dorsally and the inferior olive ventrally. The compressing artery was the PICA in 5 patients and the vertebral artery in 1. Of the 5 patients whose arteries were displaced from their brain stems, 4 experienced recovery to a normal blood pressure (although 1 was temporary), and 1 had a significant reduction but

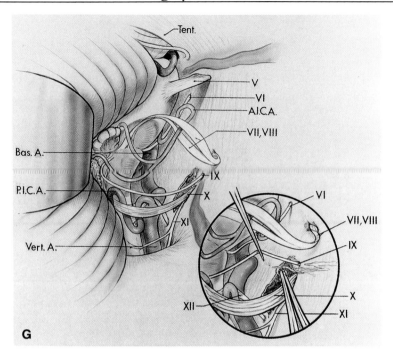

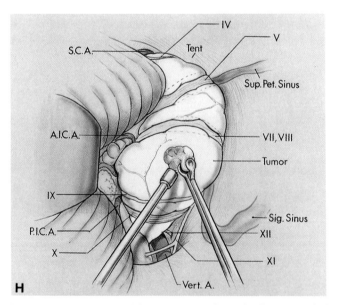

Figure 59G, H. (G) The tumor was removed by operating through the intervals between the facial and vestibulocochlear nerves above and the glossopharyngeal nerve below and between the glossopharyngeal and vagus nerves (round insert). (H) Large epidermoid tumor being removed by working through the intervals between the nerves.

not a return to a normal blood pressure.

Lesions Involving Multiple Neurovascular Complexes

Tumors in the CPA commonly involve more than one of the neurovascular complexes (Figure 59).[48] An especially difficult challenge is exposing and removing the tumors that are situated medial to the nerves. In this case, the operation must be directed through the interval between the neurovascular complexes because these tumors

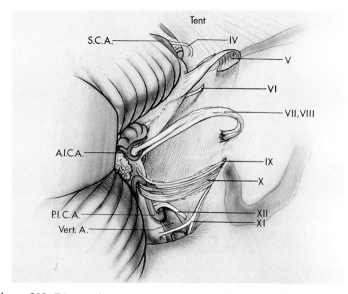

Figure 59I. Distorted nerves after the removal of the epidermoid tumor.

often will widen these intervals. High lesions may be exposed through the interval between the lower margin of the tentorium and the upper edge of the trigeminal nerve. Care is needed to protect the trochlear nerve and the SCA in this area. Further inferiorly, the medially placed tumor may be approached through the interval between the trigeminal nerve above and the facial and vestibulocochlear nerves below. If the tumor has an even lower attachment near the jugular foramen, it can be approached through the interval between the lower margin of the nerves entering the internal meatus and the upper margin of the glossopharyngeal nerve, or through the interval between the lower rootlets of the vagus nerve and the upper rootlets of the spinal accessory nerve. The intervals between the glossopharyngeal and vagus nerves, and between the individual vagal rootlets usually are too narrow to work through unless they have been opened by the tumor. Another maneuver that sometimes is used to provide access to medially placed lesions is to complete a translabyrinthine or transcochlear exposure with transposition of the facial nerve (Figure 32). In both of these approaches, however, hearing is sacrificed and transposition of the facial nerve is commonly followed by a facial palsy that slowly resolves.

References

1. Adson AW. The surgical treatment of glossopharyngeal neuralgia. *Arch Neurol Psychiatry.* 1924; 12:487-506.
2. Apfelbaum RI. Microvascular decompression for tic douloureux results. In: Brackmann DE, ed. *Neurological Surgery of the Ear and Skull Base.* New York: Raven Press. 1982:175-180.
3. Atkinson WJ. The anterior inferior cerebellar artery: its variations, pontine distribution, and significance in the surgery of cerebello-pontine angle tumours. *J Neurol Neurosurg Psychiatry.* 1949;12: 137-151.
4. Brackmann DE. Middle cranial fossa approach. In: House WF, Luetje CM, eds. *Acoustic Tumors, II: Management.* Baltimore, Md: University Park Press; 1979:15-41.
5. Dandy WE. Glossopharyngeal neuralgia (tic douloureux): its diagnosis and treatment. *Arch Surg.* 1927; 15:198-214.
6. Dandy WE. An operation for the cure of tic douloureux: partial section of the sensory root at the pons. *Arch Surg.* 1929;18:687-734.
7. Dandy WE. Concerning the cause of trigeminal neuralgia. *Amer J Surg.* 1934;24:447-455.
8. DiChiro G, Fisher RI, Nelson KB. The jugular foramen. *J Neurosurg.* 1964;21:447-460.
9. DuBois FS, Foley JO. Experimental studies on the vagus and spinal accessory nerves in the cat. *Anat Rec.* 1936; 64:285-307.
10. Emmons WF, Rhoton AL Jr. Subdivision of the trigeminal sensory root: experimental study in the monkey. *J Neurosurg.* 1971;35:585-591.
11. Fein JM, Frishman W. Neurogenic hypertension related to vascular compression of the lateral medulla. *Neurosurgery.* 1980;6:615-622.
12. Fujii K, Lenkey C, Rhoton AL Jr. Microsurgical anatomy of the choroidal arteries: fourth ventricle and cerebellopontine angles. *J Neurosurg.* 1980; 52:504-524.

13. Gardner WJ. Concerning the mechanism of trigeminal neuralgia and hemifacial spasm. *J Neurosurg.* 1962;19:947-958.

14. Gundmundsson K, Rhoton AL Jr, Rushton JG. Detailed anatomy of the intracranial portion of the trigeminal nerve. *J Neurosurg.* 1971;35:592-600.

15. Haines SJ, Jannetta PJ, Zorub DS. Microvascular relations of the trigeminal nerve: an anatomical study with clinical correlation. *J Neurosurg.* 1980; 52:381-386.

16. Hardy DG, Peace DA, Rhoton AL Jr. Microsurgical anatomy of the superior cerebellar artery. *Neurosurg.* 1980;6:10-28.

17. Hardy DG, Rhoton AL Jr. Microsurgical relationships of the superior cerebellar artery and the trigeminal nerve. *J Neurosurg.* 1978;49:669-678.

18. Harris FS, Rhoton AL Jr. Anatomy of the cavernous sinus: a microsurgical study. *J Neurosurg.* 1976; 45:169-180.

19. Horsley V, Taylor J, Coleman WS. Remarks on the various surgical procedures devised for the relief or cure of trigeminal neuralgia (tic douloureux). *Brit Med J.* 1981;2:1139-1143, 1191-1193, 1249-1252.

20. House WF. Translabyrinthine approach. In: House WF, Luetje CM, eds. *Acoustic Tumors, II: Management.* Baltimore, Md; University Park Press; 1979:43-87.

21. Hovelacque A. Osteologie, G. Doin et Cie, 1934. Osteologic (Paris). 1967;2:155-156.

22. Inoue T, Rhoton AL Jr, Theele D, et al. Surgical approaches to the cavernous sinus: a microsurgical study. *Neurosurgery.* 1990;26:903-932.

23. Jannetta PJ. Arterial compression of the trigeminal nerve at the pons in patients with trigeminal neuralgia. *J Neurosurg.* 1967;26:159-162.

24. Jannetta PJ. Microsurgical approach to the trigeminal nerve for tic douloureux. *Prog Neurol Surg.* 1976; 7:180-200.

25. Jannetta PJ. Neurovascular cross-compression in patients with hyperactive dysfunction symptoms of the eighth cranial nerve. *Surg Forum.* 1975;26: 467-469.

26. Jannetta PJ. Vascular decompression in trigeminal neuralgia. In: Samii M, Jannetta PJ, eds. *The Cranial Nerves: Anatomy-Pathophysiology-Diagnosis-Treatment.* New York, NY; Springer-Verlag. 1981: 331-340.

27. Jannetta PJ, Abbasy M, Maroon JC, et al. Etiology and definitive microsurgical treatment of hemifacial spasm: operative techniques and results in 47 patients. *J Neurosurg.* 1977;47:321-328.

28. Jannetta PJ, Gendell HM. Clinical observations on etiology essential hypertension. *Surg Forum.* 1979; 30:431-432.

29. Jannetta PJ, Møller MB, Møller AR, et al. Neurosurgical treatment of vertigo by microvascular decompression of the eighth cranial nerve. *Clin Neurosurg.* 1986;33:645-665.

30. Laha RK, Jannetta PJ. Glossopharyngeal neuralgia. *J Neurosurg.* 1977;47:316-320.

31. Lister JR, Rhoton AL Jr, Matsushima T, et al. Microsurgical anatomy of the posterior inferior cerebellar artery. *Neurosurg.* 1982;10:170-199.

32. Martin RG, Grant JL, Peace D, et al. Microsurgical relationships of the anterior inferior cerebellar artery and the facial-vestibulocochlear nerve complex. *Neurosurgery.* 1980; 6:483-507.

33. Matsushima T, Rhoton AL Jr, de Oliveira E, et al. Microsurgical anatomy of the veins of the posterior fossa. *J Neurosurg.* 1983;59:63-105.

34. Matsushima T, Rhoton AL Jr, Lenkey C. Microsurgery of the fourth ventricle, I: microsurgical anatomy. *Neurosurgery.* 1982;11:631-667.

35. Møller MB, Møller AR, Jannetta PJ, et al. Diagnosis and surgical treatment of disabling positional vertigo. *J Neurosurg.* 1986; 64:21-28.

36. Ouaknine GE, Robert F, Molina-Negro P, et al. Geniculate neuralgia and audio-vestibular disturbances due to compression of the intermediate and eighth nerves by the postero-inferior cerebellar artery. *Surg Neurol.* 1980;13:147-150.

37. Pait TG, Zeal A, Harris FS, et al. Microsurgical anatomy and dissection of the temporal bone. *Surg Neurol.* 1977;8:363-391.

38. Patridge EJ. The relations of the glossopharyngeal nerve at its exit from the cranial cavity. *J Anat.* 1918;52:332-334.

39. Paullus W, Pait TG, Rhoton AL Jr. Microsurgical exposure of the petrous portion of the carotid artery. *J Neurosurg.* 1977; 47:713-726.

40. Pelletier V, Poulos DA, Lende RA. Localization in the trigeminal root. Presented at the American Association of Neurological Surgeons, 1970. Washington, DC.

41. Rhoton AL Jr. Microsurgery of the internal acoustic meatus. *Surg. Neurol.* 1974; 2:311-318.

42. Rhoton AL Jr. Microsurgical removal of acoustic neuromas. *Surg Neurol.* 1976;6:211-219.

43. Rhoton AL Jr. Microsurgical neurovascular decompression for trigeminal neuralgia and hemifacial spasm. *J Florida Med.* 1978;65:425-428.

44. Rhoton AL Jr. Microsurgical neurovascular decompression for trigeminal neuralgia: anatomic studies and clinical results. In: Silverstein H, Norrell H, eds. *Neurological Surgery of the Ear, Volume III.* Birmingham, Ala: Aesculapius; 1979; 2:299-311.

45. Rhoton AL Jr. The surgical treatment of trigeminal neuralgia. In: Brackmann DE, ed. *Neurological Surgery of the Ear and Skull Base.* New York, NY: Raven Press; 1982:167-174.

46. Rhoton AL Jr. Microsurgical anatomy of acoustic neuromas. *Neurol Res.* 1984; 6:3-21.

47. Rhoton AL Jr. Microsurgical anatomy of the brainstem surface facing an acoustic neuroma. *Surg Neurol.* 1986;25:326-339.

48. Rhoton AL Jr. Meningiomas and other cerebellopontine angle tumors. In: Long DM, ed. *Current Therapy in Neurological Surgery - 2.* Philadelphia, Pa: BC Decker Inc.; 1989:14-19.

49. Rhoton AL Jr. Microsurgical anatomy of decompression operations on the trigeminal nerve. In: Rovit RL, Murali R, Jannetta PJ, eds. *Trigeminal Neuralgia.* Baltimore, Md: Williams and Wilkins; 1990:165-200.

50. Rhoton AL Jr. Microsurgical anatomy of acoustic neuromas. In: Jackler RK, ed. *Otolaryngologic Clinics of North America.* Philadelphia, Pa: WB Saunders Co; 1992. In press.

51. Rhoton AL Jr. Optimization of instrumentation in posterior fossa surgery. In: Apuzzo MLJ, ed. *Brain Surgery: Complication, Avoidance and Management.* New York, NY: Churchill-Livingstone; 1992. In press.

52. Rhoton AL Jr, Buza R. Microsurgical anatomy of the

jugular foramen. *J Neurosurg.* 1975; 42:541-550.

53. Rhoton AL Jr, Kobayashi S, Hollingshead WH. Nervus intermedius. *J Neurosurg.* 1968;29:609-618.

54. Rhoton AL Jr, Pulec J, Hall GM. Absence of bone over the geniculate ganglion. *J Neurosurg.* 1968; 28:609-618.

55. Saunders R, Sachs E. Accessory fibers of the fifth nerve. Presented at the American Association of Neurological Surgeons, Cleveland, Ohio, 1969.

56. Segal R, Gendell HM, Canfield D, et al. Cardiovascular response to pulsatile pressure applied to ventrolateral medulla. *Surg Forum.* 1979;30:433-434.

57. Sunderland S. Neurovascular relationships and anomalies at the base of the brain. *J Neurol Neurosurg Psychiatry.* 1948;11:243-257.

58. Tarlov IM. Structure of the nerve root. II: Differentiation of sensory from motor roots; observations on identification of function in roots of mixed cranial nerves. *Arch Neurol Psychiatry.* 1937;37: 1338-1355.

59. Tarlov IM. Section of the cephalic third of the vagus-spinal accessory complex: clinical and histologic results. *Arch Neurol Psychiatry.* 1942;47: 141-148.

60. Watt JC, McKillop AN. Relation of arteries to roots of nerves in posterior cranial fossa in man. *Arch Surg.* 1935;30:336-345.

61. Woodhall B. Anatomy of the cranial blood sinuses with particular reference to the lateral. *Laryngoscope.* 1939;49:966-1010.

CHAPTER 2

Cranial Nerve Dysfunction Syndromes: Pathophysiology of Microvascular Compression

Aage R. Møller, PhD

Vascular compression syndromes are primarily associated with trigeminal neuralgia (tic douloureux) and hemifacial spasm, but other disorders such as glossopharyngeal neuralgia and disabling positional vertigo can also be successfully treated by microvascular decompression (MVD) of the respective cranial nerve. It has also been shown, although in smaller series, that some cases of tinnitus and spasmodic torticollis can be alleviated by MVD of the vestibulocochlear (VIII) and spinal accessory (XI) nerves, respectively.

Analysis of a large series of patients who were treated for hemifacial spasm and trigeminal neuralgia during the past 10-15 years using the MVD method shows that these disorders can be treated with a high rate of success by MVD of the respective cranial nerve.[4,13,74,90] Although these rare disorders can be treated with a high success rate, the pathophysiologies of the syndromes are incompletely understood.

The primary symptoms and signs of the disorders that can be treated by MVD involve hyperactivity of the involved cranial nerve that develops over time while the sensory or motor function of the respective nerve remains essentially unchanged. Thus, patients with hemifacial spasm usually have little or no noticeable facial weakness; patients with trigeminal neuralgia have no noticeable sensory deficits of the face; and standard electro-physiologic testing of functions reveals few, if any, abnormalities.

It was probably Dandy[18,19] who first recognized and described vascular compression of the trigeminal (V) nerve as the cause of a specific disorder, trigeminal neuralgia. When Dandy[17] sectioned the trigeminal nerve in the cerebellopontine angle (CPA) to treat patients with trigeminal neuralgia, he observed vascular compression of the nerve, and later reported that he believed this compression to be the cause of tic douloureux.[19] In 1920, Cushing[16] hypothesized that trigeminal neuralgia could be caused by pressure from a tumor on the trigeminal root, but it was not until the 1950s that Taarnhøj[134] and Gardner and Miklos[39] described the beneficial effect of decompressing the trigeminal nerve root to treat trigeminal neuralgia. Later, Gardner and Sava[40] reported the presence of vascular compression of the facial (VII) nerve root in patients with hemifacial spasm.

Further work confirmed that patients with hemifacial spasm, typical trigeminal neuralgia, and glossopharyngeal neuralgia have a blood vessel that is in close contact with the respective cranial nerve, and that moving the blood vessel off the respective nerve and placing a soft implant between the vessel and the nerve (microvascular decompression, MVD) can be curative in a very large percentage of these patients. This technique, which was pioneered by Jannetta,[52,53,55-58,61-63] has been in use at many medical centers for the past decade, and has been used to treat large series of patients* with total relief of cranial nerve dysfunction in over 80% of the cases.[4,13,90,146] There are very few known recurrences of hemifacial spasm after successful MVD treatment, but the recurrence rate for trigeminal neuralgia has been estimated to be about 50% within 15 years.[13,119] It has also been shown, although in smaller series of patients, that glossopharyngeal neuralgia can be cured by MVD of the root of the glossopharyngeal (IX) nerve,[55] and more recently it has been recognized that MVD of cranial nerve VIII constitutes an effective cure of certain types of balance disturbances (disabling positional vertigo[65,104,105,107,108] and tinnitus[55,60,76,101,103]). In addition, spasmodic torticollis has been treated successfully by MVD.[31,109,110,129]

Both hemifacial spasm and trigeminal neuralgia have been treated by destructive procedures. Partial sectioning of the extratemporal branches of the facial nerve,[27,28,124] for example, has been used to treat hemifacial spasm, as has injection of phenol or alcohol.[21,22] More recently, injection of botulinum toxin into the affected muscles has been used.[77] Rhizotomy of the trigeminal nerve or selectively injuring the trigeminal ganglion can be effective in treating trigeminal neuralgia.[30,82,133]

Trigeminal neuralgia can, at least in its early stages, be controlled by drugs such as carbamazepine, phenytoin, and baclofen,[36] but the drugs that are effective in treating trigeminal neuralgia have no beneficial effect on hemifacial spasm,[2] an important difference between these disorders. Relief from hemifacial spasm has been reported in 6 patients treated with baclofen, in some cases in conjunction with imipramine.[126] In all 6 of these patients, however, the hemifacial spasm was precipitated by emotional events, such as death or marital separation. This relationship is unusual as most cases of hemifacial spasm have no known cause. Some patients with

disabling positional vertigo and certain forms of tinnitus can be treated successfully with benzodiazepines.[103,104,108]

Surgeons who have extensive experience in performing MVD of cranial nerves report finding a blood vessel in close contact with the respective cranial nerve in practically every case of trigeminal neuralgia and hemifacial spasm, and it is generally assumed that the close contact between a vessel and the respective nerve must occur at the root entry/exit zone (REZ, or Obersteiner-Redlich zone) in order to cause the pathology.[4,53,55,63,84] The REZ involves the first/last few millimeters of a cranial nerve where it enters/exits the brain stem. A cone-shaped dome of neuroglia extends outward from the central nervous system into the center of the nerve root, the nerve fibers of which are covered with central myelin (oligodendrocytes).[132,136] For cranial nerves V and VII, glia extends for 3 and 2.5 mm from the brain stem, respectively, and for cranial nerve VIII, 8 and 8.2 mm for the vestibular and cochlear portions, respectively.[130] Other investigations[78,79] have arrived at slightly different values.

It was previously assumed that only major arteries could cause vascular compression symptoms, but there is now evidence that veins and arteries of a very small caliber that are in close contact with a cranial nerve root can also be the cause.[59,76,100]

It has been reported that there are patients with trigeminal neuralgia who do not have vascular compression of the root of cranial nerve V.[1] The observation of vascular compression, however, appears to be closely related to the judgment of the individual surgeon (for hemifacial spasm 12% to 25%, and for trigeminal neuralgia 3.4% to as much as 89%).[1] Since the vast majority of surgeons have found that practically all patients with hemifacial spasm and trigeminal neuralgia have vascular compression of the respective cranial nerve, it may be assumed that vascular compression in fact is a common condition with these disorders.

The differences in the way these disorders respond to medical treatment, and the find-

---

* References 3, 4, 51-53, 55, 58, 63, 74, 76, 81, 145

ing that vascular compression of these cranial nerves also exists in asymptomatic individuals[45,73,85,116,131] have led some investigators to question whether vascular compression of cranial nerves is the real cause of these disorders.[1,7] Thus, some investigators have postulated that the high rate of success of MVD may be due, not to its relieving vascular compression, but rather to its causing a slight injury to the respective nerve.[1,7]

Despite the fact that there are effective treatments (medical and surgical) for these disorders, the pathophysiology involved is incompletely understood. Review of the literature shows two main hypotheses for the pathophysiology of trigeminal neuralgia and hemifacial spasm: one claims a peripheral cause and one claims a central cause.

The peripheral cause hypothesis claims that the symptoms and signs of these disorders are caused by facilitation of ephaptic transmission between nerve fibers at the site of the vascular compression; the central cause hypothesis claims that the symptoms and signs of these disorders are caused by anomalies (hyperactivity) of the respective nuclei. Because the two hypotheses claim different anatomic areas of involvement by the physiologic abnormalities, an important task of studies of the pathophysiology of these disorders is to identify the anatomic location of the physiologic abnormality that is causing the symptoms and signs.

In this chapter we discuss the evidence to support or deny these two hypotheses. First, it is necessary to explain how the hyperactivity that is typical of hemifacial spasm and trigeminal neuralgia develops: if a symptom is caused by hyperactivity of the respective nucleus, one must understand how such specific hyperactivity develops and what role vascular compression plays in this development. The pathophysiology of hemifacial spasm has been more extensively studied than that of trigeminal neuralgia and other vascular compression disorders, and therefore the discussion of pathophysiology will begin with the results of studies in patients with hemifacial spasm.

Pathophysiology of Hemifacial Spasm

Hemifacial spasm is a rare disease (incidence: 0.74 per 100,000 in white men and 0.81 per 100,000 in white women)[8] that has its onset relatively late in life. It is characterized by periods of facial spasm, between which there is essentially normal function of facial mimetic musculature.

Hemifacial spasm usually develops according to a specific pattern: brief periods of spasm around the eye occurs first, and over several years the intensity of this spasm gradually increases and spreads downward over the face so that 6-10 years after onset of spasm the entire half of the face is involved, including the platysma, but often excluding the forehead.[20,21] In about 8% of patients, however, hemifacial spasm is atypical in onset: the spasm begins in the buccal muscles and progresses upward over the face.[62] Spontaneous remissions are rare.[146] The two prevailing hypotheses that claim to explain the symptoms and signs of hemifacial spasm focus on (1) abnormal hyperactivity in the facial motor nucleus[26,142,143] and (2) crosstalk (ephaptic transmission) between individual nerve fibers of the facial nerve where it is compressed by a blood vessel.[37,40,83,147,148] It was assumed that the associated ectopic excitation causes the spasm in hemifacial spasm patients.

Ephaptic Transmission

For a long time the hypothesis that assumed ephaptic transmission at the site of vascular compression causes the symptoms of hemifacial spasm was favored,[37,112,113,120] but more recently the results of several studies[24,94] have provided evidence that calls this hypothesis into question and supports the hypothesis that hyperactivity of the facial motor nucleus is the cause of the disorder. Ferguson[26] was one of the first investigators to point out that ephaptic transmission between denuded facial nerve axons is not sufficient to explain the symptoms and signs of hemifacial spasm;

more recently, on the basis of preoperative studies, Esteban and Molina-Negro[24] questioned whether the ephaptic transmission hypothesis could explain hemifacial spasm because it seems unlikely that enough nerve fibers could be in contact with each other to cause the massive contractions of nearly all facial muscles seen in patients who have had hemifacial spasm for a significant period of time. Further, evidence in support of the nucleus hypothesis has accumulated from intraoperative neurophysiologic studies of patients undergoing MVD operations for hemifacial spasm,[49,50,81,91,98,99,123] as well as from preoperative neurophysiologic studies.[121,139]

Despite the fact that the facial nerve may show macroscopic deformation due to a compressing blood vessel, published studies generally show few signs of injury to the facial nerve, which makes it difficult to assess the degree of injury that is produced directly by vascular contact. Only minor changes, such as hypo- and hypermyelination of some nerve fibers are seen, and most nerve fibers are normal in the region of vascular compression.[64,122] More recently, Coad et al,[14] in a postmortem study of an individual with familial hemifacial spasm in whom there was a redundant loop of the anterior inferior cerebellar artery and an associated vein plexus compressing the facial nerve at the REZ, found signs of nerve degeneration and an increased number of corpora amylacea at the site of vascular compression. They did not, however, detect demyelination or gliosis, and demyelination has generally been regarded to be a prerequisite for ephaptic transmission.

Thus, although there seem to be histologically detectable changes in the facial nerves of individuals with hemifacial spasm which can be related to the vascular compression, the degree of demyelination noted does not seem to be sufficient to explain the spasm and synkinesis in hemifacial spasm on the basis of the ephaptic transmission hypothesis. These findings and the recent finding that close contact between the facial nerve and veins and arteries of a very small caliber can also be associated with hemifacial spasm[59,76,100] support the hypothesis that facial nerve injury

is slight in these patients.

Hyperactivity of Facial Motor Nucleus

If severe injury to the facial nerve on the affected side with substantial demyelination occurred in patients with hemifacial spasm, then one would expect that neural conduction time in that segment of the facial nerve would be measurably longer on the affected side than on the unaffected side. Such a condition could be detected by recording the blink reflex, because slowing of neural conduction in the facial nerve would give rise to a prolonged latency of the R_1 of the blink reflex. Indeed, Nielsen[113] reported that preoperatively there was a statistically significant prolonged latency of the R_1 components of the blink reflex on the affected side of patients with hemifacial spasm (12.3 ms compared to 10.8 ms on the unaffected side; 10.8 ms in controls). Such a substantial increase in neural conduction time in the facial nerve would indicate a rather severe demyelination of the facial nerve and would support the hypothesis that there is ephaptic transmission between injured nerve fibers in patients with hemifacial spasm. Nielsen[113] also found that the amplitudes of the R_1 components of the blink reflex were about twice as high on the affected side as on the unaffected side, indicating that more motor neurons than normal fire in response to stimulation of the supraorbital nerve. While other investigators[139] have confirmed the latter finding, the latency of the R_1 on the affected side has consistently been found to be normal in patients with hemifacial spasm (10.9 ms versus 11.2 ms in the involved and uninvolved side,[6] 10.3 ms versus 10.1 ms,[24] 11.3 ms versus 11.3 ms:[139] very similar results from different studies). Patients who had previously undergone destructive procedures to the facial nerve, however, have a prolonged latency of the R^1 response on the affected side (12.1 ± 1.3 ms in 26 patients).[71] These prolonged latencies should be compared with 11.1 ± 1.1 ms in 37 patients who had hemifacial spasm but had not undergone destructive procedures studied by the same investigators; the R_1 latency on the normal side was 10.8 ± 1.1 ms.

In preoperative studies of patients with hemifacial spasm, electrical stimulation of the supraorbital nerve to elicit the blink reflex gave rise to contractions not only of the muscles around the eyes but also of other muscles of the face.[6,71,113] This spread of activity to other parts of the face is in agreement with the observation that patients with hemifacial spasm often have synkinetic facial movements.

The latency of the synkinetic R_1 component of the blink response recorded from the lower face (mentalis-orbicularis oris muscle) in patients with hemifacial spasm was found to be 12.6 ± 1.3 ms;[139] this prolongation relative to the R_1 recorded from the orbicularis oculi muscle is assumed to be due to the fact that the facial nerve to the lower face is longer than that to the upper face. It is, however, interesting to note that the latency value of the R_1 from the orbicularis oculi muscle on the affected side of patients with hemifacial spasm (12.3 ms) reported by Nielsen[113] is very similar to the value of the synkinetic R_1 reported by other investigators.[139]

The finding that the latency of the R_2 component of the blink reflex is shorter when elicited from the affected side than it is when elicited from the unaffected side[24,139] is another preoperative finding regarding the blink reflex that indicates that inhibition of the blink reflex is reduced on the affected side in patients with hemifacial spasm. In addition, Roth et al[121] found evidence of hyperactivity in the facial motor nucleus in patients with hemifacial spasm, and they presented the hypothesis that the spasm in these patients is a result of an interaction between hyperactive facial motor neurons and ephaptic transmission in the facial nerve at the location of vascular compression.

The finding that the R_1 component of the blink reflex can be elicited on the affected side (but not on the unaffected side) in patients with hemifacial spasm undergoing MVD, despite the suppressive effect of general anesthesia,[98] further supports the

hypothesis that the facial motor nucleus (on the affected side) is hyperactive in patients with hemifacial spasm. These results indicate that hyperactivity of the facial motor nucleus on the affected side compensates for the suppressive action of the general anesthetic agent. (Under these circumstances the R_1 component of the blink reflex response has a latency that is slightly longer than the 10 ms latency it normally has, most likely because of the suppressive effect of anesthetic agents.)

Thus, considerable evidence exists that it is not the mechanical compression of the facial nerve that causes hemifacial spasm to develop, but more likely an as yet unknown effect of irritation of the facial nerve by a blood vessel: possibly electrical stimulation of the facial nerve via the potentials that exist on the surfaces of blood vessels that, over time, cause the facial nucleus to become hyperactive and cause the disease to develop.

The Abnormal Muscle Response

Patients with hemifacial spasm have other specific neurophysiologic signs. One is the abnormal, or delayed, muscle response that can be demonstrated by electrically stimulating one branch of the facial nerve, an action that gives rise to a response in muscles that are innervated by other branches of the facial nerve.[23,87,92,94,98,99,112] This response has a latency of about 10 ms when elicited by electric stimulation of the temporal or zygomatic branch of the facial nerve and recorded from the mentalis muscle.

This abnormal muscle response may be assumed to be caused by abnormal cross-transmission. If the anatomic location of this cross-transmission is also the location of the physiological abnormality that causes the symptoms and signs of hemifacial spasm in these patients, then studies of the abnormal muscle response can help to determine which of the two hypotheses for the pathophysiology of the disorder is correct.

If the cross-transmission occurs at the site of vascular compression, then the latency of the abnormal muscle response would be equal to the sum of the neural conduction times of

STIM. ZYGOMATIC BRANCH NVII

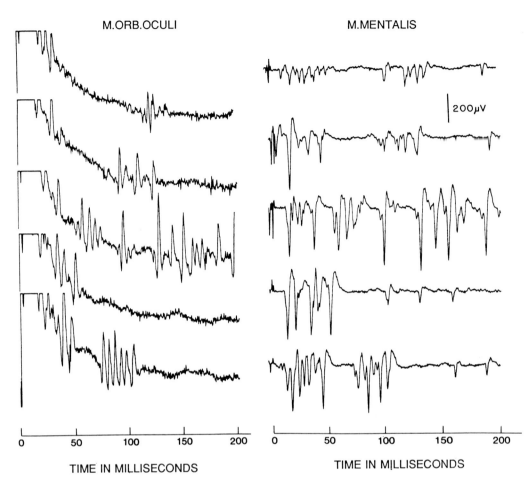

Figure 1A. *Typical electromyographic recording of the abnormal muscle response of hemifacial spasm. Recorded from the orbicularis oculi and the mentalis muscles when elicited by electric stimulation of the zygomatic branch of the facial nerve.*

the parts of the facial nerve that are involved. The abnormal muscle response can be recorded in patients under general anesthesia (provided that no paralyzing agents are used) (Figure 1A, B). It may be seen that the abnormal muscle activity consists of an initial deflection with a latency of about 10 ms followed by a burst of irregular electromyographic (EMG) activity that varies in duration.

Studies in patients undergoing MVD for hemifacial spasm have shown that the latency of the abnormal muscle response is longer than would be expected if the cross-transmission occurred at the site of vascular compression. These results were obtained by

comparing the latency of the abnormal muscle response with the sum of the neural conduction times of the paths that would be involved if the cross-transmission occurred at the location of the vascular compression (Figure 2A, B). These conduction times were determined by recording compound action potentials (CAPs) from the facial nerve near the location of the vascular compression in response to the same electrical stimulation of one branch of the facial nerve as was used to elicit the abnormal muscle response (Figure 3). EMG responses were also recorded from the same muscle from which the abnormal muscle response was recorded and elicited by

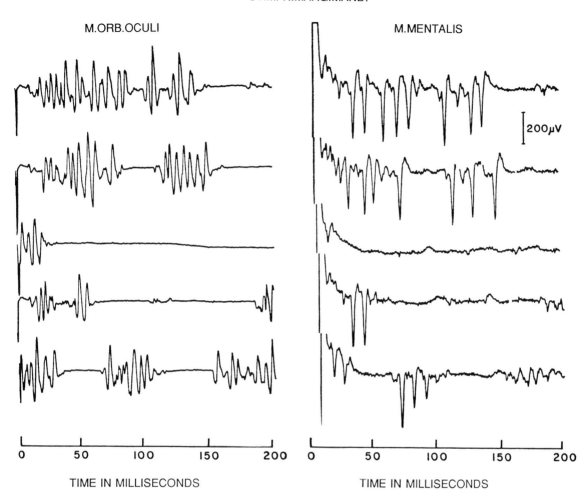

Figure 1B. Recorded from the orbicularis oculi and mentalis muscles in response to electric stimulation of the marginal mandibular branch of the facial nerve. Electrode placements are shown in Figure 2. The results were obtained in a patient undergoing an MVD operation for hemifacial spasm, after the patient was anesthetized but before the operation was begun.[96]

stimulation of the intracranial portion of the facial nerve at the location of vascular compression. The sum of the conduction times that were determined from such recordings was consistently shorter than the latency of the abnormal muscle response (by a mean value of 2.21 ms in the 16 patients when the abnormal muscle response was elicited from stimulation of the marginal mandibular nerve, and by 1.95 ms in 8 patients when the abnormal muscle response was elicited from the zygomatic branch of the facial nerve).[95] This indicates that the site of the cross-

transmission that causes this response is located proximal to the site of vascular compression, probably in the facial motor nucleus. These results confirmed those of a previous study[94] and were confirmed in later studies[87,92,98,99] and by other investigators.[49,50,123]

It has been argued that the difference in conduction times can be explained by a slowing of conduction in the facial nerve segment that was compressed by the blood vessel, because denuded axons conduct more slowly than myelinated axons.[120] Such a slowing is a prerequisite for facilitation of ephaptic trans-

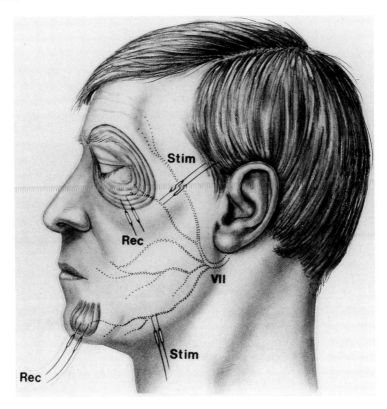

Figure 2A. Schematic illustration of the placement of recording and stimulating electrodes for recordings shown in Figure 1A, B.[97]

mission. However, as mentioned previously, there are few signs of such slowing.

While these results indicate that ephaptic transmission in the facial nerve at the REZ is unlikely to give rise to the cross-transmission that causes the abnormal muscle contraction, results in rare cases and under unusual circumstances have indeed revealed signs of ephaptic transmission in the compressed segment of the facial nerve.[87] Thus, in 3 of 50 patients in one study, an additional component appeared about 2 ms prior to the abnormal muscle response that was seen in these patients. This component arose only after extensive surgical manipulation of the facial nerve and it was present for only 1-2 minutes. The amplitude of this additional component was very small (0.3% to 3% of the amplitude of the EMG potentials evoked by intracranial electrical stimulation of the motor nerve to the muscle),[87] indicating that very few nerve fibers were involved.

These results were taken to support the hypothesis that ephaptic transmission does not normally occur in patients with hemifacial spasm, and the small amplitude of the associated EMG potentials showed that, if it was to occur, the muscle contraction would be of a very low amplitude and probably not noticeable because very few nerve fibers would be involved.

Intraoperative studies of the interaction between the blink reflex and the abnormal muscle response in patients with hemifacial spasm suggest that the abnormal muscle response is an exaggerated F-response.[92] The F-response is assumed to be the result of backfiring of motor neurons, and it is regarded as a measure of the excitability of the motor neuron pool.[29,72] An exaggerated F-response would thus be in agreement with the hypothesis that the facial motor nucleus is hyperactive in patients with hemifacial spasm.

A single-fiber EMG study by Sanders[125]

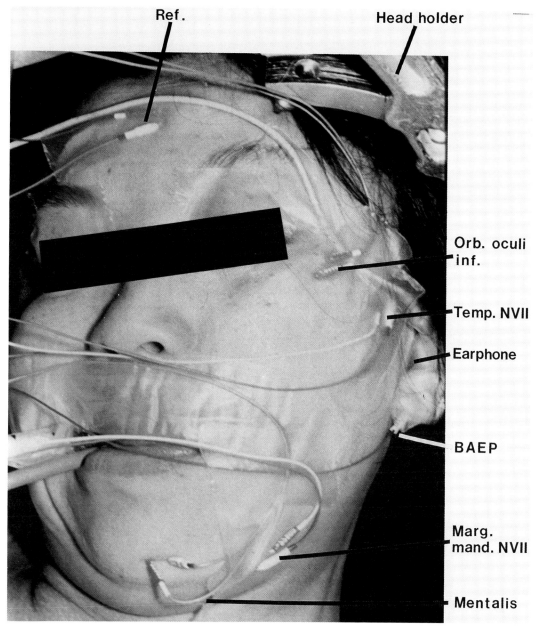

*Figure 2B. Practical arrangement of recording and stimulating electrodes for recordings as shown in Figure 1 in a patient undergoing MVD for hemifacial spasm.[87] **Ref.** = Reference; **Orb. occuli inf.** = Orbicularis occuli inferior; **Temp. NVII** = Temporal branch of VII; **Marg. mand. NVII** = marginal mandibular branch of VII; **Mentalis** = mentalis muscle.*

showed that the jitter of the abnormal muscle response recorded preoperatively in patients with hemifacial spasm was low, and he interpreted the results to support the ephaptic transmission hypothesis because they indicated that the abnormal muscle response does not depend on normal synaptic transmission. However, the value of the jitter was similar to what is seen in an F-response, which supports the hypothesis that the abnormal muscle response is an exaggerated F-response[92] and thus an indication of a hyperactive facial motor nucleus.

The late components of the compound action potentials recorded from the facial nerve intracranially (Figure 3) also indi-

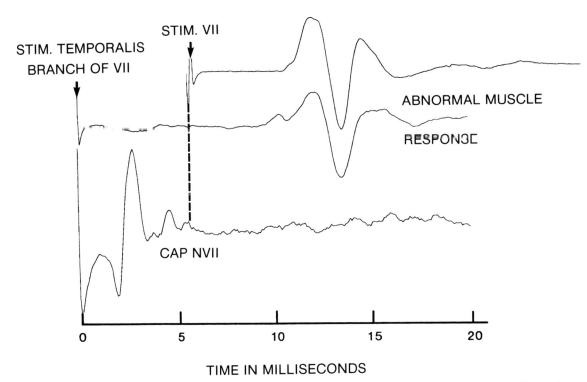

Figure 3. Middle tracing: *Recording of the abnormal muscle contraction of hemifacial spasm obtained from the mentalis muscle in response to electric stimulation of the temporal branch of the facial nerve.* **Top tracing:** *Recording from the mentalis muscle in response to electric stimulation of the facial nerve near the location of its vascular compression.* **Lower tracing:** *The compound action potentials (CAP) recorded from the facial nerve where it was compressed by a blood vessel in response to the same electric stimulation of the temporal branch of the facial nerve as used to elicit the abnormal muscle response. The response from the mentalis muscle elicited by electric stimulation of the facial nerve where it was compressed by a blood vessel was aligned in time with the abnormal muscle response; therefore, the time of stimulation to elicit the response to intracranial stimulation of the facial nerve becomes an estimate of the time when the activity in the intracranial portion of the facial nerve elicited the abnormal muscle response. Note that this response appears about 2 ms later than the compound action potentials recorded from the facial nerve. The results were obtained before the facial nerve was decompressed in a patient undergoing MVD for hemifacial spasm.*

cate that the facial motor nucleus is hyperactive and generates more than one volley of neural activity in response to antidromic stimulation.

Development of Facial Nucleus Hyperactivity

It has been proposed that the mechanisms for developing hemifacial spasm are similar to what is known as "kindling",[87,91,94,98,99] i.e. an antidromic neural activity that is gener-ated by close contact between a blood vessel that over time makes the facial motor nucleus become hyperactive.[42,140] In support of this hypothesis, experiments in animals have shown that an abnormal muscle contraction, similar to what is seen in patients with hemifacial spasm, gradually develops after daily electrical stimulation of the facial nerve for 4-6 weeks[101,128] (Figure 4), and that this muscle contraction disappears when daily stimulation is terminated. Recordings from the facial motor nucleus in such "kindled"

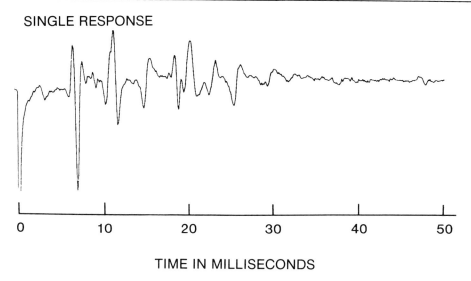

SINGLE RESPONSE

TIME IN MILLISECONDS

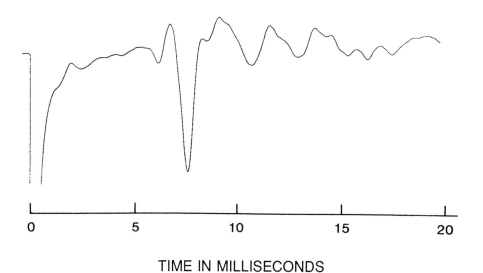

AVERAGE OF 256 RESPONSES

TIME IN MILLISECONDS

Figure 4. Recordings of the abnormal muscle response in a rat, the facial nerve of which had been electrically stimulated daily for 4 weeks. (A) Response to a single stimulus, showing after discharges in addition to the initial response. (B) Average of 256 responses similar to those in A, but shown on a faster time scale. Note that because the later discharges do not appear synchronously with the stimulus, they cancel out when many responses are summed.[128]

animals reveal an abnormal response to antidromic stimulation of the facial nerve which, in turn, indicates that the facial nucleus has been reorganized.[102]

The cross-transmission that is the basis for the abnormal muscle response, and the synkinesis of the blink reflex, cannot directly be explained by hyperactivity of the facial motor nucleus. There may be dormant synapses connecting neurons that innervate different portions of the face, and these synapses open under abnormal conditions. The

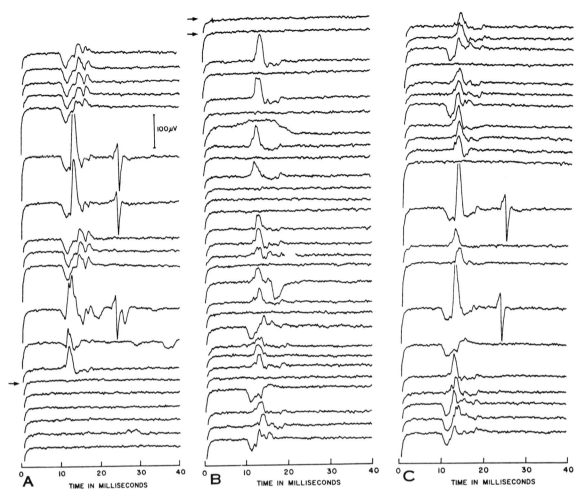

Figure 5. *Consecutive responses from the mentalis muscle elicited by stimulation of the zygomatic branch of the facial nerve in a patient undergoing MVD to relieve hemifacial spasm. Responses were obtained in a way similar to that described in Figure 1, but they are shown here on an expanded time scale. The first recording in the second column (B) was obtained 10 seconds after the last recording in the first column. The repetition rate of the stimulation was 8 pps; thus, there are 125 ms between the responses shown. Note the instant disappearance of the abnormal muscle response when the vessel that was compressing the facial nerve was moved off the facial nerve (single arrow in column A) and its gradual reappearance when the vessel was allowed to fall back on the nerve (double arrow in column B).*[96]

existence of such dormant synapses has been proposed by investigators of pain;[141] in addition, evidence has been presented of altered synaptic organization of the facial muscles after injury.[12,43]

Physiologic Effect of Microvascular Decompression

The synkinetic response of the blink reflex cannot usually be elicited postoperatively after a successful MVD operation for hemifacial spasm,[7,114] nor can the abnormal muscle response be elicited postoperatively.[114] In fact, the abnormal muscle response disappears instantly when the offending blood vessel is moved off the facial nerve[96] (Figure 5). Furthermore, the R_1 component of the blink reflex can no longer be elicited after the offending blood vessel has been moved off the facial nerve[99] (Figure 6).

The observations (1) that the abnormal

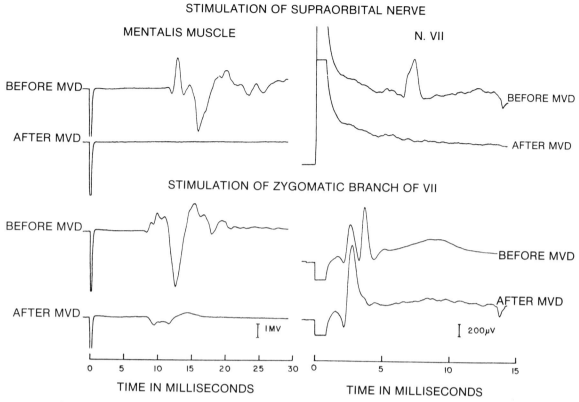

Figure 6. *Results of stimulating the supraorbital nerve and a branch of the facial nerve in a patient undergoing MVD to relieve hemifacial spasm before and after the offending blood vessel was moved off the facial nerve. **Left Column:** Responses from the mentalis muscle to stimulation of the supraorbital nerve (to elicit the blink reflex) before and after MVD of the facial nerve (upper two curves). The lower two curves show the abnormal muscle responses recorded from the mentalis muscle to stimulation of the zygomatic branch of the facial nerve before and after MVD of the facial nerve. **Right Column:** Compound action potentials recorded simultaneously from the intracranial portion of the facial nerve before and after MVD of the facial nerve in response to stimulation of the supraorbital nerve (top tracings) and the zygomatic branch of the facial nerve (bottom tracings).*[98]

muscle response disappears instantly when the offending blood vessel is moved off the facial nerve and (2) that it returns when the vessel is again allowed to touch the facial nerve (as shown in Figure 6)[98] lend considerable credence to the hypothesis that it is the close contact between a blood vessel and the facial nerve that causes the hyperactivity that gives rise to the signs of hemifacial spasm. This observation also, however, seemingly contradicts the hypothesis that hemifacial spasm is caused by the development, over time, of hyperactivity of the facial motor nucleus. One would expect that such hyperactivity would remain for a certain period of time after the irritation of the facial nerve

was removed, because the excitability of the facial motor nucleus would be expected to return gradually to normal after the offending blood vessel has been moved off the nerve. An explanation for instant abolishment of the signs of hyperactivity may be that the hyperactivity of the facial motor nucleus is only manifest in its response to the novel neural activity that is generated by close contact between a blood vessel and a nerve.[93,97,98] Indeed, in our experience, the abnormal muscle response disappears slowly (over several minutes) in patients who have had their spasm for 10 or more years; such patients may have slight spasm for several days or weeks after the operation. Although the abnormal muscle response is not noticeably suppressed by general anesthesia it may be slightly suppressed, and it therefore disappears faster during the operation than it would in an awake patient. This explanation is supported by the postoperative finding that the abnormal muscle response can be recorded in some patients for a period of time after the operation.[114]

Role of the Trigeminal System

It is also possible that excitability of the facial nucleus is increased by activity in the trigeminal nerve which is elicited by the muscle contractions (spasm). Trigeminal input from the upper face has an excitatory influence on facial motor neurons,[25,135] and such input may provide the excitatory influence on the facial motor neurons necessary for the development and maintenance of hyperactivity. Support for this hypothesis comes from the observation that the injection of alcohol into the peripheral portion of the facial nerve to alleviate the spasm in patients with hemifacial spasm also arrests the clicking sound that such patients often experience as a result of spasmodic contractions of the stapedial muscle.[46] Because the branch of the facial nerve that innervates the stapedial muscle arises from the main trunk of the facial nerve proximal to the site of alcohol injection, it cannot have been influenced directly by the nerve blockade that was produced by the alcohol injection, and it seems unlikely that the alcohol injected into the peripheral portion of the nerve could diffuse along the nerve trunk as far as the site where the stapedial nerve exits the facial nerve trunk. In fact, partial denervation of facial muscles can eliminate attacks of spasm while nearly normal facial function is attained.[27,124] This indicates that the positive feedback to the facial motor nucleus from the trigeminal stimulation from contraction of the facial muscles around the eyes increases the excitability of the facial motor nucleus to the extent that the hyperactivity of facial motor neurons causing the spasm in hemifacial spasm is maintained.

The finding that the abnormal muscle response disappears immediately when the offending blood vessel is lifted off the facial nerve[96] (see Figure 5) has led to the general practice of recording the abnormal muscle response intraoperatively to help identify the offending blood vessel and to make sure the facial nerve is adequately decompressed before the operation is ended.[44,88,100]

The fact that the abnormal muscle response seems to be specific for hemifacial spasm would make it an efficient method to distinguish hemifacial spasm from other facial spasms. Patients with blepharospasm and facial myokymia do not have this response.[112] However, to date the test for this response is not in widespread use.

Trigeminal Neuralgia

Trigeminal neuralgia is characterized by short periods of excruciating pain in specific areas of the face.[35,144] In the Western world, trigeminal neuralgia is more common than hemifacial spasm, with an estimated incidence of about 4.7 per 100,000 for both sexes in the white population in the United States, 5.9 per 100,000 in women and 3.4 per 100,000 in men.[67] The pain is usually triggered by a light touch to a specific area of the face or inside the mouth, and it does not respond to conventional analgesics.[80]

Similar to what has been suggested regarding the pathophysiology of hemifacial spasm, two different hypotheses have been put forth to explain the symptoms of trigeminal neuralgia: the first (peripheral) hypothesis assumes that the symptoms are caused by ephaptic transmission in the segment of the trigeminal nerve that is in close contact with a blood vessel;[38] the second (central) hypothesis claims that the symptoms have a central cause.[32,33,35] Recently, it has been claimed that the symptoms of trigeminal neuralgia can be explained by a peripheral etiology and a central pathogenesis.[33]

The effect of the compressing blood vessel

on the morphology of the trigeminal nerve is relatively small, as demonstrated by histologic studies of trigeminal nerve roots obtained from patients with trigeminal neuralgia during operations in which the trigeminal nerve was sectioned to treat the disorder. Such studies showed proliferation and degeneration of the myelin sheaths, with the axons preserved. These changes have been described as degenerative hypermyelination and segmental demyelination, with indications of microneuromas, abnormalities of the myelin and the axon cylinders,[9,69,70] and an irregular vacuolization in the Gasserian ganglion.[9] Similar vacuolization was found on autopsies of individuals without trigeminal neuralgia, but the anomalies in nerves from those with trigeminal neuralgia were judged to be greater than those seen in age-matched controls. The degenerative hypermyelination and segmental demyelination were similar to that seen with nerve compression injuries.

On the basis of these relatively small morphologic changes, several investigators have found it unlikely that the pain of trigeminal neuralgia is caused solely by vascular compression injury to the trigeminal nerve.

Although less experimental evidence is available regarding the pathophysiology of trigeminal neuralgia versus hemifacial spasm, one hypothesis assigning a peripheral cause for the pain of trigeminal neuralgia assumes that defects in myelin result in multiple reflections of nerve impulses. This hypothesis proposes that such reflections amplify peripheral nerve impulses which together with the dorsal root reflex may cause presynaptic depolarization that, in turn, may elicit the pain of trigeminal neuralgia.[47,48]

Howe et al[47] used chromic sutures to create focal demyelination of the trigeminal nerve and found evidence that a single spike entering the injured zone could set up a reverberation that could generate abnormal high-frequency neural spike trains. The proposal that the physiologic abnormalities causing the symptoms of trigeminal neuralgia are located in the trigeminal nucleus assumes that hyperactivity in the trigeminal nucleus

might be caused by lack of the inhibition that is normally mediated by large A-fibers of the trigeminal nerve.[32,36] However, it seems somewhat surprising that this hypothesis of the pathophysiology of trigeminal neuralgia also assumes it is stimulation of these A-fibers that elicits the pain of trigeminal neuralgia.

Fromm[33] proposed that the hyperactivity causing the pain of trigeminal neuralgia results from impaired segmental inhibition, which is caused by irritation of the trigeminal nerve root in combination with increased activity in afferent fibers of the trigeminal nerve due to ectopic spikes and possibly crosstalk (ephaptic transmission) between injured fibers. Fromm[33] also proposed that such a reduction in segmental inhibition could be caused by chronic irritation of the trigeminal nerve by a blood vessel.

The finding from experiments in animals that the drugs effective in treating trigeminal neuralgia, carbamazepine and phenytoin, increase segmental inhibition[36] supports the hypothesis that decreased segmental inhibition may be a factor in generating the pain of trigeminal neuralgia. Carbamazepine was found to be more effective than phenytoin in these experiments.[137] More recently, it has been shown that baclofen increases segmental inhibition in the trigeminal brain stem complex.[36] The effect of baclofen on the trigeminal nucleus is stereospecific. Thus levobaclofen is at least 5 times more effective than racemic baclofen, and dextro-baclofen has no effect on segmental inhibition. Clinical studies in patients with trigeminal neuralgia confirm that carbamazepine is more effective than phenytoin and that levo-baclofen gives about 5 times more therapeutic effect than racemic baclofen.[34]

These results seem to support the hypothesis that reduced segmental inhibition is involved in generating the pain of trigeminal neuralgia. However, to date it has not been possible to study this disease by electrophysiological methods to the extent that it can be shown whether ephaptic transmission at the site of compression or hyperactivity of the trigeminal nucleus causes the pain.[35]

Glossopharyngeal Neuralgia

Glossopharyngeal neuralgia is more rare than hemifacial spasm and trigeminal neuralgia, but it manifests many of the characteristics and symptoms of trigeminal neuralgia. Although there is no known medical treatment for glossopharyngeal neuralgia, it can be cured effectively by MVD.[55] Little is known about its pathophysiology.

Tic Convulsif

The term "tic convulsif" was coined by Cushing[16] to describe a combination of facial pain, trigeminal neuralgia, and hemifacial spasm. It is a very rare disorder and is assumed to be caused by vascular compression of both the facial and trigeminal nerves. Review of the literature reveals considerable disagreement as to how this disorder should be defined, and there may even be doubt as to whether this disease exists at all.

Cook and Jannetta[15] reported 11 cases of tic convulsif from a total of 900 patients with trigeminal neuralgia. When these 11 patients were treated by MVD, both the facial and the trigeminal nerves were decompressed with a success rate similar to that achieved for patients with hemifacial spasm or trigeminal neuralgia alone. Harris and Wright[46] described two cases: in each case the disorder responded to treatment of the facial nerve differently than it did to treatment of the trigeminal nerve, thus supporting the hypothesis that symptoms can arise from both nerves in the same patient.

Some reports in the literature on tic convulsif define the pain or spasm as other than the symptoms seen in patients with hemifacial spasm and trigeminal neuralgia. Thus, Yeh and Tew[149] defined tic convulsif as a combination of hemifacial spasm and geniculate neuralgia, the latter being caused by vascular compression of the nervus intermedius. The reflex muscle spasm that is often seen in connection with trigeminal neuralgia attacks in some patients may appear to be facial spasm and thus it may be mistaken for true tic convulsif.[117]

Spasm of Muscles of Mastication

Despite the relatively frequent occurrence of vascular compression of the trigeminal nerve, including compression of the portio minor, spasm of the muscles of mastication is very rare. The author is aware of only one case of "hemimasticatory spasm" alone[138] and only one of spasm in connection with hemiatrophy of face muscles[68] having been described in the literature to date. It seems odd that only the major (sensory) portion of the trigeminal nerve should be affected by the vascular compression that causes trigeminal neuralgia, and, in fact, the offending blood vessel in patients with trigeminal neuralgia has often been seen to be in close contact with the portio minor of the trigeminal nerve that is assumed to contain the motor fibers that innervate the muscles of mastication.

Spasm of Muscles Innervated by the Glossopharyngeal Nerve

As with trigeminal neuralgia, there exists no evidence that glossopharyngeal neuralgia is associated with spasm in the muscles that are innervated by the motor portion of the glossopharyngeal nerve.

Disabling Positional Vertigo

Relatively recently, it has become apparent that patients with certain forms of persistent vertigo have vascular compression of the vestibular portion of cranial nerve VIII and this vertigo can be cured by MVD.[11,54,65,104,105,108] This particular disorder was named disabling positional vertigo.[65] Disabling positional vertigo can be so incapacitating that patients are bedridden most of the time or at least unable to work or maintain normal daily activity.[65,104,105,107,108]

The pathophysiology of disabling positional vertigo has not been studied, but many of its signs and symptoms indicate that this disorder has a pathophysiology similar to that of hemifacial spasm and trigeminal neuralgia. For instance, the probability of involvement of the central nervous system in disabling positional vertigo is indicated by the finding that diazepam, which is not known to affect the function of peripheral nerves, can lessen the symptoms of disabling positional vertigo and, in some cases, can practically alleviate them.[105] Bertrand et al[11] found indications that the vestibular nuclei are hypoactive on the affected side in patients with disabling positional vertigo, but more recent studies indicate that these patients have signs of vestibular hyperactivity.[127] These recent findings indicate that disabling positional vertigo may be similar to trigeminal neuralgia and hemifacial spasm in that the symptoms are caused not by the peripheral lesion itself but by changes (perhaps a reduction in inhibition) in more central structures.

Tinnitus

There are indications that intractable tinnitus and, particularly, the hypersensitivity to sound that some patients with intractable tinnitus experience, may have causes similar to those of other disorders that can be cured by MVD. Indeed, recent evidence indicates that certain forms of tinnitus can be cured by MVD of the cochlear portions of the vestibulocochlear nerve.[60,63,76,101,103]

As is the case for disabling positional vertigo, little is known about the pathophysiology of those forms of tinnitus that can be cured by MVD. Evoked potentials that are generated by the ear, the auditory nerve, and the nuclei and fiber tracts of the ascending auditory pathway of the brain stem in patients with incapacitating tinnitus are not significantly different from those recorded from individuals with the same degree of hearing loss but no tinnitus.[93,101] On the basis of these findings it was suggested that severe tinnitus might be the result of abnormalities in more central auditory structures, and it has been hypothesized that the extralemniscal auditory system may in one way or another be involved in creating the symptoms of tinnitus.[93] The fact that injury to the peripheral auditory system can result in hyperactive changes in more central auditory structures

has been shown by Gerken et al,[41] who found that overexposure to sound can change temporal integration in the inferior colliculus. The fact that some patients with tinnitus experience hyperacusis has been taken to indicate that the physiologic abnormality is located at higher brain levels and perhaps the prefrontal cortex is involved.[66]

There is evidence that acute injury to the intracranial portion of the auditory nerve, e.g. from surgical manipulation, can result in tinnitus that occurs immediately postoperatively, and there is considerable evidence that tinnitus can be caused by cochlear injury.[86,93] This tinnitus, however, is generally not as severe as the type believed to be caused by vascular compression, and it may therefore be a different type of tinnitus with a pathophysiology that is different from the above-mentioned type.

Other indications that tinnitus can arise from injury to the cochlear nerve come from studies of patients with hemifacial spasm, some of whom experienced tinnitus in addition to hemifacial spasm. Again, the tinnitus in these patients was usually not severe. Only rarely have we seen patients who have had such severe tinnitus in addition to hemifacial spasm that they wanted to undergo an MVD operation to relieve the tinnitus.

Cyclic Oculomotor Spasm with Paresis

The pathophysiology of cyclic oculomotor spasm with paresis, which is an extremely rare disease, is similar to hemifacial spasm in that it seems to be caused by compression of a portion of the oculomotor (III) nerve while being, at the same time, a disorder of the motor nucleus of cranial nerve III.[75]

Spasmodic Torticollis

Spasmodic torticollis[118] has been assumed to be caused by either hyperactivity of central nuclei (e.g. the basal ganglia) or by vascular compression of the spinal accessory nerve and of the dorsal and ventral roots of the cervical spinal nerves—thus by mechanisms similar to those causing other disorders of cranial nerve function (trigeminal neuralgia, hemifacial spasm, and disabling positional vertigo). Although patients with spasmodic torticollis have been treated by MVD,[31,109,110,129] the results of such operations are not as encouraging as the results of MVD to treat trigeminal neuralgia and hemifacial spasm, and there are indications that two distinctly different types of spasmodic torticollis exist: one that affects the neck muscles bilaterally, and one that has a distinct unilateral pattern.[110] It has been assumed that the bilateral type of spasmodic torticollis is a result of basal ganglia hyperactivity, whereas the hyperactivity causing the symptoms of the unilateral type may be restricted to the motonuclei of one side of the head. This second type is thus likely to be caused by vascular irritation of the spinal accessory nerve. In this way the two types of spasmodic torticollis resemble blepharospasm and hemifacial spasm, respectively.

Recently, Nakashima et al[111] hypothesized that spasmodic torticollis may be caused by a reduced inhibitory influence on the spinal accessory nucleus and upper cervical motor nuclei from the nuclei of the trigeminal nerve. Such reduced inhibition may account for the significantly lower suppression, with electrical stimulation of the supraorbital nerve, of EMG activity in the sternocleidomastoid muscle in patients with spasmodic torticollis versus normal individuals. The mechanism of reduced inhibition as the cause of spasmodic torticollis may make this disorder similar to other forms of dystonia.[10] Nakashima et al[111] and Berardelli et al[10] did not, however, differentiate between bilateral and unilateral spasmodic torticollis.

Discussion

There is considerable evidence that close contact between a blood vessel and a cranial nerve is a necessary condition in the development of disorders such as trigeminal neuralgia and hemifacial spasm. There is also evidence that important signs of hemifacial spasm disappear instantly when the offending blood vessel is moved off the facial nerve, and they return when the blood vessel is allowed to fall back on the facial nerve. Additionally, some evidence suggests that the symptoms of both trigeminal neuralgia and hemifacial spasm are not caused directly by vascular compression of the respective cranial nerves but rather result from changes in the respective nuclei, changes whose development and maintenance may depend on the degree of irritation of the cranial nerve by close contact with a blood vessel(s). The changes in these nuclei are in the form of hyperactivity. However, it is not clear whether this hyperactivity is a result of reduced inhibitory input or increased excitatory input from other brain centers or of a hypersensitivity of the facial motor neurons themselves. Hypotheses that the pain in trigeminal neuralgia is caused by decreased segmental inhibition have been put forth by Fromm,[32] and early hypotheses about hyperactivity of the facial motor nucleus[26] in hemifacial spasm have been supported by the results of recent intraoperative studies.[24,92,94-100,103,139] There are also indications that the symptoms of both disabling positional vertigo and certain forms of tinnitus are the result of increased excitability of respective nuclei,[93,101,127] and some forms of spasmodic torticollis may be caused by reduced segmental inhibition.[111]

The facts that trigeminal neuralgia and hemifacial spasm are not treatable by the same medications but that MVD is equally effective in treating both of these disorders are further indications that the facial and the trigeminal nuclei respectively are involved in these disorders. These nuclei are different, which may explain why the medications that can alleviate pain in trigeminal neuralgia cannot alleviate spasm in hemifacial spasm. If the medication effective in treating one disorder acted to eliminate the effect of vascular compression, then one would expect the same medication to be equally effective in treating all the disorders that can be treated successfully by MVD.

Thus, it may be assumed that vascular compression itself does not cause the symptoms and signs of these disorders, but rather the symptoms and signs of these disorders are produced by changes in the respective nuclei, in turn, caused by vascular compression. It is not known, however, how irritation of a cranial nerve root causes changes in structures in the central nervous system. The fact that MVD is an effective treatment of these disorders,[4,53,55,63] together with the intraoperative electrophysiologic evidence that facial nerve compression causes signs in patients with hemifacial spasm,[95] points to vascular compression being a necessary condition for the development of pathophysiologic changes in the respective nuclei. Because vascular compression of cranial nerves is rather common but hemifacial spasm and trigeminal neuralgia are not, it may be concluded that vascular compression in itself is not sufficient to cause these changes. It is not known what other condition is necessary for vascular compression to cause such alterations in central neural structures. There is growing evidence that injuries to peripheral nerves, novel input to certain nuclei, or deprivation of input can result in reorganization of the nuclei in question and can cause an altered balance between inhibition and excitation. If it is assumed that irritation of a cranial nerve generates novel neural activity in the respective nerve, then it is conceivable that under certain favorable conditions such activity could cause changes in the function of nuclei.

Blood vessels can be in contact with cranial nerves without producing noticeable symptoms, which has been shown not only in studies of cadaver specimens from individuals with no sign of cranial nerve compression disorders[45,73,85,116,131] but also by intraoperative examination of patients who were undergoing MVD for cranial nerve compression syndromes. Thus, vessel(s) that compress the vestibulocochlear nerve in patients with disabling positional vertigo can indeed be in close contact with the facial nerve as well. Of a total of more than 175 patients operated upon in our institution to relieve disabling positional vertigo by MVD of the vestibulocochlear nerve, however, none has developed hemifacial spasm (M.B. Møller, personal communication, 1990). This supports the assumption that vascular compression in itself does not produce dramatic symptoms or signs. Indeed, many patients with disabling positional vertigo also have slight muscle quivering around the eyes[108] that can be seen by a trained observer but which may or may not be noticed by the patient. This quivering of the orbicularis oculi muscles may result directly from a blood vessel lying in contact with the facial nerve, but the fact that hemifacial spasm does not develop indicates that vascular compression in itself does not cause the signs and symptoms of hemifacial spasm, nor does it cause the development of hemifacial spasm over a length of time.

In like manner, patients with hemifacial spasm sometimes evidence subtle auditory nerve signs that result in small anomalies in their audiograms,[106] but they do not have disabling positional vertigo. Although these patients also may experience tinnitus, another sign of vestibulocochlear nerve irritation, it is never severe, a fact which supports the hypothesis that vascular compression in itself does not give rise to any symptoms or signs noticeable by the patient. There may be vascular compression of a nerve without any symptoms being present, which is further indicated by the observation that patients with hemifacial spasm or trigeminal neuralgia often have measurable vestibular abnormalities,[115] and observations during MVD operations on patients with hemifacial spasm or trigeminal neuralgia confirm that a blood vessel compressing the facial or the trigeminal nerve in such patients can also be in close contact with the vestibular nerve but not cause symptoms of vestibular dysfunction.[5] Thus all of these cases in which compression was present without symptoms provide evidence that vascular compression of a cranial nerve, although necessary to cause the symptoms of the compression disorder, is not sufficient to cause the disorder.

Fromm[33] recognized that vascular compression alone does not always produce the symptoms of trigeminal neuralgia when he concluded, "Vascular compression may well be the predominant, but by no means sole, cause of trigeminal neuralgia."

The author, however, finds that vascular compression is a necessary condition for these disorders to develop; it is not enough to cause the changes in the respective nuclei necessary to produce the symptoms of these disorders,[89,91] but an additional factor is necessary. This factor ("suitable substrate") could be an inborn condition or acquired at some point in life. In hemifacial spasm it could be a natural "weakness" of the facial nerve itself, but it seems more likely to be a property of the facial motor nucleus. Abnormally low membrane potentials in facial motor neurons, and/or lower-than-normal inhibition by brain stem areas that influence the facial motor neurons, and/or an abnormally high degree of excitatory input from other brain centers could all be the necessary suitable substrate, in addition to vascular compression of the facial nerve, for the development of hemifacial spasm. The fact that trigeminal input from the upper face to the facial motor nucleus is excitatory whereas input from the lower face is inhibitory[135] may explain not only why hemifacial spasm usually begins with involuntary contractions of muscles around the eye but also that an imbalance of inhibitory and excitatory trigeminal input to facial motor neurons is the suitable substrate necessary for development of hemifacial spasm in those individuals who have vascular compression of the facial nerve root.[91] This may also explain why hemifacial spasm is more common than spasm caused by vascular compression of other cranial nerves.

As in the case of vascular compression of a cranial nerve, the condition (suitable substrate) that must exist in addition to vascular compression for the symptoms and signs of a disorder to become manifest is not likely to produce noticeable symptoms or signs by itself.

Unusually low segmental inhibition in the trigeminal nucleus could cause trigeminal neuralgia, and it has been suggested that chronic irritation of trigeminal nerve fibers may lead to such decreased segmental inhibition in the trigeminal sensory nucleus and together with an abnormal afferent input to the nucleus, may cause trigeminal neuralgia.[33,34] While there is evidence that such changes may be brought about as a result of vascular compression it seems more likely that a suitable substrate, unrelated to the vascular compression, must be present for vascular compression to result in a noticeable pathology. The abnormality may be an imbalance between excitation and inhibition that could be inborn or brought about by environmental factors or the process of normal aging.

The anatomic location of the physiologic anomaly giving rise to the symptoms in cranial nerve dysfunction syndromes, such as hemifacial spasm, trigeminal neuralgia, disabling positional vertigo, glossopharyngeal neuralgia and some forms of tinnitus, may not be the site of the vascular compression but may be located in a central structure (nucleus). It seems likely that these disorders have a similar pathogenesis in which vascular compression is a necessary but insufficient condition for the manifestation of pathology (and maybe for its development) and that a suitable substrate is necessary for the development of these diseases. The assumption that vascular compression and a central abnormality are both necessary but neither one is sufficient to cause the symptoms and signs of these disorders explains why both MVD and medical treatments can be equally effective in curing these disorders.

The existence of a disorder such as tic convulsif seems to speak against the hypothesis presented in this chapter—that vascular compression is necessary but not sufficient to cause pathology. However, the fact that a combination of trigeminal neuralgia and hemifacial spasm occurs so rarely may support the assumption that another factor must be present for vascular compression to develop into a disease.

Thus, vascular compression in itself does not appear to cause any noticeable symptoms, but probably exerts its effect through changes in the respective nuclei. There is also evidence that such transformation can only take place when a second factor exists. If it is accepted that vascular compression is necessary but not enough to cause the development of cranial nerve disorders, then arguments against MVD as an effective treatment of these disorders[1] seem invalid. The documented high success rate of MVD operations can be explained because MVD removes one of two (or more) conditions necessary to the development and maintenance of the hyperactivity of the respective nuclei that produce the signs and symptoms of these disorders.

References

1. Adams CBT. Microvascular compression: an alternative view and hypothesis. *J Neurosurg.* 1989;57:1-12.
2. Alexander GE, Moses H III. Carbamazepine for hemifacial spasm. *Neurology.* 1982;32:286-287.
3. Apfelbaum RI. Surgery for tic douloureux. *Clin Neurosurg.* 1984;31:357-368.
4. Apfelbaum RI. Surgical management of disorders of the lower cranial nerves. In: Schmidek HH, Sweet WH, eds. *Operative Neurosurgical Techniques: Indications, Methods, and Results.* Orlando, Fla: Grune and Stratton; 1988;2:1097-1109.
5. Applebaum EL, Valvasori GE. Auditory and vestibular system findings in patients with vascular loops in the internal auditory canal. *Ann Otol Rhinol Laryngol.* 1984;112(Suppl):63-70.
6. Auger RG. Hemifacial spasm: clinical and electrophysiologic observations. *Neurology.* 1979;29:1261-1272.
7. Auger RG, Piepgras DG, Laws ER Jr, et al. Microvascular decompression of the facial nerve for hemi-facial spasm: clinical and electrophysiological observations. *Neurology.* 1981;31:346-350.
8. Auger RG, Whisnant JP. Hemifacial spasm in Rochester and Olmsted County, Minnesota, 1960 to 1984. *Arch Neurol.* 1990;47:1233-1234.
9. Beaver DL. Electron microscopy of the Gasserian ganglion in trigeminal neuralgia. *J Neurosurg.* 1967;26:138-150.
10. Berardelli A, Rothwell JC, Day BL, et al. Pathophysiology of blepharospasm and oromandibular dystonia. *Brain.* 1985;108:593-608.
11. Bertrand RA, Molina P, Hardy J. Vestibular syndrome and vascular anomaly in the cerebellopontine angle. *Acta Otolaryngol (Stockh).* 1977;3:187-194.
12. Bratzlavsky M, vander Ecken H. Altered synaptic organization in facial nucleus following facial nerve regeneration:an electrophysiological study in man. *Ann Neurol.* 1977;2:71-73.
13. Burchiel KJ, Clarke H, Haglund M, et al. Long-term efficacy of microvascular decompression in trigeminal neuralgia. *J Neurosurg.* 1988;69:35-38.
14. Coad JE, Wirtschafter JD, Haines SJ, et al. Familial hemifacial spasm associated with arterial compression of the facial nerve: case report. *J Neurosurg.* 1991;74:290-296.
15. Cook BR, Jannetta PJ. Tic convulsif: results in 11 cases treated with microvascular decompression of the fifth and seventh cranial nerves. *J Neurosurg.* 1984;61:949-951.
16. Cushing H. The major trigeminal neuralgias and their surgical treatment based on experience with 332 gasserian operations. *Am J Med Sci.* 1920;160:157-184.
17. Dandy WE. An operation for the cure of tic douloureux: partial section of the sensory root at the pons. *Arch Surg.* 1929;18:687-734.
18. Dandy WE. The treatment of trigeminal neuralgia by the cerebellar route. *Ann Surg.* 1932;96:787-795.
19. Dandy WE. Concerning the cause of trigeminal neuralgia. *Am J Surg.* 1934;24:447-455.
20. Digre K, Corbett JJ. Hemifacial spasm: Differential diagnosis mechanism and treatment. *Adv Neurol.* 1988;39:151-176.
21. Ehni G, Woltman HW. Hemifacial spasm: review of one hundred and six cases. *Arch Neurol Psychiatry.* 1945;53:205-211.
22. Elmquist D, Toremalm NG, Elner A, et al. Hemifacial spasm: electrophysiological findings and the therapeutic effect of facial nerve block. *Muscle Nerve.* 1982;5(suppl):S89-S94.
23. Esslen E. Der Spasmus facialis eine Parabioseerscheinung: elektrophysiologische Untersuchungen zum Entstehungsmechanismus des Facialisspasmus. *Dtsch Z Nervenheil.* 1957;176:149-172.
24. Esteban A, Molina-Negro P. Primary hemifacial spasm: a neurophysiological study. *J Neurol Neurosurg Psychiatry.* 1986;49:58-63.
25. Fanardjian VV, Kasabyan SA, Manvelyan LR. Mechanisms regulating the activity of facial nucleus motoneurones, II: synaptic activation from the caudal trigeminal nucleus. *Neuroscience.* 1983;9:823-835.
26. Ferguson JH. Hemifacial spasm and the facial nucleus. *Ann Neurol.* 1978;4:97-103.
27. Fisch U. Extracranial surgery for facial hyperkinesis. In: May M, ed. *The Facial Nerve.* New York, NY: Thieme; 1986:509-523.
28. Fisch U, Esslen E. The surgical treatment of facial hyperkinesia. *Arch Otolaryngol.* 1972;95:400-405.
29. Fisher MA, Shahani BT, Young RR. Assessing segmental excitability after acute rostral lesions, I: the F response. *Neurology.* 1978;28:1265-1271.
30. Fraioli B, Esposito V, Guidetti B, et al. Treatment of trigeminal neuralgia by thermocoagulation, glycerolization, and percutaneous compression of the gasserian ganglion and/or retrogasserian rootlets: long-term results and therapeutic protocol. *Neurosurgery.* 1989;24:239-245.
31. Freckmann N, Hagenah R, Herrmann HD, et al. Treatment of neurogenic torticollis by microvascular lysis of the accessory nerve roots: indication, technique, and first results. *Acta Neurochirur*

(Wien). 1981;59:167-175.

32. Fromm GH. Effects of different classes of antiepileptic drugs on brain-stem pathways. *Fed Proc.* 1985;44:2432-2435.

33. Fromm GH. Pathophysiology of trigeminal neuralgia. In: Fromm GH, Sessle BJ, eds. *Trigeminal Neuralgia: Current Concepts Regarding Pathogenesis and Treatment.* Boston, Mass: Butterworth Heinemann; 1991:105-130.

34. Fromm GH. Medical treatment of patients with trigeminal neuralgia. In: Fromm GH, Sessle BJ, eds. *Trigeminal Neuralgia: Current Concepts Regarding Pathogenesis and Treatment.* Boston, Mass: Butterworth Heinemann; 1991:131-144.

35. Fromm GH, Chattha AS, Terrence CF, et al. Role of inhibitory mechanisms in trigeminal neuralgia. *Neurology.* 1981;31:683-687.

36. Fromm GH, Sessle BJ. *Trigeminal Neuralgia: Current Concepts Regarding Pathogenesis and Treatment.* Boston, Mass: Butterworth Heinemann; 1991.

37. Gardner WJ. Concerning the mechanism of trigeminal neuralgia and hemifacial spasm. *J Neurosurg.* 1962;19:947-958.

38. Gardner WJ. Crosstalk: the paradoxical transmission of a nerve impulse. *Arch Neurol.* 1966;14:149-156.

39. Gardner WJ, Miklos MV. Response of trigeminal neuralgia to "decompression" of sensory root: discussion of cause of trigeminal neuralgia. *JAMA.* 1959;170:1773-1776.

40. Gardner WJ, Sava GA. Hemifacial spasm: a reversible pathophysiologic state. *J Neurosurg.* 1962;19:240-247.

41. Gerken GM, Solecki JM, Boettcher FA. Temporal integration of electrical stimulation of auditory nuclei in normal-hearing and hearing-impaired cat. *Hear Res.* 1991;53:101-112.

42. Goddard GV. Amygdaloid stimulation and learning in the rat. *J Comp Physiol Psychol.* 1964;58:23-30.

43. Graeber MB, Kreutzberg GW. Delayed astrocyte reaction following facial nerve axotomy. *J Neurocytol.* 1988;17:209-220.

44. Haines SJ, Torres F. Intraoperative monitoring of the facial nerve during decompressive surgery for hemifacial spasm. *J Neurosurg.* 1991;74:254-257.

45. Hardy DG, Rhoton AL Jr. Microsurgical relationship of the superior cerebellar artery and the trigeminal nerve. *J Neurosurg.* 1978;49:669-678.

46. Harris W, Wright AD. Treatment of clonic facial spasm: (a) by alcohol injection, (b) by nerve anastomosis. *Lancet.* 1932;1:657-662.

47. Howe JF, Calvin WH, Loeser JD. Impulses reflected from dorsal root ganglia and from focal nerve injuries. *Brain Res.* 1976;116:139-144.

48. Howe JF, Loeser JD, Calvin WH. Mechanosensitivity of dorsal root ganglia and chronically injured axons: a physiological basis for the radicular pain of root compression. *Pain.* 1977;3:25-41.

49. Itagaki S, Saito S, Nakai O. Intraoperative recording of evoked EMG in patients with hemifacial spasm-possible physiological mechanism. *Facial N Res Jpn.* 1988;8:143-146.

50. Itagaki S, Saito S, Nakai O. Electrophysiological study on hemifacial spasm: usefulness in etiological diagnosis and pathophysiological mechanism. *No To Shinkei.* 1989;41:1005-1011. English abstract.

51. Iwakuma T, Matsumoto A, Nakamura N. Hemifacial spasm: comparison of three different operative procedures in 110 patients. *J Neurosurg.* 1982;57:753-756.

52. Jannetta PJ. Arterial compression of the trigeminal nerve at the pons in patients with trigeminal neuralgia. *J Neurosurg.* 1967;26(suppl):159-162.

53. Jannetta PJ. Microsurgical exploration and decompression of the facial nerve in hemifacial spasm. *Curr Top Surg Res.* 1970;2:217-220.

54. Jannetta PJ. Neurovascular cross-compression in patients with hyperactive dysfunction symptoms of the eighth cranial nerve. *Surg Forum.* 1975;26:167-169.

55. Jannetta PJ. Observations on the etiology of trigeminal neuralgia, hemifacial spasm, acoustic nerve dysfunction, and glossopharyngeal neuralgia: definitive microsurgical treatment and results in 117 patients. *Neurochirurgia (Stutt).* 1977;20:145-154.

56. Jannetta PJ. Neurovascular compression in cranial nerve and systemic disease. *Ann Surg.* 1980;192:518-524.

57. Jannetta PJ. Vascular decompression in trigeminal neuralgia.In: Samii M, Jannetta PJ, eds. *The Cranial Nerves: Anatomy, Pathology, Pathophysiology, Diagnosis, Treatment.* New York, NY: Springer-Verlag; 1981:331-340.

58. Jannetta PJ. Hemifacial spasm. In: Samii M, Jannetta PJ, eds. *The Cranial Nerves: Anatomy, Pathology, Pathophysiology, Diagnosis, Treatment.* New York, NY: Springer-Verlag; 1981:484-493.

59. Jannetta PJ. Hemifacial spasm caused by a venule: case report. *Neurosurgery.* 1984;14:89-92.

60. Jannetta PJ. Microvascular decompression of the cochlear nerve as treatment of tinnitus. *Proceedings of III International Tinnitus Seminar.* 1987:348-352.

61. Jannetta PJ. Treatment of trigeminal neuralgia by micro-operative decompression. In: Youmans JR, ed. *Neurological Surgery: A Comprehensive Reference Guide to the Diagnosis and Management of Neurosurgical Problems.* 3rd ed. Philadelphia, Pa: WB Saunders Co; 1990:3928-3942.

62. Jannetta PJ. Cranial rhizopathies. In: Youmans JR, ed. *Neurological Surgery: A Comprehensive Reference Guide to the Diagnosis and Management of Neurosurgical Problems.* 3rd ed. Philadelphia, Pa: WB Saunders Co; 1990:4169-4182.

63. Jannetta PJ, Abbasy M, Maroon JC, et al. Etiology and definitive microsurgical treatment of hemifacial spasm: operative technique and results in 47 patients. *J Neurosurg.* 1977;47:321-328.

64. Jannetta PJ, Hackett E, Ruby JR. Electromyographic and electron microscopic correlates in hemifacial spasm treated by microsurgical relief of neurovascular compression. *Surg Forum.* 1970;21:449-451.

65. Jannetta PJ, Møller MB, Møller AR. Disabling positional vertigo. *N Engl J Med.* 1984;310:1700-1705.

66. Jastreboff PJ. Phantom auditory perception (tinnitus): mechanisms of generation and perception. *Neurosci Res.* 1990;8:221-254.

67. Katusic S, Beard CM, Bergstralh E, et al. Incidence and clinical features of trigeminal neuralgia, Rochester, Minnesota 1945-1984. *Ann Neurol.* 1990;27:89-95.

68. Kaufmann MD. Masticatory spasm in facial hemiatrophy. *Ann Neurol.* 1980;7:585-587.

69. Kerr FWL. Pathology of trigeminal neuralgia: light and electron microscopic observations. *J Neurosurg.* 1967;26:151-156.

70. Kerr FWL, Miller RH. The pathology of trigeminal neuralgia: electron microscopic studies. *Arch Neurol.* 1966;15:308-319.

71. Kim P, Fukushima T. Observations on synkinesis in patients with hemifacial spasm: effect of microvascular decompression and etiologic considerations. *J Neurosurg.* 1984;60:821-827.

72. Kimura J. Clinical uses of the electrically elicited blink reflex. In: Desmedt JE, eds. *Motor Control Mechanisms in Health and Disease.* New York, NY: Raven Press; 1983:773-786.

73. Klun B, Prestor B. Microvascular relations of the trigeminal nerve: an anatomical study. *Neurosurgery.* 1986;19:535-539.

74. Kolluri S, Heros RC. Microvascular decompression for trigeminal neuralgia: a five-year follow-up study. *Surg Neurol.* 1984;22:235-240.

75. Kommerell G, Mehdorn E, Ketelsen UP, et al. Oculomotor palsy with cyclic spasms: electromyographic and electron microscopic evidence of chronic peripheral neuronal involvement. *Neuro-Ophthalmol (Amsterdam).* 1988;8:9-21.

76. Kondo A, Ishikawa J, Yamasaki Y, et al. Microvascular decompression of cranial nerves, particularly of the 7th cranial nerve. *Neurol Med Chir (Tokyo).* 1980;20:739-751.

77. Kraft SP, Lang AE. Cranial dystonia, blepharospasm and hemifacial spasm: clinical features and treatment, including the use of botulinum toxin. *Can Med Assoc J.* 1988;139:837-844.

78. Lang J. Uber Baa, Lange and Ge fassbeziehungen der "zentralen" and "peripheren" strechen der intrazisternalen Hirnnerreno. *Zentralbl Neurochir.* 1982;43:217-256.

79. Lang J. *Clinical Anatomy of the Head: Neurocranium, Orbit, and Craniocervical Regions.* New York, NY: Springer-Verlag; 1983.

80. Loeser JD. Tic douloureux and atypical face pain. In: Wall PD, Melzack R, eds. *Textbook of Pain.* New York, NY: Churchill Livingstone; 1984:426-434.

81. Loeser JD. Long term efficacy of microvascular decompression in trigeminal neuralgia. *J Neurosurg.* 1988;69:35-38.

82. Lunsford LD, Apfelbaum RI. Choice of surgical therapeutic modalities for treatment of trigeminal neuralgia: microvascular decompression, percutaneous retrogasserian thermal, or glycerol rhizotomy. *Clin Neurosurg.* 1985;32:319-333.

83. Magun R, Esslen E. Electromyographic study of reinnervated muscles and hemifacial spasm. *Am J Phys Med.* 1959;38:79-86.

84. Maroon JC. Hemifacial spasm: a vascular cause. *Arch Neurol.* 1978;35:481-483.

85. Matsushima T, Inoue T, Fukui M. Arteries in contact with the cisternal portion of the facial nerve in autopsy cases: microsurgical anatomy for neurovascular decompression surgery for hemifacial spasm. *Surg Neurol.* 1990;34:87-93.

86. Møller AR. Pathophysiology of tinnitus. *Ann Otol Rhinol Laryngol.* 1984;93:39-44.

87. Møller AR. Hemifacial spasm: ephaptic transmission or hyperexcitability of the facial motor nucleus? *Exp Neurol.* 1987;98:110-119.

88. Møller AR. *Evoked Potentials in Intraoperative Monitoring.* Baltimore, Md: Williams and Wilkins; 1988.

89. Møller AR. Views on microvascular decompression. *J Neurosurg.* 1989;71:459-460. Letter.

90. Møller AR. The cranial nerve vascular compression syndrome, I: a review of treatment. *Acta Neurochir (Wien).* 1991;113:18-23.

91. Møller AR. The cranial nerve vascular compression syndrome, II: a review of pathophysiology. *Acta Neurochir (Wien).* 1991;113:24-30.

92. Møller AR. Interaction between the blink reflex and the abnormal muscle response in patients with hemifacial spasm: results of intraoperative recordings. *J Neurol Sci.* 1991;101:114-123.

93. Møller AR. Central processes in tinnitus. *Proceedings of IV International Tinnitus Seminar.* 1992, In Press.

94. Møller AR, Jannetta PJ. On the origin of synkinesis in hemifacial spasm: results of intracranial recordings. *J Neurosurg.* 1984;61:569-576.

95. Møller AR, Jannetta PJ. Hemifacial spasm: results of electrophysiologic recording during microvascular decompression operations. *Neurology.* 1985;35:969-974.

96. Møller AR, Jannetta PJ. Microvascular decompression in hemifacial spasm: intraoperative electrophysiological observations. *Neurosurgery.* 1985;16:612-618.

97. Møller AR, Jannetta PJ. Synkinesis in hemifacial spasm: results of recording intracranially from the facial nerve. *Experientia.* 1985;41:415-417.

98. Møller AR, Jannetta PJ. Blink reflex in patients with hemifacial spasm: observations during microvascular decompression operations. *J Neurol Sci.* 1986;72:171-182.

99. Møller AR, Jannetta PJ. Physiological abnormalities in hemifacial spasm studied during microvascular decompression operations. *Exp Neurol.* 1986;93:584-600.

100. Møller AR, Jannetta PJ. Monitoring facial EMG responses during microvascular decompression operations for hemifacial spasm. *J Neurosurg.* 1987;66:681-685.

101. Møller AR, Møller MB, Jannetta PJ, et al. Compound action potentials recorded from the exposed eighth nerve in patients with intractable tinnitus. *Laryngoscope.* 1992;102:187-197.

102. Møller AR, Sen CN. Recordings from the facial nucleus in the rat: signs of abnormal facial muscle response. *Exp Brain Res.* 1990;81:18-24.

103. Møller MB. Vascular compression of the eighth nerve as cause of tinnitus. *Proceedings of III International Tinnitus Seminar.* 1987:340-347.

104. Møller MB. Results of microvascular decompression of the eighth nerve as treatment for disabling positional vertigo. *Ann Otol Rhinol Laryngol.* 1990;99:724-729.

105. Møller MB. Disabling positional vertigo. In: Myers EN, Bluestone CD, Brackmann DE, Krause CJ, eds. *Advances in Otolaryngology—Head and Neck Surgery,* Chicago, Ill: Mosby Year Book Inc: 1990; 4:81-106.

106. Møller MB, Møller AR. Audiometric abnormalities in hemifacial spasm. *Audiology.* 1985;24:396-405.

107. Møller MB, Møller AR. Vascular compression syndrome of the eighth nerve: clinical correlations and surgical findings. *Neurologic Clinics.* 1990;8: 421-439.

108. Møller MB, Møller AR, Jannetta PJ, et al. Diagnosis and surgical treatment of disabling positional vertigo. *J Neurosurg.* 1986;64:21-28.

109. Nagata K, Matsui T, Joshita H, et al. Surgical treatment of spasmodic torticollis: effectiveness of microvascular decompression. *No To Shinkei.* 1989; 41:97-102. English abstract.

110. Nakai O, Itagaki S, Saito S. Electromyographic analysis of spasmodic torticollis. In: Program and abstracts of the 10th meeting of the World Society for Stereotactic and Functional Neurosurgery. Abstract.

111. Nakashima K, Thompson PD, Rothwell JC, et al. An exteroceptive reflex in the sternocleidomastoid muscle produced by electrical stimulation of the supraorbital nerve in normal subjects and patients with spasmodic torticollis. *Neurology.* 1989;39: 1354-1358.

112. Nielsen VK. Pathophysiology of hemifacial spasm, I: ephaptic transmission and ectopic excitation. *Neurology.* 1984;34:418-426.

113. Nielsen VK. Pathophysiology of hemifacial spasm, II: lateral spread of the supraorbital nerve reflex. *Neurology.* 1984;34:427-431.

114. Nielsen VK, Jannetta PJ. Pathophysiology of hemifacial spasm, III: effects of facial nerve decompression. *Neurology.* 1984;34:891-897.

115. Odkvist LM, Thell J, von Essen C. Vestibulo-oculomotor disturbances in trigeminal neuralgia and hemifacial spasm. *Acta Otolaryngol (Stockh).* 1988;105:570-575.

116. Ouaknine GE. Microsurgical anatomy of the arterial loops in the ponto-cerebellar angle and the internal acoustic meatus. In: Samii M, Jannetta PJ, eds. *The Cranial Nerves: Anatomy, Pathology, Pathophysiology, Diagnosis, Treatment.* New York, NY: Springer-Verlag; 1981:378-390.

117. Perkin GD, Illingworth RD. The association of hemifacial spasm and facial pain. *J Neurol Neurosurg Psychiatry.* 1989;52:663-665.

118. Podivinský F. Torticollis. In: Vinken PJ, Bruyn GW, eds. *Handbook of Clinical Neurology: Diseases of the Basal Ganglia.* New York: North Holland Publishing Co; 1968;6:567-603.

119. Pollack IF, Jannetta PJ, Bissonette DJ. Bilateral trigeminal neuralgia: a 14-year experience with microvascular decompression. *J Neurosurg.* 1988; 68:559-565.

120. Ravits J, Hallert M. Pathophysiology of hemifacial spasm: localization of the lesion in hemifacial spasm. *Neurology.* 1986;36:591. Letter.

121. Roth G, Magistris MR, Pinelli P, et al. Cryptogenic hemifacial spasm: a neurophysiological study. *Electromyogr Clin Neurophysiol.* 1990;30:361-370.

122. Ruby JR, Jannetta PJ. Hemifacial spasm: ultrastructural changes in the facial nerve induced by neurovascular compression. *Surg Neurol.* 1975;4:369-370.

123. Saito S, Itagaki S, Nakai O. Neurophysiological study on hemifacial spasm: the abnormality and origin of the electromyographic response to stimulation of the facial nerve. *No To Shinkei.* 1990; 42:621-627. English abstract.

124. Samii M. Surgical treatment of the hemifacial spasm. In: Samii M, Jannetta PJ, eds. *The Cranial Nerves: Anatomy, Pathology, Pathophysiology, Diagnosis, Treatment.* New York, NY: Springer-Verlag; 1981:502-504.

125. Sanders DB. Ephaptic transmission in hemifacial spasm: a single-fiber EMG study. *Muscle Nerve.* 1989;12:690-694.

126. Sandyk R, Gillman MA. Baclofen in hemifacial spasm. *Int J Neuroscience.* 1987;33:261-264.

127. Schwaber M, Hall JW. Cochleovestibular nerve compression syndrome, I. Clinical features and audiovestibular findings. *Laryngoscope.* 1992; 102:1020-1029.

128. Sen CN, Møller AR. Signs of hemifacial spasm created by chronic periodic stimulation of the facial nerve in the rat. *Exp Neurol.* 1987;98:336-349.

129. Shima F, Fukui M, Matsuhara T, et al. Spasmodic torticollis caused by vascular compression of the spinal accessory root. *Surg Neurol.* 1986;26: 431-434.

130. Skinner HA. Some histologic features of the cranial nerves. *Arch Neurol Psychiatry.* 1931;25:356-372.

131. Sunderland S. Neurovascular relations and anomalies at the base of the brain. *J Neurol Neurosurg Psychiatry.* 1948;11:243-257.

132. Sunderland S. Cranial nerve injury: structural and pathophysiological considerations and a classification of nerve injury. In: Samii M, Jannetta PJ, eds. *The Cranial Nerves: Anatomy, Pathology, Pathophysiology, Diagnosis, Treatment.* New York, NY: Springer-Verlag; 1981:16-23.

133. Sweet WH. Percutaneous methods for the treatment of trigeminal neuralgia and other faciocephalic pain: comparison with microvascular decompression. *Semin Neurol.* 1988;8:272-279.

134. Taarnhøj P. Decompression of the trigeminal root and the posterior part of the ganglion as treatment in trigeminal neuralgia: preliminary communication. *J Neurosurg.* 1952;9:288-290.

135. Tanaka T, Yu H, Kitai ST. Trigeminal and spinal inputs to the facial nucleus. *Brain Res.* 1971;33: 504-508.

136. Tarlov IM. Structure of a nerve root: nature of the junction between the central and peripheral nervous system. *Arch Neurol Psychitry.* 1937;37: 556-583.

137. Terrence CF, Sax M, Fromm GH, et al. Effect of baclofen enantiomorphs on the spinal trigeminal nucleus and steric similarities of carbamazepine. *Pharmacology.* 1983;27:85-94.

138. Thompson PD, Carroll WM. Hemimasticatory spasm— a peripheral paroxysmal cranial neuropathy? *J Neurol Neurosurg Psychiatry.* 1983;46:274-276.

139. Valls-Sole J, Tolosa ES. Blink reflex excitability cycle in hemifacial spasm. *Neurology.* 1989;39: 1061-1066.

140. Wada JA. *Kindling 2.* New York: Raven Press; 1981.

141. Wall PD. The presence of ineffective synapses and the circumstances which unmask them. *Philos Trans R Soc Lond (Biol).* 1977;278:361-372.

142. Wartenberg R. Associated movements in oculomotor and facial muscles. *Arch Neurol Psychiatry.* 1946;55:439-488.

143. Wartenberg R. *Hemifacial Spasm: A Clinical and Pathophysiological Study.* New York: University

Park Press; 1952.

144. White JC, Sweet WH. Facial and cephalic neuralgies: Trigeminal neuralgia (tic douloureux), trifacial neuralgia. In: White JC, Sweet WH, eds. *Pain, Its Mechanisms and Neurological Control.* Springfield, Illinois: Charles C. Thomas; 1955:433-493.

145. Wilkins RH. Hemifacial spasm: treatment by microvascular decompression of the facial nerve at the pons. *South Med J.* 1981;74:1471-1474.

146. Wilkins RH. Hemifacial spasm: a review. *Surg Neurol.* 1991;36:251-277.

147. Williams HL, Lambert EH, Woltman HW. The problem of synkinesis and contracture in cases of hemifacial spasm and Bell's palsy. *Ann Otol Rhinol Laryngol.* 1952;61:850-870.

148. Woltman HW, Williams HL, Lambert EH. An attempt to relieve hemifacial spasm by neurolysis of the facial nerves: a report of 2 cases of hemifacial spasm with reflections on the nature of the spasm, the contracture and mass movement. *Mayo Clin Proc.* 1951;26:236-240.

149. Yeh HS, Tew JM Jr. Tic convulsif, the combination of geniculate neuralgia and hemifacial spasm relieved by vascular decompression. *Neurology.* 1984;34: 682-684.

CHAPTER 3

The Physiology and Pathophysiology of Posterior Fossa Cranial Nerve Dysfunction Syndromes: Nonmicrovascular Perspective

C.B.T. Adams, MChir, FRCS

The author performs microvascular decompression (MVD) for hemifacial spasm because I believe this is the best operative procedure available for this condition.[23] About 80% to 85% of patients obtain good, long-term relief whether the author does or doesn't find a vessel adjacent to the nerve. However, usually the author does find a vessel; but the question remaining is: Does this mean such vessels *cause* hemifacial spasm?[7] At one time, neurosurgeons thought that port-wine stains in the scalp of the occipital region were associated with posterior fossa tumors. But, of course, the only time neurosurgeons shaved the scalp in this region was when they were about to operate on such a tumor! Are we in danger of the same mistake when it comes to the hypothesis of microvascular compression and posterior fossa cranial nerve dysfunction syndromes?[24]

Many neurosurgeons believe that MVD works and moreover is satisfying, even enjoyable, to perform. Certainly it does work, but how often? Is it the best treatment, and could there be better and safer methods?

Before considering the hypothesis of microvascular compression, I wish to state three facts. First, posterior fossa tumors can cause trigeminal neuralgia and hemifacial spasm. So, indeed, can some brain stem disorders; i.e. multiple sclerosis can cause classical (and sometimes nonclassical) trigeminal neuralgia, while brain stem gliomas can cause typical

(and sometimes atypical) hemifacial spasm. Second, I am not suggesting that vessels do not groove nerves—they do. Finally, I restate that I do carry out MVD for hemifacial spasm, although it is perhaps more correct to describe the procedure I do as a "wrapping" of the facial (VII) nerve adjacent to the brain stem.

The Concept of Microvascular Compression

Walter Dandy[20] first proposed that trigeminal neuralgia is caused by the nerve being compressed and distorted by the superior cerebellar artery at its point of entry into the pons. Maroon[47] noted that Schultze published an autopsy report of a patient with typical hemifacial spasm caused by a vertebral artery aneurysm compressing the facial nerve. In 1944, Campbell and Keedy[17] suggested that vascular compression in the posterior fossa was the basis of hemifacial spasm. In the 1950s and 1960s, Gardner and Miklos[27,28] advocated and extended this theory. Maroon et al[46,47] reviewed the vascular causes of hemifacial spasm and described a patient with a 6-year history of hemifacial spasm in whom a saccular aneurysm of the posterior inferior cerebellar artery was found compressing the facial nerve. In a series of papers published from 1976 on, Jannetta[33-35] has elaborated on the concept of microvascular compression. He stated that trigeminal neuralgia and hemifacial spasm are due to pulsatile compression by arteries at the root entry/exit zone (REZ) of the appropriate cranial nerve.[34,41] This zone was defined as a "junctional area between central and peripheral myelin." According to Jannetta,[35] this junctional area defines the peripheral boundary of the REZ and measures from 0.5-1 cm in length in the trigeminal (V), facial, and glossopharyngeal (IX) nerves. Møller et al,[54] stated that this area extends along the intracranial length of the vestibulocochlear (VIII) nerve. Furthermore, Janetta stressed that microvascular compression can occur only proximal to this zone, i.e. where the nerve is covered by central myelin where it is particularly susceptible to pulsatile or crossed compression; microvascular compression cannot occur peripheral to the REZ where the axons are surrounded by Schwann cells. He proposed that microvascular compression arises by the brain sagging with age, thus bringing vessels in contact with the REZ of cranial nerves and so producing vascular compression.[36] The elongation of atherosclerotic arteries accentuates this process. The corollary is that if such vessels are surgically displaced from the REZ, then the symptoms disappear. This procedure is called MVD.

Over the years, the concept has been widened in two ways.[33] First, veins, not just arteries, may cause pulsatile or cross-compression and distortion of the REZ. Presumably, veins are not subject to atherosclerotic elongation as are arteries. Although subcutaneous veins do seem to be more tortuous in the elderly, I am not aware of any such study demonstrating increasing tortuosity of intracranial veins with age. I have not noticed increasing tortuosity of intracranial veins with age during surgery and, if this is correct, then the process of venous compression depends wholly on brain sagging. Second, this mechanism is invoked as the cause of not only trigeminal neuralgia and hemifacial spasm but also glossopharyngeal neuralgia, spasmodic torticollis, disorders of the vestibulocochlear nerve function (such as tinnitus, disabling positional vertigo, and Meniere's disease), and essential hypertension.[35] These conditions

generally can be called cranial nerve dysfunction syndromes.

Mracek[56] has described five patients with trigeminal neuralgia in whom an elongated loop of the posterior inferior cerebellar artery was found to press on the descending tract of the trigeminal nerve. This variation is not in accordance with Jannetta's definition, as the REZ is not involved.

Acceptance of the REZ theory has been almost universal in the neurosurgical literature. I have looked in vain for photographs of this area in the various articles reporting microvascular compression. Lang[41] provides a diagram of the cranial nerves to show those portions lined by central glial cells, i.e. oligodendroglia as opposed to Schwann cells. All cranial nerves have such a zone: the olfactory (I) and optic (II) nerves are composed entirely of central glial cells and so is nerve VII as far as the internal auditory meatus. Jannetta[33] also described the appearances using the dissecting microscope, stating: "We found that the major sensory [trigeminal] root fibers coalesce into a soft rather gelatinous mass about 5 mm in diameter before entering the pons. This mass has a thin tough outer layer and is the 'fibrous cone' region of the portio major as described by Dandy . . . ."

Williams and Warwick,[68] in *Gray's Anatomy,* described this zone as follows:

> . . . crossing the transitional zone between the central and peripheral nervous system the sections of axons that comprise a nerve root are enclosed within a short glial segment lying close to the surface of the spinal cord or brain stem. In man the zone lies more peripherally in the sensory nerves than in motor nerves; in both cases the apex of the transitional region has been described as the "glial dome" with its convexity directed toward the periphery. Electron microscopy has shown that the centre of a dome consists of fibres showing typical central organization surrounded by an outer mantle of astrocytes. From this mantle numerous processes, the glial fringe, project into the endoneurial compartment of a peripheral nerve and inter-digitate with Schwann cells.

The author has personally looked at sections through cranial nerves and found that

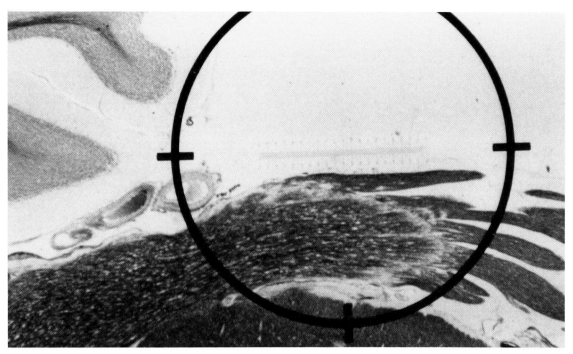

Figure 1. Photomicrograph of a section through the trigeminal sensory root showing the REZ, defined as the junction of central and peripheral myelin. A scale of 2 mm in length is superimposed to show that the REZ is no more than 3 mm in length. Note the 0.8-mm vessels adjacent to the REZ. The patient did not have trigeminal neuralgia in life.

this REZ is apparent. Staining beautifully differentiates the axon surrounded by central myelin as opposed to peripheral (Schwann cell) myelin. Figure 1 shows how the glial dome invades the peripheral nerve, reminiscent of the sea extending into an estuary as the tide comes in. There are two important points. First, this zone is only 1-3 mm in length and, as *Gray's Anatomy* indicates, it is longer in sensory nerves than in motor nerves.[68] Second, this zone can be defined only microscopically and cannot be seen by the surgeon. Thus, if microvascular compression only occurs proximal to the REZ, then such pathologic vascular compression can only exist within, at most, 3 mm of the brain stem. Those authors who state that they have seen vessels causing microvascular compression proximal to the REZ do not perhaps appreciate how short this segment is: It measures closer to 1 mm than to 1 cm.

In summary, the concept of microvascular compression is that the cranial nerves are brought into contact with arteries or veins at the REZ, which is an area of particular vulnerability, and this produces various clinical syndromes or dysfunctions of these cranial nerves by way of pulsatile or, perhaps in the case of veins, nonpulsatile compression of the cranial nerve. Brain sagging, because of atrophy, allows the cranial nerve to "drop" onto the vessels, although the increased length and tortuosity of atherosclerotic arteries aids this process.

Both mechanisms, brain atrophy and atherosclerosis of the arteries, are essentially symmetrical processes that become more severe with increasing age. Thus, if microvascular compression was the cause of these various cranial nerve dysfunction syndromes, then one would expect:

1. A high incidence of *bilateral* cranial nerve dysfunction because the underlying mechanism is symmetrical;

2. A high incidence of various cranial nerve dysfunction syndromes occurring together because if the underlying

mechanism exists for one cranial nerve it should do so for others;

3. A high incidence of cranial nerve dysfunction syndromes with senile dementia or severe atherosclerotic vascular disease; and

4. An increasing incidence of onset of cranial nerve dysfunction syndromes with each increasing decade of life.

However, the facts relating trigeminal neuralgia, hemifacial spasm, and glossopharyngeal neuralgia do not accord with these predictions. These conditions are extremely *unilateral*, only very rarely occurring in combination, and there is no evidence that cranial nerve dysfunction syndromes occur more frequently in patients with cerebral atrophy, generalized vascular disease, or with increasing age.

The Vessels

Obviously, the concept of microvascular compression depends crucially on the relationship of the vessels—arteries and veins—to the cranial nerves. The following aspects must be considered:

1. The definition of "pathologic vessels";
2. The incidence of cranial nerve dysfunction syndromes with no vessel found compressing the nerve; and
3. The incidence of vascular compression without a cranial nerve dysfunction syndrome being present.

The Definition of a Pathologic Vessel

One major difficulty facing observers of microvascular compression is the classification of vascular compression of the nerve. Jannetta[34] uses either the term *cross-compression* or *pulsatile compression* to denote the essential pathologic process. It is not clear whether these are interchangeable. Most surgeons have no difficulty recognizing grooving of the nerve by an artery, which, when displaced from the nerve, leaves a permanent groove in the nerve. Whether this is causally

significant is debatable, but certainly the nerve is compressed by the vessel if grooved in this way. When the optic nerve or chiasm is grooved by the internal carotid or the anterior cerebral artery, there is not necessarily any detectable loss of function. However, arteries often are found merely touching the nerve and when displaced leave no groove. Is this pathologic?

Presumably, in some patients with no arterial grooving or apposition, compressive veins are evoked as the pathologic mechanism.[34] Although some venous pulsation may be transmitted, as in the cerebrospinal fluid (CSF), surely veins do not pulsate sufficiently to cause pulsatile compression, although presumably cross-compression may be caused by veins. Jannetta[38] has stated that a 0.3 mm venule may cause cross-compression. There is no biomechanical data to support or refute such a statement, but it seems unlikely that such an elastic structure, the diameter of cotton thread, could seriously distort a nerve the diameter of the trigeminal sensory root. Moreover, Jannetta[33] claims that when patients are placed in the lateral decubitus position, vessels move 1-2 mm away from the nerve root and thus may not be seen to be in contact with the nerve at operation. Certainly rotating the operating table during such operations has not revealed any obvious movement of the vessels away from the individual nerve, either before or after the arachnoid has been opened and the CSF has been suctioned away. It seems tenous to say, when neither an artery nor a vein is found to be actually in contact with the nerve, that an artery is able to fall into contact with a nerve if the patient's position is moved and moreover that this contact (presumably the most delicate) is sufficient to cause cross-compression. Jannetta[35] has stated that ". . . REZ vascular compression is frequently subtle, and well-trained microsurgeons may not appreciate up to 30% of the abnormalities early on in their experience with these procedures." Of course, posterior fossa surgery does require experience, but it is hard to accept the implication in this statement: To be experienced and well trained, one needs to "see" these vessels, even 0.3 mm venules or vessels that are not actually touching the nerves but which might conceivably fall against the nerves with a change of posture.

Apfelbaum[12] has attempted to classify the degree of nerve compression. He divided his observations into "definite" arteries and veins and "possible" arteries and veins. Having analyzed his results, he carried out a partial root section for trigeminal neuralgia if he found only possible vessels, whereas he continued to perform MVD if he had found definite vessels.

Before completing this consideration of vessels, two further statements need examination.[35] First, veins having been coagulated and divided can recollateralize, causing recurrence of symptoms.[34] It is difficult to know exactly what is meant by "recollateralize"; is it really possible for a vein, having been coagulated and cut with scissors, to later redevelop or perhaps rejoin and recanalize? No laboratory evidence is given for this. Jannetta[34] states that "multiple vessels are commonly found." It already has been suggested that the underlying mechanisms of microvascular compression are bilateral and largely symmetric. It is remarkable if *multiple* pathologic vessels become bunched around a *single* cranial nerve on *one* side without affecting other cranial nerves on the same or opposite sides. No explanation has been offered for this. The fundamental problem remains about how to define nerve root compression: cross-compression, pulsatile compression, obvious grooving, touching without grooving, or not touching; the role of veins or even venules as well as more precise methods of measuring the position of these vessels in relation to the brain stem should be identified. To this end, there is a clear need for more precise clarification, classification, and correlation with or without clinical symptoms.

Another difficulty is defining not just the degree of compression of a cranial nerve by a vessel, but also the exact underlying site of compression. In one of my patients with hemifacial spasm, a vessel split the facial nerve just medial to the internal auditory meatus, well lateral to the REZ. Should this be considered pathologic? Presumably not; although most series, including my own, have included such vessels as causing vascular compression.

In summary, precise data should be recorded by surgeons claiming to find vascular compression. The degree and the exact site of compression should be recorded as well as the numbers of arteries, veins, or venules that are considered responsible. Furthermore, can veins recollateralize and can venules exert nerve root compression? How realistic is it to argue that vessels not actually touching a nerve can cause compression in other patient positions?

The Incidence of Cranial Nerve Dysfunction Syndrome with No Vessel Compressing the Nerve

Table 1 summarizes the findings in series of cranial nerve dysfunction syndromes and states the number of patients in whom no vascular compression was found. Morley[55] has stated: "it only requires one case in which a nerve is not touched by a vessel to discredit the hypothesis entirely." This may be too harsh a judgment, but clearly the proponents of microvascular compression need to provide an explanation for those patients in whom no vascular compression is found; it is not sufficient to evoke vessels that do not touch nerves but might, should the position of the patient change; nor is the implication of tiny venules convincing.

Bederson and Wilson,[14] in a series of 252 patients, found no vascular contact in 30 cases, but in 56 cases found vascular contact without grooving of the nerve. Thus, definite grooving was found in 66% of their patients with trigeminal neuralgia. Perhaps the only conclusion that can be drawn from these series is that there is a variation in incidence of vascular compression, which, no doubt, depends on the surgeon. These figures do not, I suspect, differentiate between vascular compression proximal or distal to the REZ, nor

TABLE 1
**Number of Patients with No Vascular Compression Found
During Microvascular Decompression Procedures**

Authors and Year	Condition	Cases*
Jannetta, 1980	Glossopharyngeal neuralgia	2/11
Auger et al, 1981	Hemifacial spasm	1/8
Kaye and Adams, 1981	Hemifacial spasm	4/16
Adams et al, 1982	Trigeminal neuralgia	51/57
Loeser and Chen, 1983	Hemifacial spasm	5/20
Apfelbaum, 1984	Trigeminal neuralgia	10/289
Zorman and Wilson, 1984	Trigeminal neuralgia	26/125
Burchiel et al, 1988	Trigeminal neuralgia	4/41
Bederson and Wilson, 1989	Trigeminal neuralgia	30/252

*Expressed as number of patients with no vascular compression found/total number of patients undergoing a microvascular decompression procedure in that series.

are we told in most series the degree of vascular contact—i.e. grooving—contact without grooving, or near contact that might conceivably cause contact with movement of the patient into another position. Without such a breakdown, the figures shown in Table 1 have little meaning.

The Incidence of Vascular Compression Without Cranial Nerve Dysfunction Syndrome Being Present

Observation reveals that vessels are seen in contact with nerve roots, both cranial and spinal. Jannetta refers to this but states that it is uncommon to find such vessels at the REZ; however, the 120 spinal nerve roots are ensheathed by vessels adjacent to their root entry or exit zones, yet symptoms are not described. Intracranially, most of the nerve roots are intimately in contact with arteries or veins.[2] The olfactory tract near the cribriform plate is surrounded by veins. The optic nerves or tracts are gripped by a series of arteries—the ophthalmic, internal carotid, and anterior cerebral arteries. The oculomotor (III) nerve has to pass between the superior cerebellar and posterior cerebral arteries as it leaves the midbrain, while the trochlear (IV) nerve often is intimately associated with veins and perforating arteries adjacent to the quadrigeminal plate. The abducens (VI) nerve may be in contact with the anterior inferior cerebellar artery or the internal auditory artery. Yet no microvascular compression syndrome has been described for these nerve roots. Neither hypoglossal nor hemipharyngeal spasm has yet been described as a result of compression of the hypoglossal or vagal nerves, respectively, by the vertebral artery or posterior inferior cerebellar artery. However, Møller[53] refers to the possibility of spastic dysphonia being caused by vascular compression of the vagus (X) nerve.

Sunderland[62] has studied the vascular relationships to the facial nerve and again makes the point that vascular contacts are common throughout its length, including the REZ, where such contact was found in 27 of 210 specimens.

Hardy and Rhoton[30] studied 50 trigeminal nerve roots and their vascular relationships. This was a most careful study and it is important to realize that none of these patients suffered trigeminal neuralgia in life. In that study, 60% of the nerves had vascular contacts and 20% had vascular contacts bilaterally. Often a few fascicles of the nerves were indented or distorted by the vessel. The authors also noted that "the site of vascular contact was commonly a few millimeters peripheral to the point of entry of the nerve into the pons [average 3.7 mm]." These findings are summarized in Table 2. In six cases, contact was at the point of entry of the root into the pons. Thus, this study showed that

TABLE 2
Trigeminal Nerve Roots and Their Vascular Relationships*

1. 25 cadavers, *none* having had trigeminal neuralgia in life
2. 50 trigeminal nerve roots examined
3. 50% of specimens with a vascular contact
4. Contact commonly a few millimeters peripheral to point of nerve entry into the pons (average 3.7 mm)
5. 20% of specimens with bilateral vascular contacts
6. Fascicles of nerve were often indented by the vessel

*Data from Hardy and Rhoton.[30]

in half of the nerves studied, there was vascular contact, and sometimes grooving, in *asymptomatic* persons. Because 25 patients contributed to the 50 nerves studied, on average each patient had a vessel in contact with either one or other trigeminal nerve. Furthermore, when these authors used the term *vascular contact,* they referred to arterial vascular contact only, ignoring veins and venules.

We can only conclude that it is unusual *not* to find vascular contact—arterial or venous—in asymptomatic patients at or near the REZ, depending on one's definition of the REZ. Hardy and Rhoton also saw bilateral vascular contact in 20% of their subjects.

Recently, Matsushima and colleagues[49] have carried out a most careful study of the cisternal facial nerve and the arteries in contact with it. These authors used the term *attaching point* to denote grooving of the nerve by an artery or mere contact of the nerve by an artery. Their findings are summarized in Table 3 and again it should be noted that only *arterial,* not venous, attaching points to the nerve were studied. Interestingly, the

authors conclude that "the results do aid in intraoperative orientation," referring to MVD for hemifacial spasm, yet they failed to draw perhaps the obvious conclusion from their careful work: If 97% of facial nerves have *arterial* attaching points (which when veins are considered, could easily increase to 100%) in patients who have *never* suffered hemifacial spasm, then such vascular contact may be irrelevant in the pathogenesis of hemifacial spasm! Indeed, these authors have shown that arterial contact normally is found in relation to the facial nerve; yet their belief in microvascular compression is so strong that the inevitable conclusion of their work has escaped them.

Given the symmetrical distribution of arteries in the head and the uniform nature of senile cerebral atrophy causing sagging of the brain, it is, of course, not surprising to find that at least 20% of cadavers have bilateral arterial-nerve contacts. If veins and venules are included, then this figure increases considerably. These facts also have to be reconciled to the strikingly unilateral incidence of trigeminal neuralgia and hemifacial spasm. If

TABLE 3
Arteries in Contact with Cisternal Facial Nerve*

1. 20 adult patients, *none* having had hemifacial spasm in life
2. 35 facial nerves examined
3. "Attaching points": Arterial attachment at root exit zone on 24/35 facial nerves (69%)
4. Only 1 nerve with *no* attaching point, i.e. 97% with *arterial* contacts
5. All except 1 patient with *bilateral* arterial "attaching points"
6. Up to 3 arterial contacts on some facial nerves

*Data from Matsushima et al.[49]

TABLE 4
Characteristics of
Trigeminal (V), Facial (VII), and Glossopharyngeal (IX) Nerves

Trigeminal Nerve	Facial Nerve	Glossopharyngeal Nerve
Motor root(s)	Motor root	Motor root to stylopharyngeal muscle
Sensory root	Nervus intermedius (sensory root)	Sensory root (to tonsillar fossa, tongue and pharynx)

these conditions are caused by vascular contact, then surely the frequency of these conditions occurring bilaterally should approximate the incidence of bilateral vascular contact. Most series of trigeminal neuralgia show that about 2% of patients develop bilateral trigeminal neuralgia, and if the opposite side is involved, this usually only occurs many years later.[20] Bilateral trigeminal neuralgia commencing simultaneously on both sides of the face is extremely rare. The same arguments hold for hemifacial spasm and glossopharyngeal neuralgia.

Summary

Careful studies in subjects without trigeminal neuralgia or hemifacial spasm have shown that the majority of unaffected people have vascular contacts and, moreover, a large percentage have bilateral vascular contacts. The concept of microvascular compression is incomplete without an explanation as to why such a high percentage of vascular contacts are found in asymptomatic patients; why cranial nerve dysfunction syndromes occur so unilaterally yet vascular contacts are so often found bilaterally, as indeed one would expect with a symmetrical distribution of the blood vessels and a symmetrical effect of brain sagging. Why also don't vascular contacts in relation to other cranial nerve and spinal roots fail to produce symptoms or syndromes?

Clinical Considerations

I now will consider whether the hypothesis of microvascular compression can be reconciled with the clinical features of trigeminal neuralgia, hemifacial spasm, and glossopharyngeal neuralgia. If the same pathologic process is the cause of each of these disorders, one should expect at least some common characteristics. The anatomy is again an appropriate starting point. Table 4 summarizes the anatomy of cranial nerves V, VII, and IX. Each nerve has a motor and sensory root. Table 5 highlights the salient features of the three disorders.

Jannetta et al[38,39] write: "patients with trigeminal neuralgia frequently have mild sensory loss" and, on another occasion, that signs of "vascular cross-compression of the trigeminal root include mild numbness and a slight decrease in corneal reflex." Jannetta[39] quotes three studies to support his view: Dandy,[20] Gardner,[27] and Lewy and Grant.[42] These authors do not, in fact, support Jannetta. Dandy[20] wrote that "the most delicate tests have uniformly failed to elicit any objective disturbance in the sensory or motor function of the trigeminal nerve involved in tic douloureux unless a tumor is the underlying cause." Gardner,[27] when talking generally of both trigeminal neuralgia and hemifacial spasm, stated that "although there seldom is demonstrable impairment of function of the nerve, each has been attributed to pathology of the nucleus." Gardner did not specifically say that he found impairment of trigeminal nerve function; certainly, he did not state that it was frequent. Lewy and Grant[42] began their article as follows: "It has been the general belief and part of the definition of 'neuralgia' that in major trigeminal neuralgia no objective sensory disturbance is present. This experience holds true as long as we use pin and cotton wool as means of examination." They found that the number and sensitivity of touch and pain points are reduced when tested with graduated hairs and thorns. This

TABLE 5
Summary of the Main Features of Trigeminal Neuralgia,
Hemifacial Spasm, and Glossopharyngeal Neuralgia

Feature	Trigeminal Neuralgia	Hemifacial Spasm	Glossopharyngeal Neuralgia
Nerve function (prior to any treatment)	No sensory loss ever found	Mild weakness of face common	No sensory loss ever found
Muscle spasm	Masseter/temporalis spasm not reported	Spasm always	Stylopharyngeal spasm not reported
Pain	Always: usually in second and third divisions	Neuralgia of nervus intermedius not reported (nor VIII nerve disorders)	Always
Remissions of symptoms	Almost always	Hardly ever	Common
Unilateral location	Almost always	Always	Always
Response to carbamazepine	Always initially	Never	Always initially
Effect of cutting or damaging nerve	Cure	Cure	Cure

work has not been substantiated. The late M.J. McArdle of the National Hospital for Nervous Diseases, Queens Square, London, claimed that he occasionally found a slight increase of 2-point discrimination during an actual attack of pain, but never between bouts (personal communication, 1969). Sensory testing during a bout of pain however, is unreliable. Thus, there is little, if any, support for the claim that there is sensory loss or reduction of corneal reflex in patients with idiopathic trigeminal neuralgia, irrespective of how long the condition has existed.

The reverse applies to hemifacial spasm where it is generally accepted that there is frequently a mild facial weakness, which becomes more marked the longer the condition persists. If both disorders are caused by nerve root cross-compression, then it is difficult to explain this discrepancy. All neurosurgeons know the effects of distortion of these nerves by an acoustic neuroma: The facial nerve is curiously resistant, with facial palsy occurring only late and then only with a large acoustic neuroma. Trigeminal sensory loss is an early feature and develops much earlier than facial weakness. The opposite is the case with trigeminal neuralgia and hemifacial spasm: Trigeminal sensory loss does not occur, whereas

facial weakness is seen early and progressively worsens. Yet distortion caused by an acoustic neuroma is undoubted and so one could question whether vessels do, in fact, produce trigeminal neuralgia and hemifacial spasm by distortion, as is claimed.

If hemifacial spasm is caused by microvascular compression, then one might expect to see similar spasm of the masseter and temporalis muscles with trigeminal neuralgia and also of the stylopharyngeal muscle with glossopharyngeal neuralgia. Yet one does not. One patient with hemimasticatory spasm, but without trigeminal neuralgia, has been reported.[68] One sees vessels adjacent to the motor REZ, but hemimasticatory spasm is extremely rare. I have published data showing that the first division of the trigeminal sensory root is always adjacent to the motor root and the third division occupies the opposite pole.[8] Partial root section confirms this anatomic arrangement (Figure 2). One often sees vessels passing between the motor and sensory roots, thereby affecting the motor root and the first division territory; whereas trigeminal neuralgia far more commonly affects the second and third divisions.

If trigeminal neuralgia and glossopharyngeal neuralgia are caused by microvascular

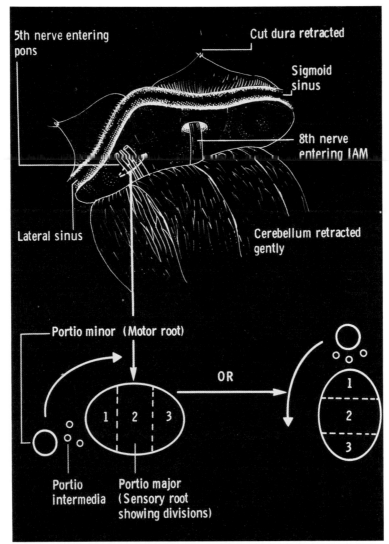

Figure 2. Diagram to illustrate the varying degree of rotation of the trigeminal roots as they enter the brain stem. The majority of sensory fibers from the third division of the trigeminal nerve maintain a constant relation to the part of the sensory root most removed from the motor root or roots.

compression, why does one not see neuralgia of the nervus intermedius with hemifacial spasm? This small nerve, the size of a thread of cotton, is presumably easily distorted or compressed, yet neuralgia of the nervus intermedius, although characteristic and extraordinarily painful, is rare.

Remissions of pain in trigeminal neuralgia are characteristic, and most doctors would hesitate to diagnose this condition in the absence of such remissions. That a patient characteristically has a remission is a fascinat-ing phenomena (although cruelly dashing the hopes of the patient upon recurrence), particularly when considering the pathogenesis. Why should the neuralgia suddenly "switch off" for weeks, months, or years and then return with ever-increasing frequency? Those who believe in microvascular compression are silent on this point. Do vessels suddenly leave the area of the trigeminal root? Are vessels able to move, and if they can, why are remissions so remarkably rare in hemifacial spasm? If there is a common mechanism, then surely one might expect remissions to be characteristic of hemifacial spasm, but remissions hardly ever occur in patients who are so afflicted.

The response to carbamazepine is a therapeutic test for trigeminal and glossopharyngeal neuralgia. Once again, most of us would hesitate to diagnose trigeminal neuralgia without the patient showing a positive response to carbamazepine. How does this work? Surely it affects the brain stem rather than altering vascular compression of the trigeminal sensory root. Again, if there is a similar pathogenesis, why doesn't carbamazepine produce relief of hemifacial spasm? It *never* does. Several further points of clinical relevance already have been mentioned, but are included here for completeness. All three conditions are extraordinarily unilateral in their expression, yet vascular contacts often are bilateral. Thus, one would not only expect a high incidence of bilateral trigeminal neuralgia, hemifacial spasm, and glossopharyngeal neuralgia, but one also would expect a high incidence of all three conditions occurring simultaneously. Surely the process of sagging cannot be confined to one small area of the posterior fossa. So why, if this concept is correct, do we not see all three conditions expressing themselves at once?

Summary

If trigeminal neuralgia and hemifacial spasm are both due to microvascular compression, then one might expect some similarity, clinically and therapeutically. This is clearly not so. Furthermore, the response of cranial nerves V and VII to overt compression, such as is caused by an acoustic neuroma, is opposite to that seen in trigeminal neuralgia and hemifacial spasm. Also, one might expect spasm of the temporalis or masseter muscle with trigeminal neuralgia or neuralgia of the nervus intermedius with hemifacial spasm; however these do not occur. Such clinical considerations do not lend any support for microvascular compression. The only common feature is that cutting or damaging the relevant cranial nerves eliminates the condition. Surely, no one would argue that the

cause of trigeminal neuralgia, hemifacial spasm, or glossopharyngeal neuralgia can be surmised from this.

The Results of Microvascular Decompression

The results of treatment by MVD require critical evaluation. They shed light on the validity of the concept of microvascular compression. The MVD operation depends on displacing or separating the compressing artery away from the nerve. If a compressing vein is found, then this is coagulated and cut, although one supposes that large veins might be treated as if they are arteries and displaced. Clearly, venous compression is much simpler to treat than arterial compression. One can easily ensure complete section and excision of the vein. Authors report differing results of MVD according to arterial or venous compression. For instance, Zorman and Wilson[69] show no difference, while Piatt and Wilkins,[60] Burchiel et al,[16] and Apfelbaum[12] all found inferior results after MVD for venous compression compared with those for arterial compression.

Therefore, if the concept of microvascular compression is correct, the results for venous vascular compression should surely be excellent. In other words, one should expect immediate and complete relief of pain without recurrence. Yet the previously mentioned authors found different results. Moreover, the proposal that veins can recollateralize is put forward to explain the recurrence of symptoms after sectioning a compressing vein. Even if this occurs, it would strongly suggest that sectioning of such a vein does not produce the dramatic result one might expect.

Few large series including long-term followup are available. One article[36] mentions complete follow-up results in 274 patients, with 32 patients having either no relief of pain or recurrent pain; however, the followup periods are not given. Such information is necessary if one is to evaluate any treatment of a condition in which there may be long periods of spontaneous remission. Apfelbaum[12]

TABLE 6
Results of Trigeminal Neuralgia Surgery*

Author and Year	Type of Operation	Initial Failure	Recurrent Pain	Pain- Free	Follow-up Period
Taarnhøj, 1961[65]	Manipulation	2%	34%	60%	78
Gardner and Miklos, 1959[28]	Manipulation	Total for both groups: 33%		67%	52.5
Ferguson et al, 1981[24]	MVD	12%	17%	71%	28
Apfelbaum, 1984[12]	MVD	5.8% (16/273)	36.2% (93/257)	63.8% (164/257)	55
Burchiel et al, 1988[16]	MVD		48% (31% major) (17% minor)	52%	102
Lichtor and Mullan, 1990[43]	Percutaneous Balloon Compression (i) 100 pts (ii) 61 pts	0% 0%	28% 20%	72% 80%	60 (12-120) 60 months +
Adams et al, 1982[8]	Selective Partial Rhizotomy	0%	12.5%	87.5%	60 months +

*MVD = Microvascular decompression. Percentages are of each total series.

reported his carefully studied series in which 289 patients underwent MVD for trigeminal neuralgia; 10 patients had tumors and 3 had arteriovenous malformations. Three patients died postoperatively. Of the remaining 273 patients, 5.8% failed to obtain complete relief initially after the operation. Of the 257 patients followed for an average of 55 months, 63.8% continued to be free of pain and 36.2% had recurrent pain varying from mild to severe. Ferguson et al[24] reported in their series of MVD for trigeminal neuralgia that 12% of the patients failed to obtain relief immediately after surgery and a further 17% developed recurrent pain; 71% remained pain-free over a 28-month followup period. The results of MVD for trigeminal neuralgia can be summarized, therefore, as follows: One-third of the patients either failed to obtain initial relief or developed recurrent pain, while two-thirds obtained longer-term relief of pain; however, the follow-up period is relatively short for both of these series. The series of Burchiel et al[16] provides a longer follow-up, but also shows a lower success rate for MVD.

Taarnhøj's series[65] is important. In 1961, he published his results of decompression of the nerve root. He made no effort to displace vessels, but he merely exposed the root and stressed the importance of manipulating the nerve root "by running a nerve hook along the root." His results and those of others are summarized in Table 6. Apparently, his results are similar to those achieved with MVD. Taarnhøj was not alone in performing manipulation of the trigeminal root. Gardner and Miklos[28] followed 100 patients for 3.25-5.50 years after decompression of the sensory root. Sixty-seven patients were painfree "after recovery from anesthesia of the operation"; of the remaining 33, 8 had mild recurrence and 25 had either no initial relief or severe recurrent pain. Gardner and Miklos stated that "the critical part of the operation appears to be a neurolysis or manipulation of the sensory root at the point where it crosses the apex of the petrous bone."[28]

The long-term results of MVD also help to evaluate the concept of microvascular compression. If MVD does, indeed, treat the underlying cause, then one would expect a cure without a significant recurrence rate. Burchiel et al[16] have published the longest follow-up after MVD for trigeminal neuralgia (average 8.5 years). They recorded a 5%

TABLE 7
Results of Hemifacial Spasm Surgery*

Operative Result	Loeser and Chen 1983	World Literature	Auger et al 1981	Adams and Kaye 1983
Number of cases	20		8	16
Good/excellent	17	84%	—	14
Recurrence	5	4%	1	—
Type of operation	MVD		MVD	Wrapping nerve

*MVD = microvascular decompression.

annual recurrence rate (3.5% major, 1.5% minor) and concluded that "MVD does not cure' trigeminal neuralgia, but simply arrests it for a prolonged period. . . ." Bederson and Wilson[14] noted a 2% late recurrence rate per year and again made the point that MVD does not "cure all patients, even though recurrent vascular compression does not account for all recurrent trigeminal neuralgia."

The results of MVD for hemifacial spasm are summarized in Table 7. Loeser and Chen[44] also provide an excellent overview of the world results. Remarkably, these results are similar, irrespective of the differing authors opinions as to the presence or absence of vascular compression. Approximately 75% to 90% of patients obtained good or excellent results, while 10% to 25% experienced recurrent spasm.

The treatment of glossopharyngeal neuralgia provides an interesting test of the surgeon's commitment to, and trust in, the concept of microvascular compression. Simple sectioning of the glossopharyngeal nerve and possibly the upper vagal rootlet provides excellent and permanent relief of pain. Janetta[34] has published results for MVD for glossopharyngeal neuralgia. Of 9 patients, 6 were painfree, while 2 experienced no relief or recurrent pain; 1 patient died. The absence of other reports in the literature suggests that other surgeons carry out nerve section rather than MVD. If surgeons who otherwise accept the concept of microvascular compression and who apparently carry out this procedure for trigeminal neuralgia and hemifacial spasm, but do not perform MVD for glossopharyngeal neuralgia, then this surely suggests a lack of conviction that the fundamental cause of glossopharyngeal neuralgia is

indeed vascular compression.

Jannetta and Møller have proposed that microvascular compression of the vestibulocochlear nerve is a cause of four conditions:[38,54] disabling positional vertigo, acoustic neuroma syndrome, Meniere's syndrome, and tinnitus. Unfortunately, it is extremely difficult to define and therefore diagnose the first two conditions, and the results were obtained in 13 of 42 patients with disabling positional vertigo and 2 of 5 with acoustic neuroma syndrome. MVD for Meniere's syndrome produced the best results by far: 5 of 6 patients so treated had excellent results, while MVD produced only 1 excellent result among 11 patients with tinnitus.

Møller et al[54] stated that previous experience in the treatment of patients with tinnitus by MVD has shown that it may take as long as 18-20 months for the symptoms to subside completely. This seems a remarkably long time and leads one to wonder how it is possible to be sure that the operative procedure is responsible for the improvement, particularly in view of the neurophysiologic observations of Møller[54] in which he observed immediate cessation of abnormal muscle response when the offending vessel was moved off the facial nerve during MVD for hemifacial spasm.

Tarlov[66] has pointed out the excellent results that can be obtained in Meniere's disease by vestibular nerve section; and it is generally recognized that auditory nerve section does not cure tinnitus. Thus, the results of MVD for nerve VIII disorders mirror those of nerve section, which suggest that microvascular compression is not an underlying mechanism in the production of these symptoms or syndromes.

Perhaps of even more significance are the results of Lichtor and Mullan[43] concerning percutaneous microcompression, which entails inflating a balloon inserted into the trigeminal ganglion. This technique is clearly designed to induce "controlled trauma" along similar lines to that of Gardner and Taarnhøj.[27,65] The results of percutaneous microcompression are extremely good and clearly better than those for MVD (Table 6).

Summary

The results of MVD for trigeminal neuralgia can be summarized as follows: First, MVD for venous compression generally is considered less effective than for arterial compression, yet removal of venous compression is technically easier and more complete because the relevant segment of vein can be excised. Second and most important, the results of MVD are no better than those of Gardner and Taarnhøj[27,66] who merely manipulated the sensory root at the petrous apex, and are clearly inferior to those of Lichtor and Mullan[43] using percutaneous microcompression. If microvascular compression was indeed the cause of trigeminal neuralgia, then one would expect the results to be far superior to mere nerve root manipulation and that a cure would occur if there was no recurrent vascular compression. That neither of these expectations are realized must cast grave doubts on the concept of microvascular compression. The results of MVD for nerve VIII disorders do not lend support for microvascular compression being the cause of these syndromes.

Complications of Microvascular Decompression

No procedure can be assessed purely on the basis of the results. If the results for one procedure were the same as for the other procedures, the incidence of complications presumably would determine which procedure should, in fact, be advised. Thus, it is appropriate to consider briefly the complications of MVD. Clearly, some procedures, such as partial root section, are associated with an inevitable loss of sensation in the face. Whether this should be considered a complication is debatable, for the patient should be counseled that he or she would be "swapping pain for some numbness." The advantage would be a reduction in the chance of recurrent trigeminal neuralgia in the future; as will be discussed later. Anesthesia dolorosa, as well as unpleasant dysesthesias, should be considered complications of the procedure as should other unexpected cranial nerve disorders, such as deafness and facial weakness. In this section, the complications of MVD for trigeminal neuralgia will be considered, for these have been more completely described than MVD for other cranial nerve dysfunction syndromes.

The exact incidence of complications for MVD is difficult to determine, for these tend to be under-reported. Hanakita and Kondo[29] described serious complications following MVD for trigeminal neuralgia and hemifacial spasm. Of 278 patients, 11 serious complications occurred, including 2 subsequent deaths, 4 hematomas, 2 cerebellar infarctions, 1 case of cerebellar swelling, and 2 patients who developed status epilepticus. Jannetta[35] reports 1 death, 4 cases of hematomas, 2 cerebellar infarctions, 3 cases of hearing loss, 2 cases of bacterial meningitis, and 6 patients with aseptic meningitis. In another publication, among 274 patients undergoing MVD, Marion and Jannetta[45] analyzed 222 patients undergoing MVD either with or without steroids. Nineteen patients developed CSF leakage, with a higher incidence if steroids were prescribed. Fritz and colleagues[26] studied 21 patients' hearing after MVD for trigeminal neuralgia; 2 patients (9.5%) developed cochlear hearing impairment, while 3 (14.3%) sustained middle ear deafness. Bederson and Wilson[14] noted that MVD was associated with a greater incidence of facial and cochlear nerve complications than partial root section. Persistent ipsilateral hearing loss occurred in 3% of the patients undergoing MVD and this incidence did not decrease with experience; this they ascribe to the "increased cerebellar retraction necessary for adequate decompression or it may be related to a vascular effect."

Sweet and Poletti[63] reported a confidential questionnaire concerning the complications of MVD for facial pain and this must be the most accurate assessment of the complications. One can do no better than to quote their conclusion from 49 departments: "from 24 services came accounts of permanently disabling sequelae or deaths in 29 cases. The 2 largest series were of 111 and circa 125 cases. The next largest series was of 50 cases. The 2 most discouraging series involved 3 technically competent distinguished neurosurgeons, who had 4 deaths in 60 patients, all in 'healthy' individuals, 3 in their 50s and 1 aged 31, all following smooth, uneventful operations. . . ." They conclude: "How to reduce the risk of microvascular decompression is not so obvious. . . ."

Summary

Clearly, MVD for trigeminal neuralgia is associated with mortality and morbidity. Although the risks are not great, they are greater than with other procedures. Unfortunately, death can occur after uneventful surgery. The complications seem mainly caused by two factors: first, the marked degree of retraction necessary to expose the REZ, and second, the manipulation and subsequent kinking of arteries or the sectioning of veins necessary for MVD. These complications, when considered in conjunction with the results of MVD in terms of pain relief, should give those surgeons who practice MVD for trigeminal neuralgia food for thought, especially when there are other equally (or more) effective and certainly safer procedures available. The evidence produced so far suggests that the concept of microvascular compression is unsustainable and, therefore, MVD does not treat the *cause* or provide a cure. Therefore, surgeons perhaps should be reluctant to advise their patients with trigeminal neuralgia to undergo MVD.

The Epidemiology of Trigeminal Neuralgia

Very little has, to my knowledge, been published on the epidemiology of cranial nerve dysfunction syndromes. One fascinating fact[5] was brought to my attention by colleagues in Africa. Trigeminal neuralgia is hardly ever seen in Africa. Yet, this is not the type of pain to be ignored and to go unreported there. On the other hand, hypertension is common and occurs early in life. So, it is inconceivable that Africans do not have "hypertensive" vessels compressing their cranial nerves. This is suggestive evidence that microvascular compression is not a cause of trigeminal neuralgia. Further studies are necessary—both epidemiologic and anatomic. For example, determination of the incidence of trigeminal neuralgia among African Americans or West Indians and anatomic studies such as those of Hardy and Rhoton[30] and Matsushima et al[49] in Africans would be of interest.

What Evidence Is There In Favor of Microvascular Compression?

Four approaches are used to support the hypothesis of microvascular compression. The first is that when there is definite vascular compression, which is relieved surgically, and there is no postoperative evidence of nerve damage, the patient obtains lasting relief.[31] The problem with this approach, however, is that "definite vascular compression" occurs in the majority of all people *without* cranial nerve dysfunction syndromes and that the results of trauma (i.e. rubbing the nerve root or balloon compression) produces as good, if not better, results that persist for as long or longer without evidence of any postoperative nerve damage. There is a view that MVD is "effective and safe,"[52] yet just how effective and how safe must be questioned.

The second approach is to claim that those who fail to find vessels have not properly exposed the nerve and looked for causative vessels[35,37] As Møller[51] states, "it is, naturally, a more serious criticism if it can be proven that not all people with these respective symptoms have vessels that are compressing their respective cranial nerves." Yet, many experienced surgeons have failed to see these vessels (Table

1), and to say that they are not capable of exposing the REZ adequately, or are incapable of seeing vessels, is an unconvincing defense of the hypothesis. Furthermore, as I have discussed, the important fact is not so much whether these vessels are or are not found in normal subjects or in patients with cranial nerve dysfunction syndromes, but what the significance of such vessels is.

The third approach in the defense of microvascular compression is the delayed therapeutic effect of MVD for hemifacial spasm, often requiring some days after surgery before the spasm ceases. This has been cited as important evidence in favor of microvascular compression. It is difficult to understand why this should favor MVD rather than trauma as the source of improvement. All surgeons who operate on acoustic neuromas are familiar with the exacerbation or onset of facial weakness that occurs days or weeks after the operation. Likewise, the delayed onset of facial weakness after a fracture of the petrous bone is well recognized. Presumably, edema of the facial nerve can spread through the nerve and, when it reaches the facial nerve canal, can produce compression and impairment of facial nerve function. Invoking "delayed cure" following MVD is unconvincing evidence to support microvascular compression as a pathologic concept.

Finally, neurophysiologic observations have been used to support microvascular compression. Indeed, Møller and Jannetta[53] have written "Electro-physiological studies have in fact been performed intra-operatively in patients with hemifacial spasm, and have demonstrated that compression of the facial nerve by a blood vessel causes the abnormal muscle responses that occur in such patients and that the responses disappear when the offending vessel is moved off the nerve (and they can be brought back if the vessel is allowed to slip back on the nerve)." Møller and Jannetta[53] state: "The EMG (electromyographic) response to antidromic stimulation disappears instantaneously when the compressing artery is removed from the facial nerve."

Some general observations can be made regarding this line of reasoning. First, intra-

operative electrophysiologic studies are difficult to carry out. There are variations that depend on anesthesia and pharmacologic agents, and it is difficult to know how much the current spreads. Second, deductions based on timing of electrophysiologic phenomena are not easy. For instance, it must be extremely difficult to argue that the lesion causing hemifacial spasm is in the brain stem, REZ, or facial nerve canal, based on conduction time differences. Considering that these sites are separated by only a few millimeters, the time difference over such distances are minute and open to error. As Schriefer et al[61] stated, "Attempts to localize the precise facial nerve stimulation site by inference from latency determinations prove difficult. A latency of only 0.3 milliseconds separates the facial nerve root exit zone from its entry through the porus acousticus. . . . With this in mind, a cautious interpretation is appropriate."

Apart from these general observations on the practical difficulties of carrying out electrophysiologic studies, Møller's results are somewhat surprising. One would hardly expect the "instantaneous" return of an electrophysiologic abnormality to normal and then sudden reversal to abnormality, with release of the vessel. Surely, nerve fibers are not going to suddenly become electrophysiologically normal on release of a vessel after years of compression.

Therefore, this author concludes that electrophysiologic techniques appear to contain such inherent variability as to make confident interpretation extremely difficult. To argue in favor of microvascular compression on the basis of such studies seems unconvincing. The techniques are difficult and, however carefully and expertly carried out, are open to different interpretations. Indeed, other neurophysiologists believe that the data support the concept that the primary lesion for hemifacial spasm lies in the brain stem or facial nerve canal.[22,57] Auger et al[13] stated that the electrophysiologic changes during surgery could reflect mild trauma, rather than microvascular compression.

More recently, Møller[51] has clarified his

views by stating:

> However, our experience in recording from more than 200 patients shows that these electromyographic recordings are very stable, and that the variabilities seen in the responses are natural fluctuations in the abnormal muscle response. Why the abnormal muscle response in patients with hemifacial spasm disappears instantaneously when the blood vessel is removed from the nerve, but may actually return when the blood vessel is allowed to touch the facial nerve again, remains a mystery; perhaps as more experience is gained and analysed objectively, the answer to this and other questions will lead to a further understanding of the pathophysiologies of these disorders.

It is significant, I think, that Møller does not claim that these neurophysiologic results prove that microvascular compression is the cause of hemifacial spasm.

Neurophysiologic observations concerning the trigeminal nerve are equally disputed. Thus, Cruccu et al[19] wrote: "The question of electrophysiologic abnormalities in trigeminal neuralgia is still a subject of controversy among authors. . . . The cause of disagreement may lie in the different methods of investigation—the first group of authors basing their opinion on testing of trigeminal reflexes and the second on cortical potentials evoked by stimulation in the trigeminal territory. Both methods are open to criticism. . ." A dispassionate observer might be forgiven if he or she concluded that both the techniques and the interpretations of neurophysiologic data are difficult and disputed, and that at present, neurophysiology does not provide clarification or support for the concept of microvascular compression. In the future, neurophysiology may provide a consensus view, either for or against microvascular compression, but as yet this consensus has not been achieved.

What Would Constitute Conclusive Evidence in Favor of Microvascular Compression?

Is there one situation that would provide conclusive and irrefutable evidence in favor

of microvascular compression? This would require MVD to cure a condition that *cannot* be remedied by sectioning the same cranial nerve. As has already been pointed out, MVD produces good results in 60% to 70% of patients with trigeminal neuralgia and hemifacial spasm. Yet, sectioning either the trigeminal or facial nerve, respectively, produces a cure as well. Inevitably, the possibility arises that the effect of MVD is by way of trauma. If there is a condition that sectioning a nerve does *not* cure, but which MVD does indeed eradicate, then the concept of microvascular compression must be valid and true.

The most obvious candidate to prove microvascular compression is spasmodic torticollis.[2] If MVD of one or both spinal accessory (XI) nerves cures spasmodic torticollis, then one has to conclude that microvascular compression is a true and valid concept. The results of MVD for spasmodic torticollis are an excellent therapeutic test for this hypothesis. This condition is well defined and easily diagnosed clinically without the need for complex neurophysiologic studies. It is agreed that the simple section of one or both spinal accessory nerves is insufficient to cure the condition. In favor of the condition being caused by microvascular compression is that it occurs in the middle-aged or elderly. Remissions are reported in one-fifth of the patients;[48] this is difficult to explain on the basis of microvascular compression, but remissions also are characteristic for trigeminal neuralgia. This disorder is essentially bilateral in its manifestations and, as has been argued previously, the clinical manifestations of any condition caused by microvascular compression should be predominantly bilateral. If MVD cures spasmodic torticollis, this would prove the concept. However, the results will have to be consistent and reproducible and with an adequate follow-up period in view of the possibility of spontaneous remission.

Spasmodic torticollis therefore, should be considered as well. Only recently has microvascular compression been proposed as the cause.[21] The condition usually occurs in the middle-aged or elderly, although in the series of Freckmann et al,[25] the average age of onset was 37 years. An unexplained and curious feature often demonstrated by these patients is the abolition or control of the spasm by a light touch of the finger to the jaw.

Freckmann et al[25] were the first to publish the results of MVD for spasmodic torticollis. The results state that "immediately post-operatively the torsion of the head was reduced in all cases. Most patients, however, still had more or less severe torsion impulses. . . . At the time of discharge from hospital six patients had improved significantly. . . . One of these patients, however, had a recurrence four weeks after operation. . . . In two patients the torsion impulses. . . were still incapacitating."[25] Thus, spasmodic torticollis was only diminished, and in no patient was it abolished. Surely, these results are what one might expect from merely cutting these nerves. They do not imply that spasmodic torticollis is caused by microvascular compression of the spinal accessory nerves. Yet Pagni et al[58] claimed that MVD produces a cure, with the obvious corollary that microvascular compression is the cause of spasmodic torticollis. They wrote: "The disorder was cured by abolishing the [vascular] compression." But elsewhere in their article they reported that the patient was "left with rare sporadic contractions." So a cure was not, in fact, achieved. Furthermore, the procedure carried out was not MVD for it was necessary to cut not only some of the lower rootlets of the left spinal accessory nerve, but also some of the C2 and C3 rootlets. It is not clear why it was necessary to cut these two cervical rootlets to relieve microvascular compression of the spinal accessory nerve by the posterior inferior cerebellar arteries. Clearly, one must await a series that has been carefully assessed for an adequate follow-up period, preferably reported by a neurologist in conjunction with a neurosurgeon. At the present time, it must be concluded that there is no evidence to suggest that MVD cures spasmodic torticollis.

Why Not Trauma?

Is it possible that the mechanism of MVD

is merely trauma to the nerve at a vulnerable site, rather than anything more profound? As Møller writes,[51] ". . . what is important is that the cranial nerves in question are covered proximal to their REZ by central myelin, which makes that part of the nerves more vulnerable to mechanical injury . . . than nerves covered with peripheral myelin." I already have discussed that those cranial nerve dysfunction syndromes that respond well to MVD also are "cured" by a section of the relevant cranial nerve, while those that do not respond are not abolished by cranial nerve section. Furthermore, the results of MVD are no better for pain relief and freedom from recurrence than procedures such as balloon compression or nerve root "rubbing" as practiced by Taarnhøj[65] and Gardner[27] via the middle fossa—procedures with no pretense of being anything except a means of applying trauma, not even in the vicinity of the REZ. The fact that these results are as good (or even better than) MVD not only raises doubts about the concept of microvascular compression, but the vulnerability of the nerve at or proximal to the REZ (depending on one's definition of the REZ).

As stated earlier, there is a definite, albeit small, incidence of vestibulocochlear nerve damage after MVD for trigeminal neuralgia and this incidence does not decrease with experience.[14] Such nerve VIII damage must reflect not inexperience or youthful clumsiness, but inevitable, indirect traction necessary to expose the REZ of the trigeminal nerve. In the hands of the less experienced this probably is more common. Thus, the very maneuver of exposing the REZ of nerve V for trigeminal neuralgia can cause traction damage to nerve VIII,[5] a nerve that is not directly in the line of retraction of the cerebellum. It is not too farfetched to argue that indirect damage must, therefore, be more likely to occur to the trigeminal nerve itself, even before dissection around the REZ has been performed. The same considerations apply to the trigeminal nerve with MVD for hemifacial spasm. In this respect, Aoki and Nagao's[11] case is of interest: They described a patient with a five-year history of hemifacial spasm. At operation, no vessel or other abnormalities were found, and no procedure of any type (other than dissection around the nerve) was carried out, yet the patient awoke completely free of spasm. Aoki[10] reported that the patient continued to remain free of spasm 3 years since the surgery and went on to describe another patient with hemifacial spasm who also had an excellent result after abandoning the proposed MVD when finding a large vein in situ. This patient remained symptomfree for 2.5 years at the time of writing, despite leaving the vein undisturbed. Sweet[64] and Parkinson[59] also have described excellent relief of trigeminal neuralgia pain after abandoned operations on the trigeminal nerve, which resulted in no more than "minimal intracranial manipulation."[64] Parkinson's[59] patient had no pain during the 35 years of followup, while Sweet's three patients remained painfree for 8, 10, and 5.5 years. Sweet[64] recommends with sadness ". . . a great reduction" in the usage of MVD for trigeminal neuralgia "because its mortality and morbidity cannot be reduced to the levels of percutaneous operations."

Surgeons have been reluctant to accept the concept that nerve trauma cannot exist without signs of postoperative nerve damage. But nerve roots do seem to be exquisitely vulnerable. It is well accepted that chronic arachnoiditis can cause permanent damage to the spinal roots even after minimal manipulation. In my opinion, the evidence is overwhelming that nerves V and VII (and indeed nerve VIII) are equally susceptible to minimal manipulation, and that MVD works by causing minimal nerve damage insufficient to cause actual cranial nerve signs postoperatively. To refute such a suggestion, Burchiel et al[15,16] have tried to show that better results occur after MVD for trigeminal neuralgia resulting in *no* postoperative sensory loss than with; but the numbers are too small and the data too incomplete for any certain conclusions to be drawn.

Summary

The results and complications of MVD,

when compared with other techniques, suggest that trauma is the basis of MVD. The vulnerability of cranial nerves allows minimal damage without overt neurologic signs developing postoperatively. But the probability that MVD works by traumatizing the nerve does not, in itself, belittle the procedure. Whether it should be done, however, must depend on how the results (and complications) of MVD compare with other available procedures.

The Probable Basis of Trigeminal Neuralgia, Hemifacial Spasm, and Glossopharyngeal Neuralgia

The etiology of cranial nerve dysfunction syndromes is unknown. Certainly, trigeminal neuralgia and hemifacial spasm can arise from brain stem disorders such as multiple sclerosis[9] or they can occur with acoustic neuromas. Even contralateral trigeminal neuralgia can occur with an acoustic neuroma as well as with other extra-axial tumors. It is surprising, however, how rare it is for these cranial nerve dysfunction syndromes to develop with intra- or extra-axial pathology: The vast majority have no associated pathology. Multiple sclerosis must provide some insight into mechanisms. Classical trigeminal neuralgia does occur in patients with multiple sclerosis, and plaques are found in these patients in a variety of areas in the brain stem—the point of entry of the trigeminal root, the main sensory root nucleus, or the descending tract.[51] Carbamazepine is a remarkably specific treatment for trigeminal neuralgia and glossopharyngeal neuralgia, but not for hemifacial spasm. It also is remarkably specific for the painless paroxysmal disorders that occasionally occur in patients with multiple sclerosis. There seems little doubt that these paroxysmal disorders arise from the brain stem, and the mode of action of carbamazepine would suggest that it acts on the central nervous system. Although the exact mechanism of action is unknown, it does seem to depress the transmission of impulses.

The rarity of trigeminal neuralgia in Africans, despite a marked tendency to develop hypertension early in life, is most interesting, particularly if one believes the suggestion that MVC can cause both essential hypertension and trigeminal neuralgia. Further epidemiologic studies are needed not only for trigeminal neuralgia but also for hemifacial spasm, which seems to be unusually common in Japan as judged by the size of some series of MVD for hemifacial spasm.

The rarity of trigeminal neuralgia in Africans does suggest a more systemic cause for this disorder. The remarkable remissions of pain also favor a noncompressive cause. Coad et al[18] have published a case report describing familial hemifacial spasm, which again suggests a more systemic factor in the genesis of this condition. They published careful histologic data of the affected patient's facial nerve complex. More such studies are required, particularly with controlled studies of nonaffected patients of a similar age. Matsushima et al[49] have shown the frequency of marked vascular compression in unaffected patients coming to postmortem.

There is an additional fact that perhaps has not received sufficient attention. It is a remarkable and unique fact that the pain of trigeminal neuralgia can be eliminated by numbing the affected area *anywhere* along the course of the trigeminal nerve. For instance, the application of an anesthetic tablet or local anesthetic injections into the appropriate mucosa or skin will stop the pain as satisfactorily as peripheral nerve or nerve root injections. This fact itself is evidence against microvascular compression at the REZ as the cause of trigeminal neuralgia. For instance, root pain caused by lumbar disk compression is not influenced one iota by local anesthetic or peripheral nerve injections in the dermatomal distribution of the pain. Indeed, I am unaware of any other pain (other than glossopharyngeal neuralgia) that has this characteristic feature. Arguably, it favors a skin or mucosal origin for the pain of trigeminal neuralgia or glossopharyngeal neuralgia, although there is little else to

support such a hypothesis. Certainly, it is a unique feature that requires an explanation in any hypothesis.

At the present time, the cause of cranial nerve dysfunction syndromes, especially trigeminal neuralgia and hemifacial spasm, is unknown. There is much evidence to suggest a primary brain stem origin, and one can only speculate that, in time, the pathobiochemical basis of these disorders will be found and probably will reside in the appropriate motor or sensory nuclei of the brain stem.

The Management of Cranial Nerve Dysfunction Syndromes

This chapter has concerned itself with evidence and debate about the cause of cranial nerve dysfunction syndromes, particularly of trigeminal neuralgia and hemifacial spasm. It seems appropriate to briefly mention my particular approach to the treatment of these conditions.

Trigeminal Neuralgia

The first line of treatment is carbamazepine. If the patient is unable to tolerate this drug or becomes resistant to it, then surgical treatment is necessary. A variety of treatments are available. What is not stressed in the literature perhaps, is that the surgeon must advise not only what is most appropriate for that particular patient (depending on the age, distribution of pain, and desire, or otherwise, for a permanent cure), but also what is most appropriate for that particular surgeon. The author (not being good at inserting needles) feels more confident using microsurgical techniques. The surgeon must pay due regard to the risks and benefits of each procedure. A few patients would be best treated by infraorbital or supraorbital nerve injections or avulsions, but these patients are comparatively few. More usually, patients have third and second division trigeminal neural-

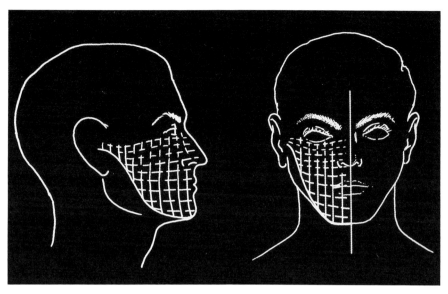

Figure 3. Typical sensory impairment following a 60% to 70% selective partial rhizotomy for second and third division trigeminal neuralgia. Vertical line = pin prick; continuous line = analgesia; dashed line, hypalgesia. Horizontal line = light touch; continuous line = anesthesia; dashed line, hypesthesia.

gia. By the time I see these patients, they usually express a wish for as permanent a cure as possible. No longer do they wish to face the future, not knowing whether or not they will wake up with trigeminal neuralgia. They wish to stop taking carbamazepine with its associated side effects.

I explain that a permanent cure would require permanent numbness, but a compromise is produced by a partial root section. This can be directed to the appropriate nerve root (Figure 2) and produce a relatively greater degree of hypalgesia than hypesthesia, a fact originally pointed out by Dandy.[20] The patient must understand that he or she is "swapping pain for numbness." Selective partial root section[8] produces an immediate cure in all cases, thus sparing the patient the trauma of being subjected to a posterior fossa operation without any relief of pain as happens sometimes after MVD, with 88% of the patients being relieved of trigeminal neuralgia for 5 years or more (Table 6). The price the patient has to pay for this more certain result is some facial numbness (Figure 3). This approach avoids the other side effects

and complications of MVD, because it is unnecessary to use excessive retraction to expose the REZ, nor is it necessary to manipulate or section "compressing" vessels with the dangers of subsequent brain stem ischemia or infarction. Selective partial root section is therefore remarkably safe and effective. Lichtor and Mullan's[43] results of percutaneous balloon compression are, in my view, striking and if confirmed, will persuade me of the advantages of this technique, given the acquisition of the necessary skills.

Hemifacial Spasm

Botulin injections would seem to be the first line of treatment for those patients who find hemifacial spasm sufficiently incapacitating or embarrassing to justify treatment of this nonfatal, painless condition. MVD or wrapping the facial nerve, in my view, is the best technique for providing long-term relief and this is, indeed, what I advise and carry out. Once again, one must question whether the retraction and vessel manipulation associated with MVD is necessary. Clearly, some believe it to be so. I am yet to be convinced and am prepared to do a "wrapping" of the facial nerve, not necessarily at the REZ, and so avoid the potential complications of MVD. The author has not personally used Aoki's technique of nerve inspection (with a little manipulation?) which has seemingly produced excellent results to date![10,11] If a patient happens to be deaf on the contralateral side, then this poses considerable difficulties: Few surgeons, if any, can *guarantee* avoidance of hearing loss following MVD for hemifacial spasm. I have resorted to thermocoagulation of the extracranial facial nerve in those circumstances.

Glossopharyngeal Neuralgia

The author does not hesitate to advise section of the glossopharyngeal nerve and the upper adjacent vagal rootlet for this condition. I explain to the patient that there may be transient dysphagia, but there is no appreciable sensory loss. To perform MVD with its uncertain long-term results, as well as the enhanced complication rate because of the greater degree of retraction necessary in vessel manipulation, seems wholly unjustified to me.

Spasmodic Torticollis

The treatment of this condition is extremely unsatisfactory. There is no medical treatment. Stereotactic thalamotomy produces unimpressive results and appreciable side effects, while the Dandy-McKenzie procedure produces alleviation by merely weakening the musculature of the neck. Too enthusiastic denervation prevents the normal physiologic extension of the neck, which is a necessary accompaniment of swallowing.[1] Consequent dysphagia may be severe with some patients requiring a cervical collar to allow them to swallow. A few patients develop catastrophic vascular (cervical cord or brain stem) complications and these have been summarized elsewhere.[1] Patients need a full and frank explanation of

the mechanism and inevitable side effects of the Dandy-McKenzie procedure preoperatively. It is a blunt weapon but one that has helped carefully selected and carefully counseled patients.

Vestibulocochlear Nerve Disorders

The author sees two groups of patients in this category: those with tinnitus and those with vertigo. It is well known that tinnitus is not helped by cochlear or auditory nerve section. Indeed, it is a troublesome symptom following the removal of acoustic neuromas, without hearing preservation and, consequently, total deafness. I would not recommend nerve section or MVD for a patient with tinnitus. There are, however, occasional patients with Meniere's disease who have sufficient preservation of hearing to make labyrinthectomy inappropriate. These patients are suitable candidates for vestibular nerve section. The author has operated on three such patients. Tarlov[66] has had considerable experience with this group of patients. (See Chapter 9.)

Conclusion: What of the Future?

This author believes the debate as to the validity of microvascular compression is important. MVD is not the perfect operation; indeed, the author believes it is not the best procedure and that it has significant complications compared with other procedures used for trigeminal neuralgia. It is the author's view that dispassionate assessment of the facts show that the concept of microvascular compression cannot be sustained and that MVD works by traumatizing the relevant cranial nerve.

The debate is important, for if the basis of MVD is trauma, then are there not other, safer and more effective methods of applying trauma without the need for the degree of retraction and vessel manipulation associated with MVD? By opening our minds to other concepts, we are more likely to produce better solutions. Furthermore, this will hopefully prevent operations from being performed for conditions which are most unlikely to be helped by MVD, such as tinnitus, spasmodic torticollis, and essential hypertension.

More work is required and epidemiologic research is needed. Careful autopsy studies with controls have yet to be done, and perhaps more understanding of the mechanism of action of carbamazepine will lead to further knowledge of the biochemical basis of trigeminal neuralgia and glossopharyngeal neuralgia.

References

1. Adams CBT. Vascular catastrophe following the Dandy McKenzie operation for spasmodic torticollis. *J Neurol Neurosurg Psychiatry.* 1984;47:990-994.
2. Adams CBT. Spasmodic torticollis resulting from neurovascular compression. *J Neurosurg.* 1987; 66:635. Letter.
3. Adams CBT. Microvascular compression: an alternative view and hypothesis. *J Neurosurg.* 1989;70: 1-12.
4. Adams CBT. Views on microvascular compression. *J Neurosurg.* 1989;71:463-464. Letter.
5. Adams CBT. Microvascular decompression. *J Neurosurg.* 1990;72:671-672. Letter.
6. Adams CBT. Microvascular decompression. *Surgical Neurology.* In Press 1991. Letter.
7. Adams CBT, Kaye AH. Hemifacial spasm: treatment by posterior fossa surgery. *J Neurol Neurosurg Psychiatry.* 1983;46:465-466. Letter.
8. Adams CBT, Kaye AH, Teddy PJ. The treatment of trigeminal neuralgia by posterior fossa microsurgery. *J Neurol Neurourg Psychiatry.* 1982;45: 1020-1026.
9. Ambrosetto P. Views on microvascular compression. *J Neurosurg.* 1989;71:462-463. Letter.
10. Aoki N. Views on microvascular compression. *J Neurosurg.* 1989;71:462. Letter.
11. Aoki N, Nagao T. Resolution of hemifacial spasm after posterior fossa exploration without vascular decompression. *Neurosurgery.* 1986;18:478-479. Letter.
12. Apfelbaum RI. Surgery for tic douloureux. *Clin Neurosurg.* 1984;31:351-368.
13. Auger RG, Piegras DG, Laws ER Jr, et al. Microvascular decompression of the facial nerve for hemifacial spasm: clinical and electrophysiological observations. *Neurology.* 1981;31:346-350.
14. Bederson JB, Wilson CB. Evaluation of microvascular decompression and partial sensory rhizotomy in 252 cases of trigeminal neuralgia. *J Neurosurg.* 1989;71:359-367.
15. Burchiel KJ. Microvascular decompression. *J Neurosurg.* 1990;72:671-672. Letter.
16. Burchiel KJ, Clarke H, Haglund M, et al. Long-term efficacy of microvascular decompression in trigeminal neuralgia. *J Neurosurg.* 1988;69:35-38.
17. Campbell E, Keedy C. Hemifacial spasm: a note on the aetiology of two cases. *J Neurosurg.* 1947;4: 342-347.
18. Coad JE, Wirtschafter JD, Haines SJ, et al. Familial hemifacial spasm associated with arterial compression of the facial nerve: case report. *J Neurosurg.* 1991;74:290-296.
19. Cruccu G, Inghilleri M, Manfredi M, et al. Intracranial stimulation of the trigeminal nerve in man, III: sensory potentials. *J Neurol Neurosurg Psychiatry.* 1987;50:1323-1330.
20. Dandy WE. Surgery of the brain. In: Lewis D, ed. *Practice of Surgery.* Hagerstown, Md: WF Prior; 1945;12:167-187.
21. Dyck P. Spasmodic torticollis. *J Neurosurg.* 1986; 65:726. Letter.
22. Esteban A, Molina-Negro P. Primary hemifacial spasm: a neurophysiological study. *J Neurol Neurosurg Psychiatry.* 1986;49:58-63.
23. Fabinyi GCA, Adams CBT. Hemifacial spasm: treatment by posterior fossa surgery. *J Neurol Neurosurg Psychiatry.* 1978;41:829-833.
24. Ferguson GG, Brett DC, Peerless SJ, et al. Trigeminal neuralgia: a comparison of the results of percutaneous rhizotomy and microvascular decompression. *Can J Neurol Sci.* 1981;8:207-214.
25. Freckmann N, Hagenah R, Herrmann HD, et al. Treatment of neurogenic torticollis by microvascular lysis of the accessory nerve roots—indication, technique, and first results. *Acta Neurochir Wien.* 1981;59:167-175.
26. Fritz W, Shafer J, Klein HJ. Hearing loss after microvascular decompression for trigeminal neuralgia. *J Neurosurg.* 1988;69:367-370.
27. Gardner WJ. Concerning the mechanism of trigeminal neuralgia and hemifacial spasm. *J Neurosurg.* 1962;19:947-958.
28. Gardner WJ, Miklos MV. Response of trigeminal neuralgia to "decompression" of sensory root: discussion of cause of trigeminal neuralgia. *JAMA.* 1959;170:1773-1776.
29. Hanakita J, Kondo A. Serious complications of microvascular decompression operations for trigeminal neuralgia and hemifacial spasm. *Neurosurgery.* 1988;22:348-352.
30. Hardy DG, Rhoton AL Jr. Microsurgical relationship of the superior cerebellar artery and the trigeminal nerve. *J Neurosurg.* 1978;49:669-678.
31. Heros RC. Views on microvascular compression. *J Neurosurg.* 1989;71:460-461. Letter.
32. Jannetta PJ. Gross (mesoscopic) description of the human trigeminal nerve and ganglion. *J Neurosurg. Suppl.* 1967;26:109-111.
33. Jannetta PJ. Treatment of trigeminal neuralgia by suboccipital and transtentorial cranial operations. *Clin Neurosurg.* 1977;24:538-549.
34. Jannetta PJ. Neurovascular compression in cranial nerve and systemic disease. *Ann Surg.* 1980;192: 518-525.
35. Jannetta PJ. Treatment of trigeminal neuralgia by micro-operative decompression. In: Youmans JR, ed. *Neurological Surgery VI.* 2nd ed. Philadelphia, Pa: WB Saunders, Co.; 1982:3589-3603.
36. Jannetta PJ. Hemifacial spasm: treatment by posterior fossa surgery. *J Neurol Neurosurgery Psychiatry.* 1983:46:465. Letter.
37. Jannetta PJ. hemifacial spasm caused by a venule: case report. *Neurosurgery.* 1984;14:89-92.
38. Jannetta PJ, Møller MB, Møller AR, et al. Neurosurgical treatment of vertigo by microvascular

decompression of the eighth cranial nerve. *Clin Neurosurg.* 1986;33:645-665.

39. Jannetta PJ, Zorub DS. Microvascular decompression for trigeminal neuralgia. In: Buckheit WA, Truex RC, eds. *Surgery of the Posterior Fossa.* New York, NY: Raven Press; 1979:143-154.

40. Kaye AH, Adams CBT. Hemifacial spasm: a long-term follow-up of patients treated by posterior fossa surgery and facial nerve wrapping. *J Neurol Neurosurg Psychiatry.* 1981;44:1100-1103.

41. Lang J. *Clinical Anatomy of the Head: Neurocranium, Orbit and Craniocervical Region.* New York, NY: Springer-Verlag; 1983:184.

42. Lewy FH, Grant FC. Physiopathologic and pathoanatomic aspects of major trigeminal neuralgia. *Arch Neurol Psychiatry.* 1938;40:1126-1134.

43. Lichtor T, Mullan JF. A 10-year follow-up review of percutaneous microcompression of the trigeminal ganglion. *J Neurosurg.* 1990;72:49-54.

44. Loeser JD, Chen J. Hemifacial spasm: treatment by microsurgical facial nerve decompression. *Neurosurgery.* 1982;13:141-146.

45. Marion DW, Jannetta PJ. Use of perioperative steroids with microvascular decompression operations. *Neurosurgery.* 1988;22:353-357.

46. Maroon JC. Hemifacial spasm: a vascular cause. *Arch Neurol.* 1978;35:481-483.

47. Maroon JC, Lunsford LD, Deeb ZL. Hemifacial spasm due to aneurysmal compression of the facial nerve. *Arch Neurol.* 1978;35:545-546.

48. Marsden CD. Movement disorders. In: Weatherall DJ, Ledingham JGG, Warrell DA, eds. *Oxford Textbook of Medicine.* New York, NY: Oxford University Press; 1983;R:21.100-121.

49. Matsushima T, Inoue T, Fukui M. Arteries in contact with the cisternal portion of the facial nerve in autopsy cases: microsurgical anatomy for neurovascular decompression surgery of hemifacial spasm. *Surg Neurol.* 1990;34:87-93.

50. McAlpine D, Lumsden CE, Acheson ED. Multiple sclerosis: a reappraisal. 2nd ed. Baltimore, Md: Williams & Wilkins; 1972:167.

51. Møller AR. Views on microvascular compression. *J Neurosurg.* 1989;71:459-460. Letter.

52. Møller AR. Courtesy in medical and scientific writing. *J Neurosurg.* 1987;67:627-628. Letter.

53. Møller AR, Jannetta PJ. Microvascular decompression in hemifacial spasm: intraoperative electrophysiological observations. *Neurosurgery.* 1985;16:612-618.

54. Møller MB, Møller AR, Jannetta PJ, et al. Diagnosis and surgical treatment of disabling positional vertigo. *J Neurosurg.* 1986;64:21-28.

55. Morley TP. *Current Controversies in Neurosurgery.*

Philadelphia, Pa: WB Saunders Co; 1976:433.

56. Mracek Z. (Compression of the spinal trigeminal tract due to pressure of the inferior posterior cerebellar artery as the causative factor of facial neuralgia) *Rohzl Chir.* 1982;61:116-119. (Cze). English abstract.

57. Nielson VK, Jannetta PJ. Pathophysiology of hemifacial spasm, III: effects of facial nerve decompression. *Neurology.* 1984;34:891-897.

58. Pagni CA, Naddeo M, Faccani G. Spasmodic torticollis due to neurovascular compression of the 11th nerve: case report. *J Neurosurg.* 1985;63:789-791.

59. Parkinson D. Microvascular compression: decompression; a recollection. *J Neurosurg.* 1989;70:819. Letter.

60. Piatt JH, Wilkins RH. Treatment of tic douloureux and hemifacial spasm by posterior fossa exploration: therapeutic implications of various neurovascular relationships. *Neurosurgery.* 1984;14:462-471.

61. Schriefer TN, Mills KR, Murray NMF, et al. Evaluation of proximal facial nerve conduction by transcranial magnetic stimulation. *J Neurol Neurosurg Psychiatry.* 1988;51:60-66.

62. Sunderland S. Neurovascular relations and anomalies at the base of the brain. *J Neurol Neurosurg Psychiatry.* 1948;11:243-257.

63. Sweet WH, Poletti CE. Complications of percutaneous rhizotomy and microvascular decompression operations for facial pain. In: Schmidek HH, Sweet WH, eds. *Operative Neurosurgical Techniques: Indications, Methods and Results, II. 2nd ed.* Orlando, Fl: Grune & Stratton Inc; 1988:1139-1143.

64. Sweet WH. Trigeminal neuralgia: problems as to cause and consequent conclusions regarding treatment. In: Wilkins RH, Rengachary SS, eds. *Neurosurgery Update III.* New York, NY: McGraw-Hill 1991:366-372.

65. Taarnhøj P. The place of decompression of the posterior root in the treatment of trigeminal neuralgia. *J Neurol Neurosurg Psychiatry.* 1961;24:295-296. Abstract.

66. Tarlov EC. Microsurgical vestibular nerve section for intractable Meniere's syndrome—technique and results. *Clin Neurosurg.* 1986;33:667-684.

67. Thompson PD, Carroll WM. Hemimasticatory spasm—a peripheral paroxysmal cranial neuropathy? *J Neurol Neurosurg Psychiatry.* 1983;46:274-276.

68. Williams PL, Warwick R. *Gray's Anatomy.* 36th ed, Brit. Philadelphia, Pa: WB Saunders Co;1980:846.

69. Zorman G, Wilson CB. Outcome following microsurgical vascular decompression or partial sensory rhizotomy in 125 cases of trigeminal neuralgia. *Neurology.* 1984;34:1362-1365.

CHAPTER 4

Cranial Nerve Dysfunction Syndromes: Evidence for Microvascular Compression

Robert H. Wilkins, MD

There can no great smoke arise, but there must be some fire.
Lyly, *Euphues,* 1579.[4]

Historical Background

The existence of the cranial nerves has been known for at least 2,000 years, although their classification has varied over that time.[15] As recently as 1830, Sir Charles Bell listed as the seventh pair, the facial and auditory nerves on each side.[9,15,78] This is especially interesting because Bell was the first to distinguish the sensory and motor roles of the trigeminal (V) and facial (VII) nerves.[15,78] Between 1821 and 1829, he established that the trigeminal and facial nerves have separate functions,[6-8] thereby enabling physicians to localize tic douloureux (so named by André in 1756[2]) to the trigeminal nerve.[76]

This not only resulted in a second name for the illness, trigeminal neuralgia, but also focused the search for its cause(s) on conditions affecting the trigeminal nerve. Over the subsequent years, some patients with tic douloureux were found to have a process affecting the ipsilateral trigeminal system. Such processes included multiple sclerosis, various types of neoplasms, arterial ectasia, arteriovenous malformations, Paget's disease of the skull, etc.[75] Yet in the majority of cases, the cause remained unclear.

Walter E. Dandy, MD

During the 1920s, Dandy developed an operative treatment for tic douloureux that involved sectioning the sensory root of the trigeminal nerve within the posterior fossa.[12,13,56] As his experience with this procedure grew, Dandy noted that adjacent vessels were frequently in contact with the nerve. By 1934, he had found such a relationship in 45% of 215 cases and postulated that such vascular compression could be a cause of trigeminal neuralgia.[14] Dandy stated:

> In the routine treatment of trigeminal neuralgia by division of the posterior root, either totally or subtotally, and using the sub-cerebellar approach, I have been impressed with the frequency of certain anatomical findings which, I believe, must have a bearing upon the production of this pain. From a series of 215 cases, in which I have personally made the operative notes, the following findings are presented:
>
> In 12 cases (5.6 per cent), there has been a gross lesion impinging upon the trigeminal nerve. Six of these tumors were the ordinary acoustic neuromas; one was a neuroma of an entirely different type arising from the eighth nerve; 4 were pearly body tumors (cholesteatomas). The remaining case was an osteoma arising from the base of the skull alongside the porus acusticus.
>
> In 6 cases (2.8 per cent) aneurysms of the basilar artery pressed upon the sensory root. The frequency of aneurysms of the basilar artery has not been appreciated, and it is only through operations in the posterior fossa that their

number can be realized. Increasing age, arterio-sclerosis, and frequently associated hypertension, cause elongation of the basilar artery, which becomes s-shaped, and the bulge of the s reaches the trigeminal nerve.

In 5 cases (2.3 per cent) there were cavernous angiomas which surrounded and obscured, in large part, the sensory root. There can, I think, be no question whatever concerning the relationship of these three groups of tumors to the production of trigeminal neuralgia. Together they represent 10.7 per cent of the total number of cases.

Other findings which, perhaps, are less impressive to casual inspection, are, I believe, no less responsible for the production of trigeminal neuralgia; these are the arteries and veins which impinge upon and frequently distort the sensory root.

In the region of the sensory root the superior cerebellar artery usually sends out a branch which dangles freely in the lateral cistern before reaching its destination. This is easily seen in specimens of cadavers and at operation. Frequently this arterial branch forms a loop; but regardless of its formation, the branch passes either beneath the trigeminal root, that is between the root and the brain stem, or along the lateral surface of the sensory root, and in either case, as the artery hardens from advancing age, the nerve becomes indented by the arterial branch. . . . In 66 cases (30.7 per cent) the artery in some way affected the nerve.

It may well be asked why a contiguous artery should produce pain in the trigeminal nerve and not produce disturbances in other nerves. There are, I think, two answers: one, that similar arterial loops are not contiguous to other cranial nerves, and secondly, there are no other cranial nerves that begin to have the supply of pain fibers that obtain in the trigeminal nerve. Aside from the glossopharyngeal nerve there are no other cranial nerves in which this unique pain is found (possibly the facial nerve may be a very rare exception).

It may also be asked why in those cases in which the nerve is not distorted, the artery may be looked upon as the cause of the pain. If one examines the actual tumors which are causing trigeminal neuralgia one usually finds that the nerve is barely reached by the tumor and rarely much deformed by it. Another question which demands answer is: are not such findings frequently present without the production of tic douloureux? The answer unquestionably is yes, and for exactly the same reason that only a few

acoustic tumors produce trigeminal neuralgia, though when an acoustic tumor is present there can be no doubt that it is the actual cause. Just as one sees many cases of gallstones without pain, so one sees lesions attacking the sensory root in the angle without the actual production of pain, but when the patient has pain and gallstones are present, the gallstones are unquestionably the cause.

Another group of cases presented in which a branch of the petrosal vein crosses the sensory root or passes directly through it. In 30 cases of the series (14 per cent) such a finding was noted. I feel less willing to ascribe relationship to this finding, although it is difficult to believe that it is not the actual causal factor. These venous branches frequently indent the nerve, or are quite firmly attached to it, or may lie lightly against it.

In 2 additional cases (1 per cent) there were congenital malformations at the base of the skull. In both cases the base of the skull was markedly concave and in compensating for the reduced intracranial room, the eighth nerve had been pushed anterior to the plane of the fifth nerve. I feel that with such a strong congenital anomaly the trigeminal neuralgia was probably related thereto. Both occurred in young individuals in which a congenital malformation is always suspected.

In 7 cases the sensory root was tightly adherent to the brain stem. Whether this should be included among the probable causes of trigeminal neuralgia, I do not know.

In one case the patient had multiple sclerosis. The relationship of multiple sclerosis to trigeminal neuralgia has been frequently commented upon in the literature, and while representing but a small percentage of the cases of multiple sclerosis, the incidence is sufficiently high to denote a direct bearing upon tic douloureux.

In 87 cases (40 per cent) no gross findings of any kind were noted. It will be remembered, of course, that the entire extent of the sensory root is not visible from the operative approach, so that quite probably some of these cases may have had gross findings which could not be seen. Then too, perhaps arterial branches were present, especially among the earlier cases, and were not regarded as significant . . . .

From the latter cases one can only conclude that there must be an intrinsic disturbance of the sensory root . . . , and since it has been shown that one-half of the sensory root can be sectioned without the loss of function, such extensive intrinsic disturbance of the root can certainly exist without actual loss of sensory function. This, of course, is a purely hypothetical explanation of the cases in which no gross finding is observable.[14]

W. James Gardner, MD

Gardner carried Dandy's idea a step further. In 1959, Gardner and Miklos reported exploring the trigeminal nerve in the posterior fossa in a patient with tic douloureux: ". . . an anomalous arterial loop was found lying against the nerve; the pain was completely relieved after separating this vessel from the nerve root by the interposition of a piece of absorbable gelatin sponge (Gelfoam)."[17]

Following their assessment of 200 patients with tic douloureux, these authors concluded as follows. "Trigeminal neuralgia is a symptom—not a disease. It may constitute a symptom of multiple sclerosis, of basilar impression, or of a tumor located either in the middle or in the posterior fossa. . . . The only portion of the trigeminal sensory system that is common to both the middle and the posterior cranial fossae is the sensory root. The cause of trigeminal neuralgia, therefore, presumably lies in the sensory root."[17]

As the initial knowledge about trigeminal neuralgia was being accumulated, another cranial nerve dysfunction syndrome, hemifacial spasm, gradually became recognized as a clinical entity and also was found on occasion to be caused by compression or distortion of the nerve (the facial nerve in this case) by a pathologic process such as a neoplasm, arterial ectasia, an arteriovenous malformation, Paget's disease of the skull, etc.[77] Of historic interest, Schultze in 1875 presented the pathologic evidence at autopsy of a vertebral artery aneurysm that had caused ipsilateral hemifacial spasm during life.[66] And in 1947, Campbell and Keedy reported two patients whose hemifacial spasm seemed to be caused by compression of the facial nerve by a cirsoid aneurysm of the basilar artery.[11]

In 1962, Gardner and Sava presented a series of 19 patients with hemifacial spasm who had undergone surgical exploration of the cerebellopontine angle.[18] In seven of these patients, there was compression of the facial nerve by an obvious pathologic process such as a cirsoid aneurysm of the basilar artery or an arteriovenous malformation. In another seven patients, the facial nerve was compressed and distorted by a redundant anterior inferior cerebellar or internal auditory artery. In only five cases were no abnormalities found.

Later the same year, in a paper entitled "Concerning the mechanism of trigeminal neuralgia and hemifacial spasm," Gardner wrote:

> Despite the fact that one is a sensory and the other a motor phenomenon, trigeminal neuralgia and hemifacial spasm have many features in common: each occurs in spontaneous paroxysms that resemble the effect of electrical stimulation of the nerve; each is limited to the distribution of the nerve involved; occurs only in adults, predominantly in women; is subject to remissions; and . . . there seldom is demonstrable impairment of function of the nerve. . . . Both types of paroxysms are precipitated by facial movements on some occasions but not on others. They also occur during sleep. There is a tendency for the opposite side to become involved, in which case the attacks are neither synchronous nor symmetric. . . .
> Hemifacial spasm is the motor counterpart of tic douloureux. Both are expressions of an unstable and reversible pathophysiologic state caused by a mild compression of the nerve root which permits transaxonal excitation while not interfering with axonal conduction. . . .
> . . . the paroxysms of hemifacial spasm, like trigeminal neuralgia, may be stopped immediately, and with no impairment of function, by a *nontraumatic* manipulation of the nerve root.[16]

Concerning the last statement, Gardner and Sava treated their 19 patients with hemifacial spasm by neurolysis of the facial nerve in the cerebellopontine angle.[18] In 18 of the 19 operations, the facial nerve was gently manipulated with a nerve hook, and in several instances, the nerve also was irrigated forcefully with a stream of Ringer's solution. Gardner and Sava stated:

> [In the seven cases] in which the nerve was compressed and distorted by a loop of a normal artery, the causal relationship may be questioned in view of Sunderland's . . . finding that a large

loop of the anterior inferior cerebellar artery was related intimately to the 7th and 8th nerves in 64 per cent of routine autopsies. . . . Despite the incidence of such vessels, it is difficult to argue with the fact that, in these 7 cases of hemifacial spasm, freeing of the nerve from the vessel and the interposition of a bit of Gelfoam where feasible, was followed by relief in every case and at the cost of mild and transient weakness in only 1 instance. It must be noted however that in the last 3 cases, in addition to this manipulation, a bundle of fibers believed to be nervus intermedius, was divided.[18]

Peter J. Jannetta, MD

In the mid-1960s, Jannetta worked with Rand to develop a transtentorial microsurgical approach to the trigeminal nerve for the treatment of tic douloureux.[23] In five consecutive patients, the trigeminal nerve was found to be mildly to severely compressed and distorted by one or more small tortuous arteries that appeared to be branches of the superior cerebellar artery. Jannetta noted:

> In four of the five patients, the artery could be freed from the fine to dense arachnoidal membranes, thus allowing the vessel to assume a new position away from the nerve. We carried out partial to total section of the portio major in all cases, with resultant hypalgesia to analgesia in the corresponding area of the face. . . . On one patient with first division tic and a decrease in the corneal reflex, we freed the artery and did a small inferolateral section of the portio major. . . . This possibly definitive procedure, namely, release of the artery without nerve section, is planned in a future series of patients. . . . It is of interest that in none of the 56 fresh cadavers that we studied did we see any evidence of trigeminal nerve compression by blood vessels at or near the pons. For several years we have inspected the trigeminal nerve in patients undergoing suboccipital craniectomy for other reasons, and have found no vascular compression at the pons.[23]

In 1966, these authors began to perform microvascular decompression (MVD) for the treatment of tic douloureux. Rand described a 58-year-old woman for whom:

> . . . the original operative plan was to perform

a partial section of the portio major of the trigeminal nerve by approaching the root by a subtemporal transtentorial operation. An arterial loop of the ipsilateral superior cerebellar artery was found to be causing severe distortion and compression of the trigeminal root. The husband came to the operating room during surgery to discuss performance of microneurosurgical transposition of the arterial loop from the distorted and compressed trigeminal nerve. The microneurosurgical vascular decompression operation was subsequently performed, with displacement of two arteries that looped back over the trigeminal nerve and coagulation of a vein adjacent to the trigeminal nerve. Adhesions were found between the trigeminal nerve and the arterial loop. These were cut and released so that the artery could be pushed gently away, and a 5-mm space was left between the nerve and the arterial loop. An important observation was that the segment of the trigeminal root that was compressed had a more grey appearance than the usually bright white appearance of the trigeminal root. The offending arteries were permanently separated from the nerve by a small piece of Ivalon sponge. . . . This gave relief of the trigeminal neuralgia without sensory loss during the 5-year follow-up period.[57]

Based on his collaborative studies of tic douloureux with Rand, Jannetta postulated that the crucial point of vascular compression as the cause of hemifacial spasm is at the zone of exit of the facial nerve from the brain stem, where the central myelin changes to peripheral myelin. His first operation to decompress the facial nerve was in February 1966. In 1970, Jannetta reported:

> In the first patient . . . the 7th and 8th cranial nerves looked normal until the brain stem was approached; at this point a small vein along the surface of the pons above the facial nerve was found compressing and distorting this nerve. . . . The vein was coagulated and divided. . . . In the second patient . . . a tortuous left vertebral artery was found compressing the facial nerve at the point just adjacent to the brain stem. This was mobilized and held away from the brain stem by placing gelfoam between the vessel and the brain stem away from the facial and auditory nerves. . . . Five more patients have been operated upon, all with classical hemifacial spasm. All had vascular compression-distortion of the facial nerve at the brain stem. Three patients in whom the facial nerve was not traumatized awoke with hemifacial

spasm which gradually disappeared postoperatively. They have remained free of spasms and without facial weakness.[24]

Since 1966, Jannetta has accumulated a vast experience with MVD as treatment of a variety of lower cranial nerve dysfunction syndromes. For example, in 1991 he and his associates analyzed the results of a selected series of 1,117 patients with trigeminal neuralgia who had been treated by MVD between 1971 and 1989 (Larkins MV, Jannetta PJ, Janosky JE, et al. Microvascular decompression for recurrent trigeminal neuralgia. Presented at the 59th Annual Meeting of the American Association of Neurological Surgeons, New Orleans, Louisiana, April 23, 1991). And in 1990, Jannetta reported the outcome of 366 patients treated in similar fashion for hemifacial spasm.[32] In addition, he has documented his experience with glossopharyngeal neuralgia, essential hypertension, certain vestibulocochlear (VIII) nerve dysfunction syndromes, spontaneous facial palsy, atypical trigeminal neuralgia, and trigeminal neuropathy.[28-30,32,33,35-38,42]

Hypotheses

From the foregoing and additional evidence, Jannetta and others have postulated that the following pathophysiologic steps occur in the development of a posterior fossa cranial nerve dysfunction syndromes caused by vascular compression (with the recognition that such dysfunction syndromes also may result from other causes):

1. The appropriate nerve is compressed by one or more adjacent arteries or veins.[20,23-38] Normally, there are close associations of vessels and nerves in the posterior fossa.[19,21,22,40,43-53,58-63,69-71,74] In an aging individual, these relationships change because of arterial elongation and/or ectasia, brain sagging, changes in the bony configuration of the skull base, etc. As this occurs, one or more vessels are brought into direct contact with the nerve. Jannetta has proposed that the important point of compres-

sion in certain of these syndromes such as tic douloureux and hemifacial spasm is at the point of junction between central and peripheral myelination of the nerve,[43,53,68] ordinarily within a few millimeters of the brain stem (except for the acoustic nerve).[27,28,32] In other syndromes, such as atypical trigeminal neuralgia[29] and spontaneous facial palsy,[32,33] the important point of compression seems to be further lateral.

2. Vascular compression of the nerve leads to demyelination at the point of contact.

3. This compression and demyelination causes ephaptic transmission of nerve action potentials between adjacent axons. Alternatively, it has been postulated that such ectopic excitation of the nerve causes crucial electrophysiologic changes centrally (e.g. within the facial nucleus in the case of hemifacial spasm), or that injury to the nerve leads to aberrant regeneration.[77]

4. Whatever the exact pathophysiologic mechanism, hyperactive dysfunction of the nerve results. For the trigeminal and facial nerves, such hyperactive dysfunction would be expressed as trigeminal neuralgia and hemifacial spasm, respectively.

5. With long-standing and marked vascular compression, some reduction of nerve function also may develop.[27] For the trigeminal nerve this is manifest as mild hypesthesia in some area supplied by that nerve, and for the facial nerve this occurs as mild paresis of some of the ipsilateral facial muscles.

Corollary Expectations

Based on the previous hypotheses, certain consequences might be expected.

1. If nerve compression by one or more vessels at the nerve root entry or exit zone is the major cause of the syndromes under discussion, then nerve compression should be found in every

patient in whom there is not some other obvious cause such as a tumor in the cerebellopontine angle. This is most often the case, but not always. For example, in my initial experience with 48 operations for hemifacial spasm, I identified arterial contact with the facial nerve at its exit zone from the brain stem in 46 (96%), but no abnormality of any type could be seen in one patient.[55] Among 105 operations for tic douloureux, I found arterial contact in 74 (70%), but in 21 there was no recognized abnormality or only minor venous contact.[55] Other surgeons also have reported that vascular compression is not present in 100% of the cases.* Jannetta has commented that surgeons with limited experience with this procedure may not expose or recognize important points of contact between vessels and nerves,[28] but in my personal experience with more than 250 operations for tic douloureux and more than 80 operations for hemifacial spasm, the initial trends cited previously have continued. Even so, some vascular compression may remain hidden from the surgeon's view, especially on the opposite side of the nerve, and crucial nerve-vessel relationships may be altered during the process of surgical exposure (e.g. the nerve may be pulled away from the vessel by retraction).

2. Any posterior fossa cranial nerve with a central-peripheral myelin junction near the brain stem should be involved at times in an appropriate vascular compression dysfunction syndrome. Yet this seldom or never occurs in the case of certain nerves such as the trochlear (IV), abducens (VI), spinal accessory (IX), and hypoglossal (XII). The reason for this discrepancy is still unknown.

3. Vascular nerve compression adjacent to the brain stem should not be seen in asymptomatic individuals. Again, this is often but not always the case. Various investigators have commented on the fact that occasionally vessel-nerve contacts, and even distortion of the nerve by the vessel, can be identified after death in subjects who were asymptomatic during life.[19,21,22,40,46,47,51,58,59] Perhaps some, but certainly not all, of these observations might be explained by the fact that they were made postmortem, on fixed brains usually having been removed from the skull before study. Jannetta has responded to this line of evidence against the etiologic importance of microvascular compression by noting that just as some cadaver brains have apparently significant vascular compression without a history of symptoms during life, some individuals with significant lumbar or cervical disk disease or spondylosis may remain asymptomatic during life, without evidence of radiculopathy.[28]

4. If nerve compression at the brain stem requires arterial elongation, arterial ectasia, brain sagging, or bony remodeling to bring the vessel into contact with the nerve, the condition produced should occur preferentially in older individuals. This certainly is the case for tic douloureux, hemifacial spasm, and glossopharyngeal neuralgia.

5. If vascular compression leads to demyelination, biopsy of the nerve at the point of compression should demonstrate this change. Such biopsies, however, have not often been performed.[65] The surgeon ordinarily chooses MVD as the operative procedure to avoid nerve injury and does not want to complicate the procedure.

6. The evaluation of the electrophysiologic changes found in patients with a vascular compression syndrome should shed light on its etiology and pathophysiology. This topic is discussed in Chapter 2.

7. If vascular compression of a cranial nerve is an important cause of a syndrome, MVD should provide relief without the necessity of injuring the nerve.

*References 1, 3, 5, 10, 21, 39, 41, 54, 64, 67, 73

Although in many such operations, the nerve is mildly traumatized during the dissection, this is not uniformly true. Jannetta has observed that in patients with minimal or no operative trauma, the syndrome may persist for a while before gradually subsiding—an argument against the idea that MVD achieves its effect through mild trauma to the involved nerve.[25-27]

8. When adequate decompression is achieved, relief should occur and should persist. Most patients do experience lasting relief, yet initial relief does not always occur, and the syndrome may recur. The initial failure rate after MVD for tic douloureux is about 7%,[72] and the rate of major recurrence is about 3.5% per year.[10] Regarding hemifacial spasm, about 10% of patients have persistence or recurrence of sufficient severity to require a second operation.[77] Jannetta has stressed that when symptoms recur after initial relief by MVD there often is a mechanical explanation such as slippage of the surgical implant with recurrent nerve compression by the initially responsible vessel, new nerve compression by a previously uninvolved vessel, or nerve compression by a firm implant.[34] In the most recent review of Jannetta's experience with tic douloureux, among 116 patients reoperated upon following an initial MVD at the same institution, compression by one or more arteries was identified in 65.5%, compression by one or more veins in 69.8%, and compression by an implant in 5.2%; only 3.4% of the patients had a negative exploration (Larkins MV, Jannetta PJ, Janosky JE, et al. Microvascular decompression for recurrent trigeminal neuralgia. Presented at the 59th Annual Meeting of the American Association of Neurological Surgeons, New Orleans, Louisiana, April 23, 1991). In contrast, among the patients I have re-explored for persistent or recurrent tic douloureux or hemifacial spasm, I rarely have found an obvious cause.

In explanation of the fact that a repeat MVD for tic douloureux has only about a 50% chance of success (Larkins MV, Jannetta PJ, Janosky JE, at al. Microvascular decompression for recurrent trigeminal neuralgia. Presented at the 59th Annual Meeting of the American Association of Neurological Surgeons. New Orleans, Louisiana, April 23, 1991), Jannetta has stated: "Several mechanical factors may be functional in . . . lack of improvement. Scar formation and gliosis, although mild, may be such as to prevent reformation of normal myelin and axis cylinders; the intrinsic disease within the nerve may be too extensive for repair of the damage. Still other vascular compression may be missed. Secondary changes may have occurred more centrally in the trigeminal system."[34]

Conclusion

The theory of vascular compression of cranial nerves in the posterior fossa is built on various pieces of evidence, some strong and some weak. It is an attractive idea that provides an encompassing view of several syndromes. Seen through the eyes of the believer, the exceptions prove the rule. Seen through the eyes of the skeptic, the exceptions disprove the rule. Yet no matter how the theory will be viewed a century from now, it has provided a helpful framework for investigating certain types of neural dysfunction and has resulted in a valuable approach to treatment, especially for hemifacial spasm and tic douloureux.

References

1. Adams CBT, Kaye AH, Teddy PJ. The treatment of trigeminal neuralgia by posterior fossa microsurgery. *J Neurol Neurosurg Psychiatry.* 1982;45: 1020-1026.
2. Andre. *Observations Pratiques sur les Maladies De L'Urethre, etc.* Paris: Chez Delaguette; 1756.
3. Apfelbaum RI. Surgical management of disorders of the lower cranial nerves. In: Schmidek HH, Sweet WH, eds. *Operative Neurosurgical Techniques: Indications, Methods and Results. II.* 2nd ed. Orlando, Fl: Grune & Stratton Inc; 1988:1097-1109.
4. Bartlett J, Beck EM, ed. *Familiar Quotations: A Collection of Passages, Phrases and Proverbs Traced to*

Their Sources in Ancient and Modern Literature. 15th ed. Boston, Mass: Little, Brown; 1980:160.

5. Bederson JB, Wilson CB. Evaluation of microvascular decompression and partial sensory rhizotomy in 252 cases of trigeminal neuralgia. *J Neurosurg.* 1989;71:359-367.

6. Bell C. On the nerves: giving an account of some experiments on their structure and functions, which lead to a new arrangement of the system. *Philos Trans R Soc Lond.* 1821;111:398-424.

7. Bell C. On the nerves which associate the muscles of the chest in the actions of breathing, speaking and expression: being a continuation of the paper on the structure and functions of the nerves. *Philos Trans R Soc Lond.* 1822;112:284-312.

8. Bell C. On the nerves of the face; Second part. *Philos Trans R Soc Lond.* 1829;119:317-330.

9. Bell C. *The Nervous System of the Human Body.* 2nd ed. London: Longmans; 1830.

10. Burchiel KJ, Clarke H, Haglund M, et al. Long-term efficacy of microvascular decompression in trigeminal neuralgia. *J Neurosurg.* 1988;69:35-38.

11. Campbell E, Keedy C. Hemifacial spasm: a note on the etiology in two cases. *J Neurosurg.* 1947;4:342-347.

12. Dandy WE. Section of the sensory root of the trigeminal nerve at the pons: preliminary report of the operative procedure. *Bull Johns Hopkins Hosp.* 1925;36:105-106.

13. Dandy WE. An operation for the cure of tic douloureux: partial section of the sensory root at the pons. *Arch Surg.* 1929;18:687-734.

14. Dandy WE. Concerning the cause of trigeminal neuralgia. *Am J Surg.* 1934;24:447-455.

15. Flamm ES. Historical observations on the cranial nerves. *J Neurosurg.* 1967;27:285-297.

16. Gardner WJ. Concerning the mechanism of trigeminal neuralgia and hemifacial spasm. *J Neurosurg.* 1962;19:947-958.

17. Gardner WJ, Miklos MV. Response of trigeminal neuralgia to "decompression" of sensory root: discussion of cause of trigeminal neuralgia. *JAMA.* 1959;170:1773-1776.

18. Gardner WJ, Sava GA. Hemifacial spasm—a reversible pathophysiologic state. *J Neurosurg.* 1962;19:240-247.

19. Haines SJ, Jannetta PJ, Zorub DS. Microvascular relations of the trigeminal nerve: an anatomical study with clinical correlation. *J Neurosurg.* 1980;52:381-386.

20. Haines SJ, Martinez AJ, Jannetta PJ. Arterial cross compression of the trigeminal nerve at the pons in trigeminal neuralgia: case report with autopsy findings. *J Neurosurg.* 1979;50:257-259.

21. Hamlyn PJ, King TT. Neurovascular compression in trigeminal neuralgia: a clinical and anatomical study. *J Neurosurg.* 1992;76:948-954.

22. Hardy DG, Rhoton AL Jr. Microsurgical relationships of the superior cerebellar artery and the trigeminal nerve. *J Neurosurg.* 1978;49:669-678.

23. Jannetta PJ. Arterial compression of the trigeminal nerve at the pons in patients with trigeminal neuralgia. *J Neurosurg.* 1967;26(suppl):159-162.

24. Jannetta PJ. Microsurgical exploration and decompression of the facial nerve in hemifacial spasm. *Curr Top Surg Res.* 1970;2:217-220.

25. Jannetta PJ. Trigeminal neuralgia and hemifacial spasm—etiology and definitive treatment. *Trans Am Neurol Assoc.* 1975;100:89-91.

26. Jannetta PJ. Microsurgical approach to the trigeminal nerve for tic douloureux. *Prog Neurol Surg.* 1976;7:180-200.

27. Jannetta PJ. Observations on the etiology of trigeminal neuralgia, hemifacial spasm, acoustic nerve dysfunction and glossopharyngeal neuralgia: definitive microsurgical treatment and results in 117 patients. *Neurochirurgia.* 1977;20:145-154.

28. Jannetta PJ. Neurovascular compression in cranial nerve and systemic disease. *Ann Surg.* 1980;192:518-525.

29. Jannetta PJ. Cranial nerve vascular compression syndromes (other than tic douloureux and hemifacial spasm). *Clin Neurosurg.* 1981;28:445-456.

30. Jannetta PJ. Posterior fossa neurovascular compression syndromes other than neuralgias. In: Wilkins RH, Rengachary SS, eds. *Neurosurgery.* New York, NY: McGraw-Hill; 1985:1901-1906.

31. Jannetta PJ. Treatment of trigeminal neuralgia by micro-operative decompression. In: Youmans JR, ed. *Neurological Surgery: A Comprehensive Reference Guide to the Diagnosis and Management of Neurosurgical Problems.* 3rd ed. Philadelphia, Pa: WB Saunders Co; 1990:3928-3942.

32. Jannetta PJ. Cranial rhizopathies. In: Youmans JR, ed. *Neurological Surgery: A Comprehensive Reference Guide to the Diagnosis and Management of Neurosurgical Problems.* 3rd ed. Philadelphia, Pa: WB Saunders Co; 1990:4169-4182.

33. Jannetta PJ, Bissonette DJ. Bell's palsy: a theory as to etiology. Observations in six patients. *Laryngoscope.* 1978;88:849-854.

34. Jannetta PJ, Bissonette DJ. Management of the failed patient with trigeminal neuralgia. *Clin Neurosurg.* 1985;32:334-347.

35. Jannetta PJ, Møller MB, Møller AR. Disabling positional vertigo. *N Engl J Med.* 1984;310:1700-1705.

36. Jannetta PJ, Møller MB, Møller AR, et al. Neurosurgical treatment of vertigo by microvascular decompression of the eighth cranial nerve. *Clin Neurosurg.* 1986;33:645-665.

37. Jannetta PJ, Robbins LJ. Trigeminal neuropathy—new observations. *Neurosurgery.* 1980;7:347-351.

38. Jannetta PJ, Segal R, Wolfson SK Jr. Neurogenic hypertension: etiology and surgical treatment: I. Observations in 53 patients. *Ann Surg.* 1985;201:391-398.

39. Klun B. Neuro-vascular relationships in trigeminal neuralgia. *Zentralbl Neurochir* 1981;42:123-126.

40. Klun B, Prestor B. Microvascular relations of the trigeminal nerve: an anatomical study. *Neurosurgery.* 1986;19:535-539.

41. Kolluri S, Heros RC. Microvascular decompression for trigeminal neuralgia: a five-year follow-up study. *Surg Neurol.* 1984;22:235-240.

42. Laha RK, Jannetta PJ. Glossopharyngeal neuralgia. *J Neurosurg.* 1977;47:316-320.

43. Lang J, Über Bau, Länge und Gefässbeziehungen der "zentralen" und "peripheren" Strecken der intrazisternalen Hirnnerven. *Zentralbl Neurochir.* 1982;43:217-256.

44. Lang J. *Clinical Anatomy of the Posterior Cranial Fossa and Its Foramina.* Stuttgart, Germany: Thieme; 1991.

45. Martin RG, Grant JL, Peace D, et al. Microsurgical relationships of the anterior inferior cerebellar artery and the facial-vestibulocochlear nerve complex. *Neurosurgery.* 1980;6:483-507.

46. Matsushima T, Fukui M, Suzuki S, et al. The micro-

surgical anatomy of the infratentorial lateral supra-cerebellar approach to the trigeminal nerve for tic douloureux. *Neurosurgery.* 1989;24:890-895.

47. Matsushima T, Inoue T, Fukui M. Arteries in contact with the cisternal portion of the facial nerve in autopsy cases: microsurgical anatomy for neurovascular decompression surgery of hemifacial spasm. *Surg Neurol.* 1990;34:87-93.

48. Matsushima T, Rhoton AL Jr, de Oliveira E, et al. Microsurgical anatomy of the veins of the posterior fossa. *J Neurosurg.* 1983;59:63-105.

49. Mehta L, Fatani J, Rao G. Superior cerebellar artery in the pontine zone. *Saudi Med J.* 1981;2:213-216.

50. Milisavljevic M, Marinkovic S, Lolic-Draganic V, et al. Oculomotor, trochlear, and abducens nerves penetrated by cerebral vessels: microanatomy and possible clinical significance. *Arch Neurol.* 1986;43:58-61.

51. Murali R, Chandy MJ, Rajshekhar V. Neurovascular relationships of the root entry zone of lower cranial nerves: a microsurgical anatomic study in fresh cadavers. *Br J Neurosurg.* 1991;5:349-356.

52. Newton TH, Potts DG. *Radiology of the Skull and Brain.* Vol 2, *Angiography;* Book 2, *Arteries;* Book 3, *Veins.* St. Louis: CV Mosby; 1974.

53. Ouaknine GE. The arterial loops of the pontocerebellar angle: microsurgical anatomy and pathological consideration. *Adv Otorhinolaryngol.* 1982;28:121-138.

54. Petty PG, Southby R, Siu K. Vascular compression: cause of trigeminal neuralgia. *Med J Aust.* 1980;I:166-167.

55. Piatt JH Jr, Wilkins RH. Treatment of tic douloureux and hemifacial spasm by posterior fossa exploration: therapeutic implications of various neurovascular relationships. *Neurosurgery.* 1984;14:462-471.

56. Pinkus RL. Innovation in neurosurgery: Walter Dandy in his day. *Neurosurgery.* 1984;14:623-631.

57. Rand RW. The Gardner neurovascular decompression operation for trigeminal neuralgia. *Acta Neurochir (Wien).* 1981;58:161-166.

58. Rhoton AL Jr. Microsurgical anatomy of the posterior fossa cranial nerves. *Clin Neurosurg.* 1979;26:398-462.

59. Rhoton AL Jr. Microsurgical neurovascular decompression for trigeminal neuralgia: anatomic studies and clinical results. In: Silverstein H, Norrell H, eds. *Neurological Surgery of the Ear. II.* Birmingham, Ala:Aesculapius; 1979:299-311.

60. Rhoton AL Jr. Microsurgical anatomy of decompression operations on the trigeminal nerve. In: Rovit RL, Murali R, Jannetta PJ, eds. *Trigeminal Neuralgia.* Baltimore, Md: Williams & Wilkins; 1990:165-200.

61. Rhoton AL Jr, Buza R. Microsurgical anatomy of the jugular foramen. *J Neurosurg.* 1975;42:541-550.

62. Rhoton AL Jr, Buza RC. Microsurgical anatomy of the jugular foramen. In: Rand RW, ed. *Microneurosurgery,* 3rd ed. St. Louis, Mo: CV Mosby; 1985:692-704.

63. Rhoton AL Jr, Martin RG, Grant JL, et al. Microsurgical relationships of the anterior inferior cerebellar artery and the facial-vestibulocochlear nerve complex. In: Brackmann DE, ed. *Neurological Surgery of the Ear and Skull Base.* New York, NY: Raven Press; 1982:23-37.

64. Richards P, Shawdon H, Illingworth R. Operative findings on microsurgical exploration of the cerebello-pontine angle in trigeminal neuralgia. *J Neurol Neurosurg Psychiatry.* 1983;46:1098-1101.

65. Ruby JR, Jannetta PJ. Hemifacial spasm: ultrastructural changes in the facial nerve induced by neurovascular compression. *Surg Neurol.* 1975;4:369-370.

66. Schultze F. Linksseitiger Facialiskrampf in Folge eines Aneurysma der Arteria vertebralis sinistra. *Virchows Arch.* 1875;65:385-391.

67. Sindou M, Szapiro J. Prognostic factors implicated in the microsurgical treatment of trigeminal neuralgia. In: Samii M, ed. *Surgery In and Around the Brain Stem and the Third Ventricle.* New York, NY: Springer-Verlag; 1986:273-279.

68. Skinner HA. Some histologic features of the cranial nerves. *Arch Neurol Psychiatry.* 1931;25:356-372.

69. Stopford JSB. The arteries of the pons and medulla oblongata. *J Anat Physiol.* 1916;50:131-164, 255-280.

70. Sunderland S. The arterial relations of the internal auditory meatus. *Brain.* 1945;68:23-27.

71. Sunderland S. Neurovascular relations and anomalies at the base of the brain. *J Neurol Neurosurg Psychiatry.* 1948;11:243-257.

72. Sweet WH. Trigeminal neuralgia: problems as to cause and consequent conclusions regarding treatment. In: Wilkins RH, Rengachary SS, eds. *Neurosurgery Update II.* New York, NY: McGraw-Hill; 1991:366-372.

73. van Loveren H, Tew JM Jr, Keller JT, et al. A 10-year experience in the treatment of trigeminal neuralgia: comparison of percutaneous stereotaxic rhizotomy and posterior fossa exploration. *J Neurosurg.* 1982;57:757-764.

74. Watt JC, McKillop AN. Relation of arteries to roots of nerves in posterior cranial fossa in man. *Arch Surg.* 1935;30:336-345.

75. Wilkins RH. Trigeminal neuralgia: introduction. In: Wilkins RH, Rengachary SS, eds. *Neurosurgery.* New York, NY: McGraw-Hill; 1985:2337-2344.

76. Wilkins RH. Historical perspectives. In: Rovit RL, Murali R, Jannetta PJ, eds. *Trigeminal Neuralgia.* Baltimore, Md: Williams & Wilkins; 1990:1-25.

77. Wilkins RH. Hemifacial spasm: a review. *Surg Neurol.* 1991;36:251-277.

78. Wilkins RH, Brody IA. Neurological classics XXVI: Bell's palsy and Bell's phenomenon. *Arch Neurol.* 1969;21:661-669.

CHAPTER 5

Operative Positioning and Perioperative Management

Harry R. van Loveren, MD, John M. Tew, Jr., MD, and Patricia Fernandez, MD

This chapter is dedicated to the concept that proper patient positioning enhances the limits of surgical exposure, the ease of exposure, and the surgeon's comfort so that the surgical outcome will improve. Improper positioning results in diminished success, avoidable complications, and surgical fatigue affecting judgment. In surgery of the posterior fossa, the stakes are high. "Position yourself for success!"

Proper positioning for surgery of the cranial nerves of the posterior fossa must achieve certain minimum standards which include the following[8]:

- Adequately exposing the cranial nerves with minimum retraction of the cerebellum or brain stem;
- Facilitating respiratory mechanics and cardiovascular function;
- Avoiding severe distortion of the cervical anatomy which might cause injury to the spinal cord and nerves, or might compromise blood flow to or from the brain;
- Minimizing the risk of air embolism; and
- Providing comfort for the surgeon.

Patient positions traditionally used for this surgery include prone (Concorde), lateral oblique ("park bench") (Figure 1A), and sitting. No one position fulfills every requirement, but the lateral oblique position has evolved as the preferred one. This position is more easily established than the others; it provides the surgeon with adequate surgical access and with the ability to operate while sitting. The risk of air embolism in the park bench position is lower when compared with the sitting position, although it is not totally eliminated. Orthostatic hypotension under anesthesia is not a problem, but a patient in the right lateral decubitus position may show a mean arterial pressure lower than when compared with the supine position prior to positioning. The movement of the ribs and diaphragm of the downside hemithorax are restricted, causing a 10% reduction in vital capacity. With controlled ventilation under general anesthesia, this restriction will not become a limiting factor. Limiting factors to the application of this position may include instability of the thoracic cage, massive obesity, or late pregnancy.

Preoperative Preparation

In a standing patient (with the head and neck in a neutral position), the suboccipital bone is nearly parallel with the floor. Access to the posterior fossa by the infratentorial route therefore requires significant cervical flexion to bring the suboccipital bone parallel to the spine. Patients, especially those with foramen magnum compromise, should be tested by active cervical flexion for at least 5 minutes. Significant neurologic symptoms warn of imminent neurologic damage if cervical flexion is maintained during prolonged surgery.[5]

In cases when the sigmoid sinus may be injured or sacrificed, the adequacy of contralateral venous drainage must be assessed by angiography. If the surgeon anticipates a need to assess the circulation intraoperatively during posterior fossa vascular surgery, a femoral artery sheath must be placed in the upside leg while the patient is still supine and must be maintained by continuous pressure irrigation with heparinized saline.

Appropriate hemodynamic monitoring includes adequate venous access and an arterial line for continuous monitoring of blood pressure. Urine output is measured by an indwelling Foley catheter. A catheter may be avoided in young, hemodynamically stable patients undergoing relatively brief (less than 1½ hours) functional procedures, such as posterior fossa exploration for trigeminal microvascular decompression.[7] Lumbar cerebrospinal fluid (CSF) drainage is contraindicated in patients with mass lesions. If the cisterna magna is exposed during the approach, drainage of CSF will be achieved rapidly by opening the arachnoid layer. Small superior craniotomies, such as those used for trigeminal nerve exploration, will not expose the cisterna magna, but we routinely perform lumbar puncture after anesthetic induction prior to the posterior fossa exploration.

Although the patient's risk of air embolism is reduced well below that associated with the sitting position, embolism can occur when a gradient of greater than or equal to 5 cm exists between the right atrium of the heart and the upper pole of the wound.[1,7] Under these conditions, negative pressure causes an ingress of air to the sectioned veins rather than an egress of blood. This phenomenon intensifies if the veins are encased in bone or by fibrous tissue, thus preventing their collapse. Accumulation of air within the right atrium can be monitored by transcutaneous Doppler and can be removed by a catheter placed in the right atrium prior to surgery. We do not routinely monitor for air embolism when using the lateral oblique position.

Intubation is accomplished using an armored endotracheal tube, which prevents kinking of the tube with cervical flexion and increasing ventilation pressures. Electrocardiographic monitoring is particularly critical in posterior fossa operations because manipulation of the brain stem or cranial nerves produces cardiac arrhythmias in 25% to 50% of adult patients.[1,2,9]

Critical to preoperative preparation is a detailed discussion with the anesthesia personnel regarding patient positioning and potential complications as noted previously. If cranial nerve stimulation or evoked potential monitoring will be used during positioning or later in the operation, the use of various anesthetic agents that will not suppress these parameters must be agreed upon.

Positioning
The Room

Although there are logical principles for positioning each person and piece of equipment in the operating room, at times these principles will be compromised. Compromise will be most notable when using the left lateral oblique position. Throughout this chapter, the assumption is that the surgeon is right-hand dominant and that the patient is in a right lateral oblique position (Figure 1).

The surgeon sits at the patient's back (level with the shoulders), facing the posterior fossa. In principle, the scrub nurse stands at the surgeon's right, thus passing instruments without crossing the operative field (a maneuver most distracting during microsurgery). The assistant surgeon stands at the surgeon's right. The surgeon's left hand generally is stationary for either suction or retraction and poses a constant barrier to the assistant's entry into the operative field. The assistant surgeon has greater access around the more mobile right hand of the surgeon; however, in the right lateral oblique position, this principle is compromised. By using specialized tubing that diminishes dead space, the anesthesiologist may overcome the desire to see the endotracheal tube entering the

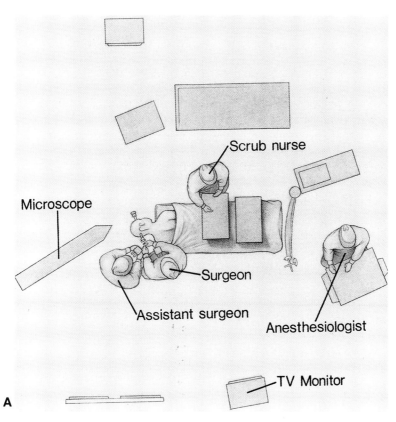

Figure 1. (A) *Room setup for the right lateral oblique position.* (B) *Modified room setup for the left lateral oblique position. (From Tew JM, Jr, van Loveren H.* Operative Microneurosurgery: Atlas of Neurosurgical Procedures. *W.B. Saunders. In press; with permission.)*

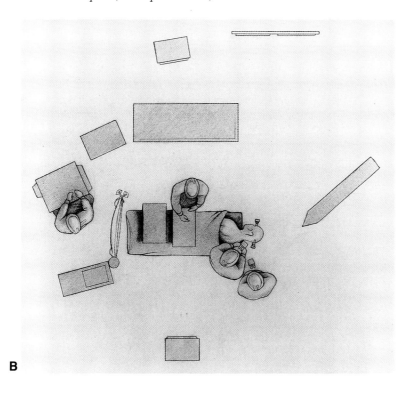

patient's mouth and may assume a position at the foot of the table.

The primary purpose of a television monitor is to allow the scrub nurse to follow the operation and anticipate the needs of the surgeon. The monitor is positioned to the nurse's advantage rather than for other observers in the room. The surgical microscope is used directly over the patient's head. The instrument table and the back table are at the same height. If access to the lower body is anticipated for either intraoperative angiography or tissue grafting, the instrument table should be portable and removable without breaking the sterile field of either the table or the patient.

The Patient

General anesthesia is induced and the patient is intubated in the supine position. All necessary lines are inserted, including the Foley catheter. Pneumatic compression boots applied to the calves are inflated just prior to inducing general anesthesia to prevent venous stasis. If intraoperative angiography is anticipated, a femoral catheter sheath is placed in the groin. The Mayfield three-pin head holder (Ohio Medical Instruments) is applied while the patient is still supine, using 40 lbs/inch^2 pressure with the two-pin lever arm on the downside of the head for support.[6]

The patient is turned on his or her side, guiding the head and neck with the Mayfield head holder. In the classic lateral oblique position, the patient is slightly oblique with the chest angled approximately 10° toward the floor. A gelatin axillary roll is placed beneath the chest wall just below the axilla to prevent brachial plexus compression by the shoulder or occlusion of the axillary artery. The bottom leg is flexed at the hip and knee to stabilize the patient on the table, while the top leg should be kept relatively straight. A pillow between the patient's knees will prevent pressure sores. The patient is secured to the table with a 3-inch cloth tape across the body just below the iliac crest and

across the knee, which is first padded with a folded blanket. Tape also is used to retract the shoulder down and expand the operative field (Figure 2A).

The thorax is elevated 15° to enhance venous drainage while keeping the venous pressure gradient between the cervical veins and right atrium at a minimum. If indicated, a lumbar puncture may be performed or a lumbar drain may be inserted at this point in the positioning process.

The Head

Beginning with the patient's head and neck in a neutral position, the neck is flexed until the chin rests within 3-finger breadths of the sternum. This maneuver rotates the suboccipital bone from its oblique position in neutral to a more vertical position and increases the distance between the inion and atlas, thus facilitating exposure of the posterior fossa. Extreme flexion is avoided because it can cause jugular vein compression with elevation of intracranial pressure, cerebellar engorgement, and/or venous hemorrhage (Figure 2B). An armored endotracheal tube prevents kinking, which results in high ventilation pressures.

The Incision

There are three basic incisions for posterior fossa surgery: linear paramedian, linear midline, and hockey stick (lateral hemispheral) (Figure 3).

Linear Paramedian Incision

The linear paramedian incision is preferred for exposure of the lateral cerebellopontine angle (CPA), functional neurosurgery (e.g. microvascular decompression, rhizotomy) of cranial nerves V-X, and small CPA tumors. The incision is centered 1 cm medial to the mastoid notch and extends 4 cm above and below the mastoid notch. The incision may be

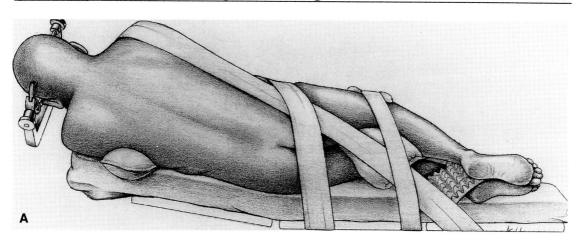

Figure 2. (A) Patient position on the table; right lateral oblique position. (B) Close-up of head position; right lateral oblique position. (From Tew JM, Jr, van Loveren H. Operative Microneurosurgery: Atlas of Neurosurgical Procedures. W.B. Saunders. In press; with permission.)

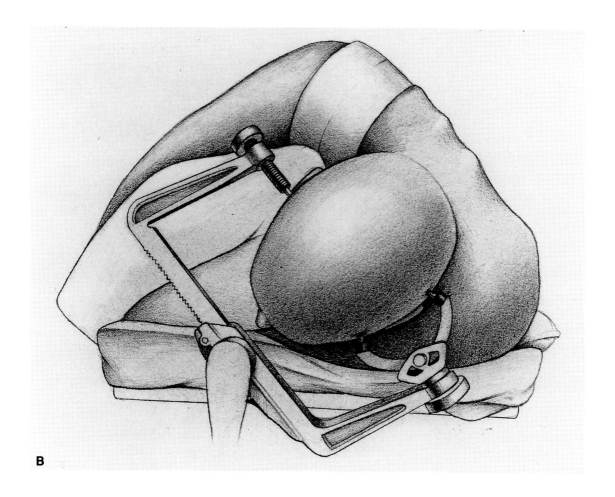

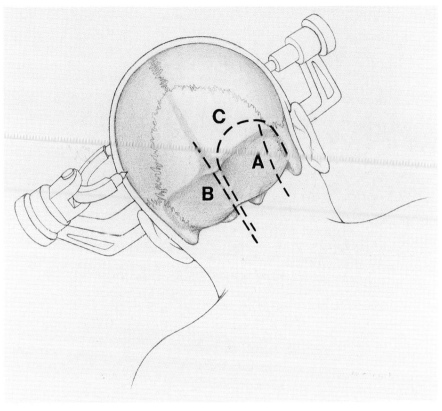

Figure 3. Preferred incisions for posterior fossa surgery: *(A)* linear paramedian incision, *(B)* linear midline incision, and *(C)* lateral hemispheral incision. *(From Tew JM, Jr, van Loveren H.* Operative Microneurosurgery: Atlas of Neurosurgical Procedures. *W.B. Saunders. In press; with permission.)*

modified superiorly 1 cm for decompression of the trigeminal root and inferiorly 1 cm for vagoglossopharyngeal neurectomy. The muscles are split along the same line of incision down to the periosteum of the occipital bone. The surgeon must exercise caution to avoid injuring the vertebral artery at the inferior pole of the muscle-splitting incision.

Linear Midline Incision

The linear midline incision is preferred for a bilateral suboccipital craniotomy to expose midline lesions. The skin incision, extending from the spinous process of C2 cephalad across the foramen magnum and occipital bone, ends 2 cm above the superior nuchal line. The cutaneous flap is developed to both sides of the midline at the superior

nuchal line. The myofascial flap is incised transversely at the superior nuchal line, leaving a superior myofascial cuff for reattachment. The cervical muscles are split in the avascular midline.[4]

Lateral Hemispheral "Hockey-Stick" Incision

The lateral hemispheral incision is preferable to expose tumors of the cerebellar hemisphere and large tumors of the CPA. The skin incision begins at the midpoint of the mastoid bone, turns medially above the superior nuchal line, and continues inferiorly along the midline down to the spinous process of C2. The cutaneous flap is developed superiorly so that the myofascial flap can be incised transversely at the superior nuchal line, leaving a superior myofascial flap for

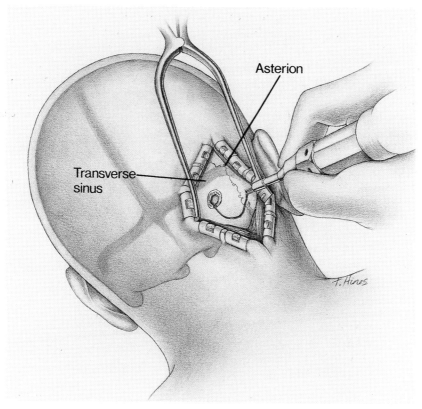

Figure 4. *Entry burr hole 1 cm below and medial to the asterion. Unilateral suboccipital craniotomy for exposure of the upper and lateral cerebellopontine angle. (From Tew JM, Jr, van Loveren H.* Operative Microneurosurgery: Atlas of Neurosurgical Procedures. *W.B. Saunders. In press; with permission.)*

reattachment. The cervical muscles are split in the avascular midline.

The Craniotomy

The surgeon must be able to project the planned craniotomy onto the occipital bone based on surface landmarks. Only the classic suboccipital craniotomy is described in this chapter as a method illustrating the concept of "positioning the craniotomy."

The asterion lies just medial and inferior to the transverse sigmoid sinus junction. A single burr hole is made 1 cm medial and inferior to the asterion. After dissection of the dura surrounding the burr hole, a free bone flap is turned with a power-driven craniotome. Further bone is removed with a rongeur laterally to expose the medial edge

of the sigmoid sinus (Figure 4). Open mastoid air cells are sealed with bone wax to prevent CSF rhinorrhea (or otorrhea if the tympanic membrane is incompetent). For a superior exposure, the occipital bone is removed to expose the inferior edge of the transverse sinus. Inferior exposure is maximized by resecting the bone of the foramen magnum.

Postoperative Care

The primary management of postoperative complications is prevention. The most common complications are infection, CSF leakage, and delayed formation of hematoma, causing mass effect or obstructive hydrocephalus. Infection may be prevented by using sterile techniques and perioperative antibiotics. While there is no statistical evidence that perioperative antibiotics prevent infection, some evidence suggests that they will not alter normal flora leading to superinfection if used in a single dose administered prior to skin incision. Antibiotics are continued beyond 24 hours postoperatively only if a significant break in sterility occurred during the operation.

CSF leakage can be prevented by using a proper closure technique. The dura is closed in watertight fashion with absorbable sutures. The authors maintain a low threshold for using a fascial or synthetic patch graft covered with fibrin glue to achieve a watertight closure. The bone edges are rewaxed before closure to seal any overlooked open mastoid air cells. The craniotomy bone flap or fragments are replaced to decrease the epidural dead space. Fragments of bone can be applied over the dura as a malleable "bone pâte." If there is no postoperative mass effect, daily lumbar punctures sometimes are performed to decrease CSF pressure on the dural and myofascial closure.

The most dreaded complication of posterior fossa surgery is delayed hematoma formation or cerebellar swelling that can lead to both mass effect or obstructive hydrocephalus. Resection of the lateral one-third of the cerebellar hemisphere is preferable to over-retraction or closing over a "tight" cerebellum. If a large tumor or vascular malformation has been resected, an emergency burr hole is placed prior to closing (6 cm above and 4 cm lateral to the inion) for emergency postoperative ventricular cannulation and aspiration of CSF. A bedside sterile ventricular needle should accompany these patients.

The patient is managed by the neurosurgical critical care team in the neurosurgical intensive care unit for the first 24 hours. Extubation is delayed if swelling is anticipated, if surgery exceeds 6 hours, or if the patient emerges slowly from anesthesia. Parameters monitored include neurologic function, blood pressure by arterial line, pulse by electrocardiogram, arterial O_2 saturation, urine output, and, if indicated, pulmonary wedge pressure by Swan-Ganz catheter. Arterial pressure is maintained within the range of auto-regulation (less than 160 mm Hg systolic) by titration with a nitroprusside infusion. Oxygen tension is maintained above 100 mm Hg.

The Foley catheter is discontinued as soon as possible to avoid urinary tract infection. Pneumatic compression boots are maintained until the patient is weight-bearing. If the corneal reflex (cranial nerve V) is diminished or absent, artificial tears and lubricant are prescribed. Facial motor function is tested (cranial nerve VII). If eyelid closure is weak or absent, then artificial tears, lubricant, and nighttime eyelid closure with a gentle patch or tape are prescribed. The combination of poor eyelid closure and diminished corneal reflex may necessitate a temporary lateral tarsorrhaphy for corneal protection. If the gag reflex (cranial nerves IX and X) is absent or diminished, oral feeding is delayed and nutrition is provided through a nasogastric tube. Hematocrit, serum chemistries, and arterial blood gas tensions are routinely monitored.

Neurologic deterioration tends to be precipitous. Warning signs include a decreased level of consciousness, altered respiratory pattern, hypertension, tachycardia, or bradycardia. The first concern is respiratory arrest. An immediate decision must be made whether to intubate the patient for airway protection or proceed with evaluation. Evaluation includes emergency computed tomography (CT) scan to detect hematoma or obstructive hydrocephalus. If the patient's condition is judged too critical to delay intervention until the CT scan, the ventricle is cannulated, and CSF pressure is decreased. If the patient's condition improves, a CT scan is obtained. If the patient's condition fails to improve, an emergency exploratory surgery of the posterior fossa is performed. More patients have been injured while the need for exploration was debated than by the surgery itself.[3]

References

1. Albin MS, Babinski M, Maroon JC, et al. Anesthetic management of posterior fossa surgery in the sitting position. *Acta Anaesth Scand.* 1976;20:117-128.

2. Artru AA, Cucchiara RF, Messick JM. Cardiorespiratory and cranial-nerve sequelae of surgical procedures involving the posterior fossa. *Anesthesiology.* 1980;52:83-86.

3. Horwitz NH, Rizzoli HV. *Postoperative Complications of Intracranial Neurological Surgery.* Baltimore, Md: Williams & Wilkins; 1982.

4. Kempe LG. *Operative Neurosurgery; Volume 2: Posterior Fossa, Spinal Cord, and Peripheral Nerve Disease.* New York, NY: Springer-Verlag; 1970.

5. Kurze T. The surgical removal of acoustic tumors. In: Ransohoff J, ed. *Modern Technics in Neurosurgery.* Mount Kisco, NY: Futura Publishing Co; 1984;30:1-16.

6. Martin JT. *Positioning in Anesthesia and Surgery.* 2nd ed. Philadelphia, Pa: WB Saunders Co; 1987.

7. Newfield P. Anesthesia for posterior fossa procedures. In: Cottrell JT, Turndorf FL, eds. *Anesthesia and Neurosurgery,* 2nd ed. St. Louis, Mo: Mosby, 1986:131-149.

8. Stewart DH, Krawachenko J. Patient positioning. In: Wilkins RH, Rengachary SS, eds. *Neurosurgery.* New York, NY: McGraw-Hill; 1985:452-457.

9. Whitby JD. Electrocardiography during posterior fossa operations. *Brit J Anaesth.* 1963;35:624-630.

CHAPTER 6

Intraoperative Neurophysiologic Monitoring of Cranial Nerves

Aage R. Møller, PhD

Purpose and Goals of Intraoperative Monitoring of Cranial Nerves

It has recently become evident that using relatively common neurophysiologic techniques in the neurosurgical operating room is valuable in (1) reducing complications in the form of neurologic deficits and (2) aiding the surgeon in the operation.

The principals underlying uses of intraoperative neurophysiologic recordings to reduce neurologic complications are (1) that it is possible to detect, before they become permanent, changes in function of the systems being surgically manipulated by recording electrical potentials and (2) that reversal of the surgical manipulation can prevent the induced change from resulting in permanent neurologic deficits.

One might assume that the results of intraoperative neurophysiologic monitoring would be used to warn the surgeon when manipulations have caused changes that could result in permanent deficits, and such warning of imminent disaster is no doubt one use of neurophysiologic intraoperative monitoring. Such monitoring can be of wider usefulness, however. For example, when any change in the recorded potentials greater than the normal variations is communicated to the surgeon, the surgeon can use that information to help carry out the operation so the risk of injury is kept at a minimum. In some cases, intra-operative neurophysiologic monitoring can also help the surgeon achieve optimal therapeutic benefit for the patient.

When the results of intraoperative neurophysiologic monitoring are used in this way, they can play an active role in helping avoid the risk of neurologic deficits. If information about changes in intraoperative responses is communicated when the changes are first detected, the surgeon is provided information about what manipulations caused the changes and has the option to remedy the problem immediately or to wait and see if the changes continue or become worse. To provide the surgeon this option, the monitoring team must communicate promptly all changes in the recorded potentials that can be assumed to be a result of surgical manipulations.

If the only information conveyed to the surgeon implies an imminent risk of permanent neurologic deficit, an important advantage of intraoperative monitoring is missed: only when all changes in the recorded potentials are reported promptly can the surgeon identify what manipulation caused the change in the physiologic response. If the surgeon is not informed when the changes begin to affect the function of the system being monitored, the opportunity to reverse the step that led to the change is lost.

When the surgeon is informed only when the recorded potentials indicate a high risk of neurologic deficit, the surgeon in many cases has only two options: (1) to terminate the operation to avoid the neurologic deficit, or (2) to proceed cautiously and hope that the deficit incurred will be mild. If the intraoperative monitoring team stays in close communication with the surgeon, this situation can usually be avoided.

The subject of "false positive" responses in intraoperative monitoring has been much discussed. However, changes reported to the surgeon, even though they are not likely to lead to permanent neurologic deficits, are not really "false positive" responses because when intraoperative monitoring is used optimally it provides the surgeon all information available to prevent placing the patient at any risk of deficit.

Even though the operating room is a rather different environment than the clinical neurophysiology testing laboratory, relatively standard neurophysiologic recording techniques can be used with one important difference, namely, that the results of intraoperative monitoring must be available instantaneously in order to be of value. This places considerably greater responsibility on the personnel who perform intraoperative monitoring compared with those who perform clinical testing for diagnostic purposes. The person responsible for interpreting intraoperative monitoring must be able to interpret the results immediately and must have enough experience to make judgments about the nature and implications of observed changes in sensory evoked potentials and electromyographic (EMG) potentials. To make such judgments, the neurophysiologic monitoring personnel must have basic knowledge about how neuroelectrical potentials are generated and must understand the physiology of the systems being monitored.

It is also important that the people responsible for intraoperative monitoring of evoked potentials know about the recording equipment they use and have practical experience in troubleshooting equipment used to obtain neurophysiologic recordings. In this way they can identify and resolve promptly the technical problems that may arise in a modern operating room with its multitude of sources of electrical interference. The neuro-physiologist in charge of intraoperative neurophysiologic monitoring must also be knowledgeable about the surgical procedures being monitored and know the basics of modern anesthesia techniques. This will enable him to evaluate whether changes in recorded electrical potentials are related to harmless surgical maneuvers such as irrigation with hypothermic fluid or changes in the anesthesia regimen.

For intraoperative monitoring of the function of neural systems to be successful, a suitable anesthesia regimen must be used. Therefore, the anesthesia team must be made aware of specific requirements related to neurophysiologic monitoring in individual cases. For example, when motor nerves are monitored by recording EMG potentials, the anesthesia regimen must exclude muscle relaxants; and the cortical components of, for example, somatosensory evoked potentials (SSEPs) are greatly affected by inhalation anesthesia. Potential problems with anesthesia for intraoperative monitoring can usually be solved or avoided by the neurophysiologic monitoring team and the anesthesia team communicating their needs to one another both before and during the operation.

Another prerequisite for successful use of intraoperative neurophysiologic monitoring techniques is that the surgeon understand and be able to interpret the information presented by the neurophysiologic monitoring team, and that the surgeon be prepared to make the appropriate changes in the surgical procedure.

It has, for various reasons, been difficult to quantify the benefits of intraoperative monitoring. However, it is generally agreed that proper use of neurophysiologic monitoring techniques can help reduce the incidence of permanent neurologic deficits. It is also widely recognized that this monitoring during neurosurgical procedures can help the surgeon (1) identify important neural structures when the anatomy has been distorted by disease processes or injury and (2) detect when specific neural pathways have been manipulated. Such information can help the surgeon carry out the operation in an optimal way, and it can facilitate the development of better surgical methods. For example, intraoperative recordings of the abnormal muscle response characteristic for patients with hemifacial spasm can directly aid the surgeon in achieving the therapeutic goal of a microvascular decompression (MVD) operation, i.e. to relieve the spasm. When intraoperative neurophysiologic recordings show the absence of the abnormal muscle response, the surgeon can be assured that the cause of hemifacial spasm has been removed.[31]

Intraoperative neurophysiologic monitoring has contributed to improvements in surgical methods because monitoring allows, for the first time, direct identification of exactly which surgical manipulations cause injuries. Intraoperative monitoring is also of benefit in teaching because it gives direct feedback to the surgeon regarding some of the adverse effects of surgical manipulations. However, intraoperative neurophysiologic monitoring is still in its infancy, and methods need to be standardized and norms defined for the qualifications necessary in the personnel who perform such monitoring.

General Information on Electrophysiologic Methods in the Operating Room

Techniques to monitor sensory cranial nerves have been most successful for monitoring the vestibulocochlear nerve (VIII) to reduce the incidence of impairment of hearing.[7,8,10,17,25,33,37] Technological problems associated with presentation of efficient stimuli have so far made it impossible to make optimal use of monitoring the vestibular portion of the vestibulocochlear nerve or the optic nerve (II).[17,39]

Intraoperative neurophysiologic monitoring of cranial motor nerves has been particularly effective for the facial nerve (VII)[26] and the nerves that control the extraocular muscles, oculomotor (III), trochlear (IV), and abducens (VI).[16,17,40] For these nerves, monitoring has been shown to decrease the incidence of reduced or lost function as a complication of such operations, mainly by making it possible

to identify these nerves during the operation and detect when surgical manipulations are causing injuries to these nerves. These nerves are located by the surgeon probing tissue with an electrical nerve stimulator while EMG responses are recorded from each of the extraocular muscles. Some institutions have monitored intraoperatively the part of the vagal nerve (X) that innervates the laryngeal muscles, and other institutions have monitored the motor portion of the glossopharyngeal nerve (IX). The hypoglossal nerve (XII) has been monitored by recording EMG responses from the tongue, and the spinal accessory nerve (XI) has been monitored by recording EMG potentials from the trapezoid muscles.[17]

Monitoring Auditory Function

Auditory function is most often monitored for the purpose of preserving function of cranial nerve VIII, which is at risk in operations to remove acoustic tumors or other skull base tumors and in MVD operations to treat such cranial nerve dysfunctions as trigeminal neuralgia, hemifacial spasm, glossopharyngeal neuralgia, disabling positional vertigo, or tinnitus.[5-8,17,32,33,35] In some cases in which the brain stem is manipulated it is of value to monitor brain stem auditory evoked potentials (BAEPs) because such monitoring has been found to detect changes in the function of the nuclei and fiber tracts of the ascending auditory pathway.[17]

Function of the vestibulocochlear nerve can be monitored either by recording BAEPs in response to transient stimuli such as click sounds, or by recording the compound action potentials (CAPs) by placing the recording electrode directly on the exposed vestibulocochlear nerve or in its vicinity.[17,25,42]

Brain Stem Auditory Evoked Potentials

BAEPs and SSEPs were among the first modalities routinely monitored during neurosurgical operations.[3,6-8,10,37] The BAEP is characterized by a series of 5-7 vertex-positive

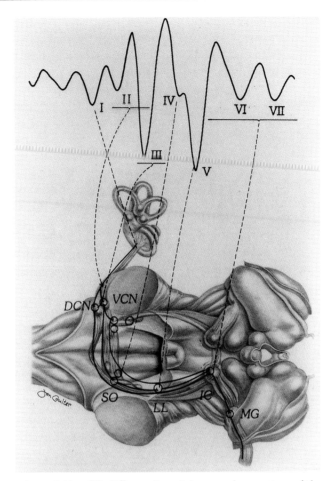

Figure 1. Simplified illustration of the neural generators of the brain stem auditory evoked potentials, based on the results of intracranial recordings in patients undergoing neurosurgical operations. Note that the vertex-positive peaks are shown as downward deflections in accordance with common practice for displaying neuroelectrical potentials. Some authors, however, prefer to display the brain stem auditory evoked potentials with the vertex-positive peaks as upward deflections.[27]

peaks that occur between 2 ms and 10 ms after the presentation of a high-intensity transient sound such as a click or a short, high-intensity tone burst. These peaks, usually given Roman numerals, are generally assumed to reflect successive activations of the vestibulocochlear nerve and the nuclei and fiber tracts of the ascending auditory pathway (cochlear nucleus, superior olivary complex, lateral lemniscus, and inferior colliculus).[11,20,22-24,32] This pathway crosses the midline at the level of the superior olivary complex, so that the responses from the lateral lemniscus and inferior colliculus are from the side opposite the stimulated ear.[20,24] Because of the great complexity of the ascending auditory pathway, each peak, except peaks I and II, in the human BAEP receives contributions from more than one structure, and in addition each structure contributes to more than one peak.[27] (A simplified illustration of the main neural generators of the earliest 5 peaks of the BAEP is shown in Figure 1.) The two earliest peaks (I and II) in the human BAEP are generated by the distal and proximal portions of the vestibulocochlear nerve, which together have a length of about 2.5 cm.[12,13] The BAEP is little affected by general anesthesia, but hypothermia results in prolongation of the latencies by an amount that becomes noticeable when the patient's temperature is lowered by 2.5⁰ to 3.0⁰ C.[15,41]

Practical Aspects of Intraoperative BAEP Monitoring

Although BAEPs can be recorded in the operating room using techniques similar to those used in the clinic, several variations should be considered. The vertex-earlobe placement used in the clinic can be used for recording BAEPs intraoperatively, but it is often more suitable to use needle electrodes such as subdermal platinum needles rather than the surface electrodes that are commonly used in the clinic. This is because needle electrodes can be applied more quickly than surface electrodes, and when secured by a good-quality "micropore" adhesive tape, reliable recordings can be obtained for many hours. There is, however, a slight risk that a burn can occur at the electrode site if faulty electrocautery equipment is used or if the return electrode is faulty. Faulty return electrodes from the electrocautery equipment to the patient can lead to high frequency electrocautery energy returning to the cautery equipment via the recording electrodes. More severe burns may occur when needle electrodes are used rather than surface electrodes because of the smaller surface area of needle electrodes. However, most state-of-the-art electrocautery devices have automatic checks of the return (ground) electrode, so occurrence of such burns is highly unlikely.

Click sounds are as suitable for stimuli in the operating room as they are in the clinic, but the large earphones that are often used in the clinic are not suitable for use in the operating room. The author and colleagues have used miniature stereo earphones in intraoperative monitoring for more than 7

years with good results.[17] Such earphones fit into the outer ear with the sound-generating (front) part of the earphone facing the ear canal. When secured in a watertight fashion by the same type of adhesive tape as is recommended for securing the electrodes, they will remain in place despite manipulations during the operation and fluid will not reach the earphone. Other earphones suitable for use in the operating room are those that connect the sound transducer to the ear by a plastic tube.

It is common for intraoperative monitoring to use clicks of alternating polarity because this cancels the stimulus artifact. Alternating click stimuli give satisfactory results in patients with normal hearing because the responses have very little dependence on the polarity of the stimuli. However, the response to clicks of opposite polarity can be rather different in patients who have hearing loss,[34] and therefore clicks of only one polarity should be used in such patients. Rarefaction clicks are probably preferable. The stimulus artifact can be reduced by other means, such as by using the type of earphones mentioned above and by using suitable filter settings on the recording amplifier in connection with zero-phase digital filtering applied after averaging the responses.[18]

When BAEPs are used to monitor function of the vestibulocochlear nerve, the results must be interpreted with as little delay as possible so that changes in the recorded potentials can be detected as soon as possible after they occur. Early detection is important because if too much time elapses between the occurrence of a change in the evoked potentials and the detection of the change, it may be difficult to determine what surgical manipulation caused the change and, therefore, what to do to reverse the change. Thus to prevent permanent injury, changes in recorded potentials should be communicated to the surgeon as soon as possible after the change has occurred.

Signal averaging has been the prevailing method for improving the quality of recorded potentials so they can be interpreted, but this implies that it takes a certain time to obtain an interpretable record. Spectral filtering of the recorded potentials, however, can improve the signal-to-noise ratio and thereby facilitate the interpretation of recorded potentials without causing any delay. Spectral filtering therefore should be maximally utilized. The use of zero-phase digital filtering of recorded potentials is optimal because this technique permits aggressive filtering but does not shift the peaks of the response in time.[18] Figure 2 shows examples of BAEPs recorded in the operating room, before and after they were subjected to zero-phase digital filtering. The various peaks are much clearer after the filtering, so much so that computerized routines can be used to identify the various peaks and to print out their latencies totally automatically (rather than by using a manually operated cursor).[17,18]

It is notable that the stimulus artifact in Figure 2 is small and of short (0.5 ms) duration. This is because these records were obtained using miniature stereo earphones to deliver the stimuli for obtaining intraoperative BAEPs. Although the earphones and their leads were not shielded in any way, the stimulus artifacts do not overlap in time with the response and they can easily be removed automatically by using computer routines.

In the operating room, a baseline BAEP should be obtained after the patient has been anesthetized but before the operation begins. That baseline should be used for comparison with the responses obtained during the operation.

It is important that the ears and hearing of patients in whom auditory evoked potentials are to be obtained intraoperatively are examined preoperatively. Cerumen, if present, must be removed from the ear canal. Also, a complete audiogram and preferably BAEP recordings should be obtained preoperatively. If the patient is deaf before the operation it is obviously not meaningful to attempt to monitor BAEPs intraoperatively. It is also of importance to know preoperatively if the patient has a hearing loss because that can result in an abnormal BAEP.

Compound Action Potentials Recorded Directly from the Exposed Vestibulocochlear Nerve

Even when optimal recording parameters and optimal spectral filtering are used, it takes considerable time to obtain an interpretable BAEP record. The time necessary to detect changes in neural conduction time in the vestibulocochlear nerve may be an obstacle in certain situations to the use of neurophysiologic monitoring of evoked potentials. In operations where the vestibulocochlear nerve becomes exposed, recording CAPs directly from the exposed nerve can solve some of these problems. CAPs recorded from the vestibulocochlear nerve can be viewed directly on an oscilloscope, and therefore these potentials do not need to be averaged; or only a few responses need to be averaged in order to obtain an interpretable record.[17,25] This naturally reduces the time necessary for obtaining an interpretable record.

The intracranial portion of the vestibulocochlear nerve is more fragile than other cranial nerves of the posterior fossa because the transition zone between peripheral and central myelin (Obersteiner-Redlich zone) is located inside the internal auditory meatus.[12,13] It is covered by myelin that originates from oligodendrocytes; both perineurium and epineurium are absent and the endoneurium is finer than it is in a peripheral nerve.[43] Since this intracranial portion of the vestibulocochlear nerve is very fragile, when recording CAPs directly from the vestibulocochlear nerve, great care must be taken not to injure the nerve with the recording electrode. We use a fine, malleable, multistrand Teflon-coated silver wire with a small cotton wick sutured to the uninsulated tip with 5-0 silk (Figure 3A). This electrode can be placed on the exposed vestibulocochlear nerve (Figure 3B) and it will stay in place when the wire is fixed in the edge of the wound, for example, by tucking it under a dural suture.

In addition to being interpretable instantly, the potentials (CAPs) that are recorded di-

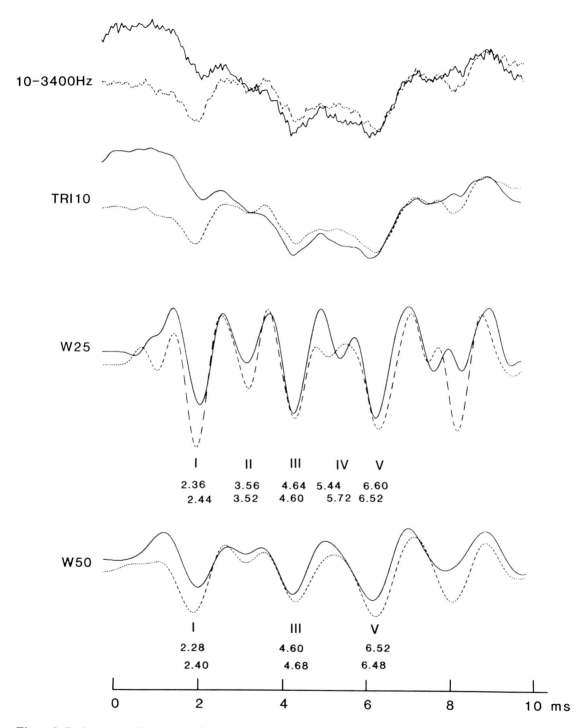

10-3400Hz

TRI10

W25

I	II	III	IV	V
2.36	3.56	4.64	5.44	6.60
2.44	3.52	4.60	5.72	6.52

W50

I	III	V
2.28	4.60	6.52
2.40	4.68	6.48

0   2   4   6   8   10 ms

Figure 2. Brain stem auditory evoked potential recordings typical of those obtained in the operating room. The upper tracings are averaged responses to 2048 stimulus presentations (rarefaction clicks, solid lines; condensation clicks, dashed lines). The recordings were made via electrodes placed on the vertex and the ipsilateral earlobe. The lower tracings represent the same data as the upper tracings but after zero-phase digital filtering and removal of the stimulus artifact. The data were obtained in a patient with normal hearing who was undergoing a microvascular decompression operation.

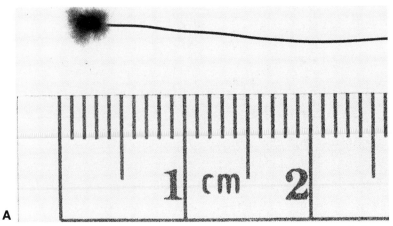

Figure 3. *(A) Electrode used to record compound action potentials from the vestibulocochlear nerve. (B) Electrode in place on the exposed vestibulocochlear nerve.*[17]

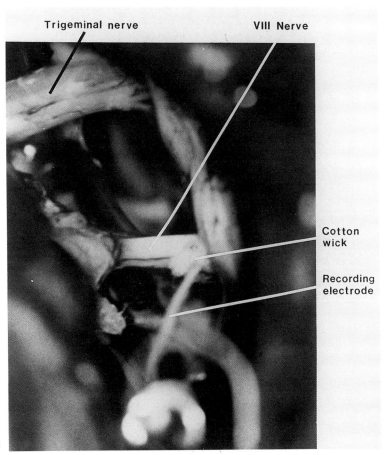

rectly from the vestibulocochlear nerve contain more information than the BAEP recorded from electrodes placed on the scalp. Thus it is possible to determine from the CAP whether a specific change is the result of stretching the vestibulocochlear nerve or of a partial or complete conduction block. When the vestibulocochlear nerve is stretched moderately, for example by retraction, the latency of the negative peak will increase with little change in the waveform of the recorded CAP (Figure 4). Heating of the auditory nerve (as can occur with nearby electrocoagulation) can result in a change of CAP waveform. This change in CAP waveform recorded from the vestibulocochlear nerve takes the form of a decrease in amplitude of the negative peak or of total obliteration of this peak so that only a single positive peak remains (Figure 5). Because the negative peak occurs when the volley of neural activity passes under the recording electrode, and the initial positive peak reflects the approaching volley,[14] a decrease in the amplitude of the negative peak indicates partial conduction block in the vestibulocochlear nerve. Likewise, obliteration of the negative peak indicates that the neural volley in the vestibulocochlear nerve approaches the recording electrode but never reaches it, and thus that there is a total conduction block distal to the location of the recording electrode. Such changes in the CAP therefore indicate that the heat from coagulation has blocked neural transmission in a larger or smaller number of vestibulocochlear nerve fibers.[17]

Use of BAEPs in Monitoring Brain Stem Manipulations

Many large acoustic tumors distort the brain stem, and removal of such tumors involves further manipulation of the brain stem. Brain stem manipulations are traditionally detected through their effects on cardiovascular function, but we have found it of value to use BAEPs as well to monitor brain stem manipulations during operations to remove acoustic tumors. In this context, we monitor the BAEP evoked by stimulating the ear contralateral to the tumor. We monitor these BAEPs, and not for instance SSEPs, because the ascending auditory pathway has several nuclei located in the brain stem and it may be assumed that these nuclei are more sensitive to mechanical manipulation of the brain stem than fiber tracts. Monitoring SSEPs is likely to detect changes in the long fiber tract (the medial lemniscus) in the part of the brain stem that is at primary risk for manipulations, but monitoring BAEPs is more likely to lead to detection of more significant changes in the nuclei. There is also reason to expect that monitoring of BAEPs is a more sensitive means than monitoring cardiovascular parameters to detect the effect of manipulations or compression of the brain stem. The cardiovascular system has a complex set of control systems that tend to keep blood pressure and heart rate within narrow limits, and the operation of these systems may keep heart rate and blood pressure within the normal range for some time after changes occur in the brain stem cardiovascular control centers. These mechanisms would thus delay detection of changes in cardiovascular parameters due to brain stem manipulations. These hypotheses regarding the relative utility of monitoring brain stem function with BAEPs, SSEPs, or cardiovascular parameters have not been tested extensively. However, the results of a recent study (Richard Angelo, unpublished data, 1992) in which we recorded BAEPs in patients who were operated upon to remove large acoustic tumors support the assumption that monitoring BAEPs provides valuable information about brain stem manipulations (Figure 6).

In the patient whose BAEP and cardiovascular function values are shown in Figure 6, there was little change in the latencies of peak III while there were noticeable changes in the latency of peak V of the BAEP. This is in agreement with the assumption that peak III originates mainly from the ipsilateral cochlear nucleus, thus, in this case, from a structure that is located contralateral to the tumor. Peak V is generated by the (contralat-

BEFORE MANIPULATION

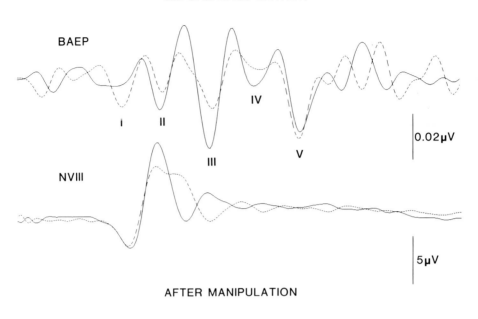

AFTER MANIPULATION

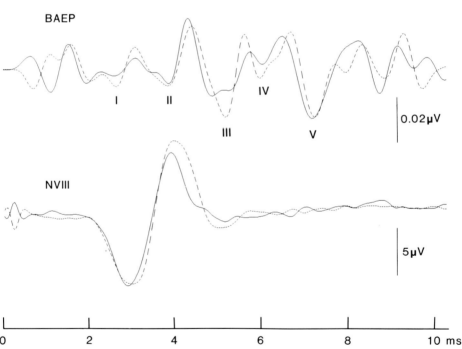

Figure 4. Brain stem auditory evoked potentials and responses recorded directly from the vestibulocochlear (VIII) nerve (compound action potentials, CAPs) before and after manipulation (stretching) of the vestibulocochlear nerve. The brain stem auditory evoked potentials were recorded differentially between vertex and neck and subjected to zero-phase digital filtering similar to that used on the recordings shown in Figure 2. The CAPs were recorded from the midportion of the vestibulocochlear nerve, a location similar to that shown in Figure 3B, and the opposite earlobe was used as reference. The CAPs recorded from the exposed nerve are shown with negativity as an upward deflection. The results were obtained in a patient with normal hearing who was undergoing a microvascular decompression operation.

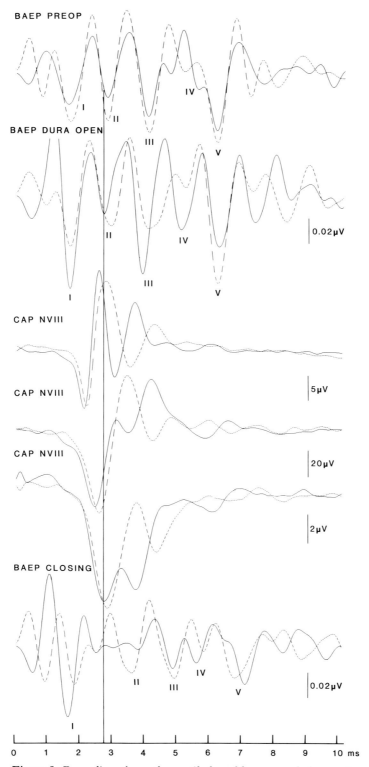

Figure 5. *Recordings from the vestibulocochlear nerve before and after the nerve was subjected to heat from electrocoagulation. The results were obtained in a patient with normal hearing who was undergoing a microvascular decompression operation to relieve disabling positional vertigo.*

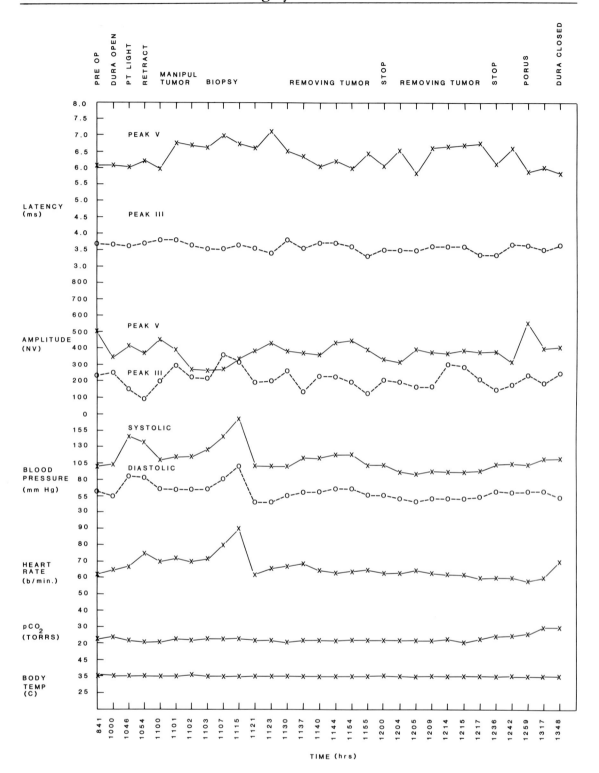

Figure 6. *Changes in the latencies and amplitudes of peaks III and V of the brain stem auditory evoked potentials as a function of time, displayed together with cardiovascular changes, during an operation to remove a large acoustic tumor. The brain stem auditory evoked potentials were elicited by stimulating the ear opposite the side of the tumor (from Richard Angelo, unpublished data, 1992).*

eral) lateral lemniscus, and is affected by changes in the function of the lateral lemniscus as well as all structures of the ascending auditory pathway located caudal to the lateral lemniscus, such as the trapezoid body located in the center of the brain stem and the superior olivary complex located on both sides of the brain stem.[17,20,23] There is considerable evidence that the inferior colliculus does not produce any noticeable farfield potentials.[21] A prolongation of the latency of peak V with the latency of peak III unchanged may thus be assumed to indicate that structures of the ascending auditory pathway located between the cochlear nucleus and the inferior colliculus are affected, i.e. the superior olivary complex, trapezoidal body, or lateral lemniscus.

It is presently believed that it is the shift of the peaks in the BAEP (prolongation of their latency) that is the most important indication that neural conduction has been affected, although the amplitudes of the potentials are probably also important in detecting injuries to the vestibulocochlear nerve or ascending auditory nervous system. If the changes are caused by manipulations of the vestibulocochlear nerve, all peaks except peak I will shift and many neurophysiologists then prefer to monitor the latency of peak V because that peak is usually easier to identify than peak III. We do not know exactly how much the latency or amplitude of the BAEP can change before there is a significant risk of permanent postoperative hearing loss.

Criteria for Acceptable Changes in Auditory Evoked Potentials

It has been debated at which point the surgeon should be notified of changes in the recorded potentials: when the changes have reached a level where they are just larger than the normal small variations or when they have changed to an extent where one could expect a significant risk of a permanent impairment of hearing. The criteria adopted in different institutions with regard to how much the BAEP must change to be indicative of a noticeable risk for a permanent neuro-

logic deficit varies widely. Thus, some surgeons do not regard changes less than total obliteration of the BAEP to be indicative of a significant risk of postoperative hearing loss, whereas others assume that changes of 1.5-2.5 ms indicate a significant risk.[8,38,45] It is advantageous to make the surgeon aware of any change greater than the normal small fluctuations in the latencies, and the author's adoption more than 10 years ago of this principle for intraoperative monitoring has provided good results. The latencies of the various peaks in the BAEP show very little spontaneous variation, and a change of 0.25-0.5 ms represents a clear indication that the system under test has been affected. One major advantage of reporting even small changes is that if the surgeon is aware of when the changes began, he/she will be able to determine what caused the change. This is important if the changes should increase to a level where action must be taken. The situation where it must be decided how large a change can be tolerated will therefore occur rarely.

Although the present level of knowledge and experience does not allow us to state exactly how much the latency can be allowed to change before a measurable hearing loss might occur, this author is convinced that a shift of 1-1.5 ms indicates that action needs to be taken, and a shift in latency of 2-2.5 ms indicates that the risk of postoperative hearing loss is high. Many factors probably influence the threshold for changes in latency associated with a high risk for permanent postoperative hearing deficit, including the patient's general state of health and the temperature of the patient during the operation. For example, it has been reported that mild hypothermia significantly reduces the risk of permanent injury to the nervous system.[1,2] The length of time during which the BAEP is changed is also most likely an important factor.

It is important to remember that not all changes in recorded evoked potentials are caused by surgical manipulations. Irrigation with a fluid of below-body temperature will cause prolongation of the latency of peaks in the BAEP,[15,41] and slow changes can be caused by a slow decrease in the patient's body temperature. A rapid change is most likely caused by manipulation of the vestibulocochlear nerve.

Monitoring Facial Nerve Function in Acoustic Tumor Operations

Locating the facial nerve is critical to attempts to preserve facial function in operations to remove acoustic tumors. Electrical stimulation has been used for many years to probe the tumor and tissues in its vicinity in order to find the facial nerve. Contractions of the facial musculature that occur with such probing are taken as an indication that the tissue probed is the facial nerve.

Different Methods for Recording Muscle Contractions

For many years facial muscle contractions were identified by simple visual monitoring of the face by an assistant. Then 10 to 15 years ago, various devices came into use for recording facial muscle contractions electrically or using mechanotransducers. Sugita and Kobayashi[44] introduced the use of accelerometers placed on the face, and another device that makes use of other mechanical recordings of movements of the facial musculature was described by Silverstein et al.[42] Delgado et al[4] were among the first to use recordings of EMG potentials to monitor facial muscle contractions intraoperatively. Methods that make it possible to listen to the recorded EMG without disturbance from the stimulus artifact in addition to having the EMG displayed on an oscilloscope have been described.[17,26] Recording of EMG is now the most common method for detecting facial muscle contractions, and making the EMG audible, in addition to oscillographic display, is now widely practiced. Several models of equipment are commercially available that make use of this principle.

Use of Electromyographic Potentials to Detect Stimulus-Evoked and Nonstimulus-Evoked Facial Muscle Contractions

Electrodes for recording facial EMG can be placed in individual muscle groups and the potentials can be amplified and displayed separately so that contractions of different muscle groups can be detected. However, since the purpose of recording facial EMG is to identify when any portion of the facial nerve has been stimulated, there is no obvious reason to discriminate between EMGs from different muscle groups. Recording separately from different muscle groups only adds complexity to the recording, so recording the EMG potentials from the entire face on only one channel is recommended (Figure 7). To do this, place one of two differential recording electrodes in the upper face and the other in the lower face.

Needle electrodes, such as subdermal platinum needles, are suitable for recording EMG potentials and are more practical to use in the operating room than surface electrodes. Needle electrodes can be placed in less time than can surface electrodes, and needle electrodes tend to stay in place better than do surface electrodes, when they are secured by a good quality adhesive tape.

Selection of Methods of Stimulating the Facial Nerve

A handheld, monopolar stimulating electrode that is electrically insulated except for about 1 mm at the tip is suitable for probing the tumor and surrounding tissue for the purpose of finding the facial nerve in operations for acoustic tumors (Figure 7B). Bipolar electrodes are more specific stimulators of the nerve and may therefore help to identify the nerve more accurately, but since it is only the negative phase of the stimulation impulse that is effective, the orientation of a bipolar electrode is critical to its ability to stimulate a

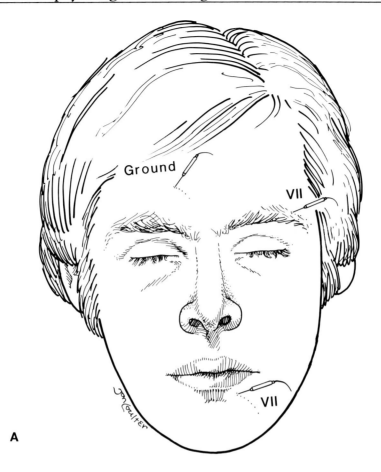

A

Figure 7. *(A) Electrode placement for recording facial muscle electromyograph for the purpose of monitoring the facial nerve. (B) Handheld stimulating electrode for intracranial nerve stimulation (Grass Instrument Co.). The all-metal hypodermic needle is placed in the wound near the opening in the bone and is used as a return electrode.*[17]

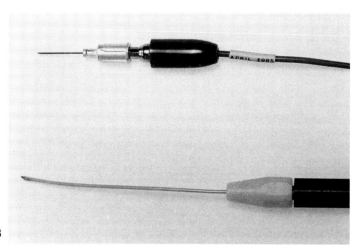

B

nerve. Checking for proper orientation of a bipolar stimulating electrode may thus add unnecessary complexity to detecting the facial nerve, which increases the risk that the nerve may be damaged because the surgeon cannot detect the nerve's presence.

Short (100-200 μs) negative (cathodal) rectangular pulses are suitable for driving a monopolar stimulating electrode. Constant-voltage (or nearly constant-voltage) impulses, rather than the more often used constant-current impulses, are preferable for probing in the cerebellopontine angle because constant-voltage stimulators deliver almost the same electrical current to a nerve regardless of the degree of electrical shunting that occurs. Shunting of current is variable in the cerebellopontine angle because the amount of cerebrospinal fluid present at the location of stimulation varies. If the stimulating electrode is driven by a constant current instead of constant voltage, the amount of current that passes through tissues will be directly dependent on the degree of shunting, which is uncontrollable.

A monopolar electrode can also be used conveniently to probe a large tumor to identify areas of the tumor where no facial nerve is present, so such portions can be removed safely without risk of injuring the facial nerve. When electrical stimulation is used for that purpose, the current delivered must be as independent as possible of such factors as electrical shunting. Monopolar electrodes driven by nearly constant voltage, as were just described, have proven to be effective for that purpose. Using a nerve stimulator to identify portions of a tumor that can be removed without risk of injury to the facial nerve can markedly decrease the time necessary for removal of particularly large tumors.

Recording and Display of the Recorded Potentials

EMG potentials can be amplified using any physiologic amplifier that has a current-limiting interface to protect the patient from electrical shock.[17] A filter setting of 10-3000 Hz is suitable. The recorded potentials should be made audible by connecting the output of the amplifier to an audioamplifier and a speaker. It is useful to have as part of this system a circuit that silences the speaker when the stimulus artifact occurs.[17,26]

Interpreting the Recorded Potentials

The recording electrodes shown in Figure 7 will record not only the EMG activity from all facial muscles but also the EMG potentials from the masseter and temporalis muscles, which are innervated by the motor portion (portio minor) of the trigeminal nerve. Stimulation of the trigeminal nerve will therefore also give rise to recorded EMG potentials when the electrode configuration shown in Figure 7B is used. When the recorded potentials are displayed on an oscilloscope in addition to being made audible, it is easy to distinguish between the potentials from stimulation of the facial nerve and those that originate from stimulation of the trigeminal nerve, because the latency of the EMG potentials that are generated by facial muscles is 5-6 ms whereas the EMG response from the muscles innervated by the trigeminal nerve is only 1.5-2 ms (Figure 8).[17]

There are other reasons why it is useful to observe facial EMG responses on an oscilloscope. The amplitude (or, rather, the area) of the recorded EMG potentials when the facial nerve is stimulated supramaximally is a measure of how many nerve fibers are activated. A reduction in the amplitude of the EMG potentials indicates that there is a conduction block in part of the facial nerve. Should the amplitude of EMG potentials remain low, the patient is likely to have facial weakness postoperatively.

Recording of facial EMG is also effective in detecting injuries to the facial nerve from surgical manipulations such as those that occur when tumor is scraped off the exposed facial nerve. If such manipulations injure the facial nerve, the nerve usually gives rise to characteristic and more-or-less sustained EMG

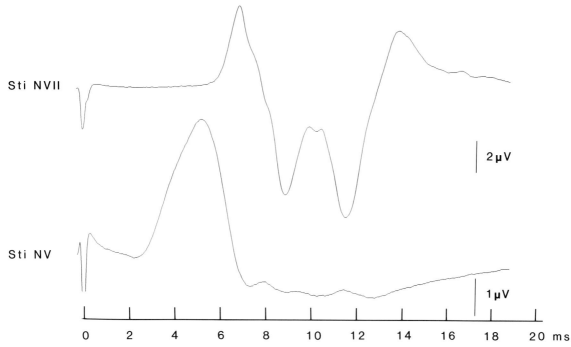

Figure 8. Recordings of electromyographic activity typical of those obtained from electrodes averaged as shown in Figure 7, when the intracranial portion of the facial nerve is stimulated electrically with rectangular impulses of 100-µs duration and a voltage of about 0.8 V and when the trigeminal nerve (portio minor) is stimulated.

activity that can easily be detected by listening to the recorded EMG potentials.[17,26,36] Listening to EMG activity is important in avoiding permanent injuries to the facial nerve during an operation for acoustic tumors. Such EMG activity is likely to occur when a severely injured facial nerve is being manipulated or when tumor tissue is being scraped off an injured nerve. Although there is no definite evidence regarding the exact meaning of such activity, experience shows that it is beneficial to halt the operation until such activity has subsided.

Monitoring Nerves of the Extraocular Muscles

Although the oculomotor (III), trochlear (IV), and abducens (VI) nerves are not located in the posterior cranial fossa, they are often affected by tumors that invade the cavernous sinus, and such tumors may originate in the posterior cranial fossa. During removal of such skull base tumors there is a risk of injuring the nerves that innervate the extraocular muscles.[16,17,40] As is the case for preserving the facial nerve in operations for acoustic tumors, it is important to find ways to identify these cranial nerves because the anatomy is usually distorted by the tumor. Electrical probing of the tumor in connection with recording of EMG potentials from the muscles innervated by these nerves is the method of choice for identifying these nerves. It is often of even greater importance than when operating near the facial nerve to be able to ensure that specific regions of a tumor do not contain the oculomotor, trochlear, or abducens nerves so these portions of the tumor can be removed safely. The techniques used for identification of these cranial nerves are similar to those described above for identifying the facial nerve when removing an acoustic tumor.

Electrode Placement

Subdermal platinum needle electrodes similar to those used for recording facial EMG

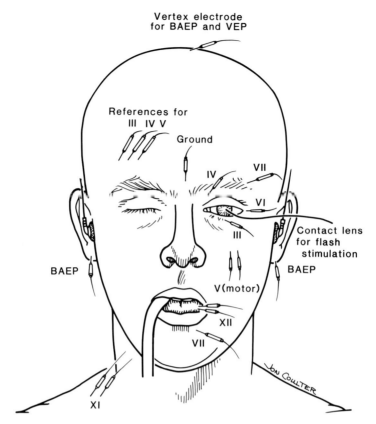

Figure 9A. Schematic illustration of the placement of electrodes for recording electromyographic activity from the extraocular muscles as well as from the facial muscles, the masseter muscle, and the tongue.[19]

are also suitable for recording EMG potentials from the extraocular muscles.[19] These electrodes can be placed percutaneously, aimed at the respective muscles (Figure 9). To monitor the oculomotor nerve, one electrode should be placed in the inferior medial rectus muscle, and to monitor the abducens nerve, a needle electrode should be placed in the lateral rectus muscle. The trochlear nerve can be monitored by placing an EMG recording electrode in the superior oblique muscle. Only one electrode is placed in each muscle, and the respective reference electrodes are placed on the opposite side on the forehead, to avoid contaminating the recording with EMG activity from the ipsilateral facial muscles.

Utmost care should be exercised when the needles are placed in the extraocular muscles that the eye is not injured and the risk of bleeding into the orbit is minimized. It is important that the electrodes are well secured by high-quality adhesive tape so that manipulations and pulling on the electrode wires during the operation will not cause the needles to move.

Recording and Display of Potentials

The potentials recorded from the extraocular muscles should be connected to separate amplifiers via suitable interfaces to protect the patients from electrical hazards. Suitable filter settings would be 30-3000 Hz. As was mentioned regarding monitoring of the facial nerve, it is practical to make the EMG potentials recorded from the extraocular muscles audible so the operating surgeon can hear the responses. The potentials should also be displayed on an oscilloscope, with a separate channel allotted to responses from

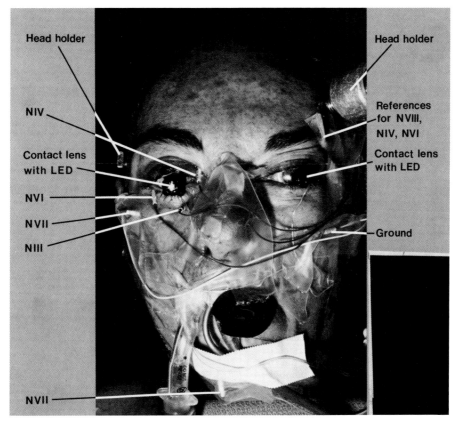

Figure 9B. *Illustration of placement of electrodes shown in (A), in a patient undergoing an operation for removal of a skull base tumor.*[17]

each different muscle. Even though the recording needle electrodes will most likely be placed in the vicinity of the respective muscles rather than directly into the respective muscles, these EMG potentials have amplitudes large enough to be viewed either directly on an oscilloscope or after only a few responses have been averaged (Figure 10).

Monitoring of Cranial Motor Nerves V, IX, XI, and XII

Other cranial motor nerves can be monitored in ways similar to those just described, by recording EMG potentials from their respective muscles. The masseter muscle is suitable for recording the response from the motor portion of the trigeminal nerve. The glossopharyngeal nerve can be monitored by placing EMG electrodes in the pharyngeal muscles that are innervated by that nerve. The spinal accessory nerve can be monitored by placing pairs of needle electrodes in the sternocleidomastoid muscle or the upper part of the trapezius muscle. The hypoglossal nerve can easily be monitored by placing two EMG electrodes in the tongue to record EMG potentials (see Figure 9). Because the hypoglossal nerve is small and often difficult to locate in patients with tumors extending to the lower medulla and upper spinal cord, being able to monitor this nerve can make a difference in the success of operations for such tumors.

Caution should be exercised when electrical stimulation is used on nerves that innervate large muscles. Supramaximal stimulus strength may cause injury because it over-

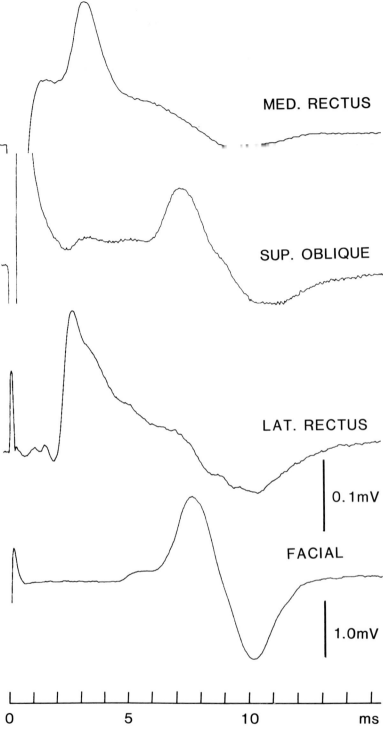

MED. RECTUS

SUP. OBLIQUE

LAT. RECTUS

0.1mV

FACIAL

1.0mV

0   5   10   ms

Figure 10. Recordings typical of those obtained from the extraocular muscles and facial muscles in response to electrical stimulation of the respective motor nerves intracranially. For these recordings, stimuli were rectangular impulses of 150-μs duration and a strength of 0.8-1.5 V. Stimulation was performed with the handheld electrode shown in Figure 7B.[17]

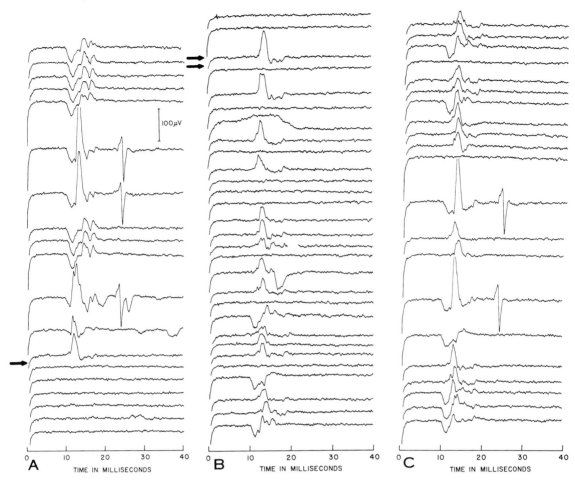

Figure 11. Consecutive recordings of the abnormal muscle response in a patient undergoing a microvascular decompression operation to relieve hemifacial spasm. At single arrow the offending vessel was moved off the facial nerve and at the double arrow the vessel fell back on the facial nerve (modified from reference 28).

rides the feedback mechanism that normally limits the strength of voluntary contractions and causes the entire muscle to contract very strongly. Therefore, the stimulus intensity should initially be set low and should only be increased while a muscle contraction is observed.

Hemifacial Spasm

Monitoring the Abnormal Muscle Contraction

During MVD operations for hemifacial spasm, it can be of benefit to monitor the abnormal muscle contraction that seems to be specific to patients with hemifacial spasm.[31]

This abnormal (or delayed) muscle contraction can be elicited by electrical stimulation of a branch of the peripheral portion of the facial nerve while recording EMG potentials from muscles innervated by other branches of the facial nerve.

When recorded from the mentalis muscle as the temporal or zygomatic branch of the facial nerve is stimulated electrically, this abnormal muscle contraction appears as brief EMG activity that may be followed by a long burst of irregular EMG activity (Figure 11). While the initial component of the response has a relatively constant latency of about 10

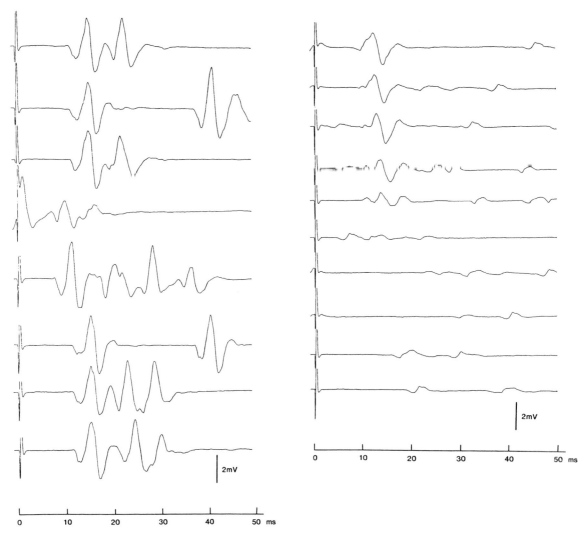

Figure 12. *Responses recorded from the mentalis muscle to electrical stimulation of the temporal branch of the facial nerve in a patient undergoing microvascular decompression to relieve hemifacial spasm. The recordings shown on the left were obtained before the beginning of the operation, but after the patient was anesthetized. The recordings shown on the right were obtained after the arachnoid membrane over the facial nerve was opened. The lower portion of the right-hand column shows recordings that were obtained after the offending vessel was moved off the nerve.*[31]

ms, the pattern of the following EMG activity is variable.

The use of intraoperative monitoring of the abnormal (or delayed) muscle response is based on the finding that the muscle response disappears instantaneously when the offending vessel is moved off the facial nerve[28] (see Figure 11). Observing this muscle response therefore helps the surgeon identify which blood vessel is causing the symptoms of hemifacial spasm and makes it possible for the surgeon to be assured that the facial nerve has been adequately decompressed before the operation is ended. This ability to determine during the operation that the facial nerve has been adequately decompressed is also an important quality control feature.

Electrode Placement for Recording and Stimulation

Placement of electrodes for electrical stimulation of individual branches of the facial

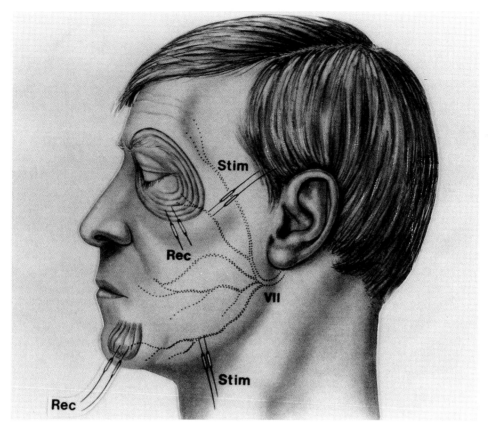

Figure 13. Placement of recording and stimulating electrodes for monitoring the abnormal muscle contraction in patients who are operated on to relieve hemifacial spasm.[29]

nerve and for recording EMG potentials are shown in Figure 12. Platinum needle electrodes similar to those used for recording and stimulation in other situations can be used for both recording and stimulation to monitor the abnormal potentials of hemifacial spasm.

Interpretation of Results

Normally, the abnormal muscle response will disappear instantaneously when the offending vessel is lifted off the facial nerve and will reappear if the vessel is allowed to fall back on the facial nerve.[28,29] This makes it possible to accurately identify the vessel that is causing the symptoms. It is often seen that the prolonged EMG activity that follows the initial component at 10-ms latency disappears as the operation proceeds, even before the dura mater is opened, and only a brief

potential with a latency of 10 ms remains when the MVD procedure begins (Figure 13). The small unsynchronized EMG potentials that were present at the end of the operation in this case are indications of a slight (temporary) injury to the facial nerve.

In some patients, particularly patients who have had hemifacial spasm symptoms for a relatively short time, it may be necessary to activate the abnormal muscle response by stimulating at a high rate. The initial component of EMG activity elicited during monitoring of the abnormal muscle response in hemifacial spasm follows a rapid rate of stimulation (at least up to 50 pps).[30] Such rapid stimulation rates activate the abnormal muscle response so that its amplitude increases. Stimulation at these rates may also reactivate the activity that follows the initial 10-ms component, when such activity has disappeared. Stimulation at a high rate should also be performed whenever the abnormal muscle contraction is monitored as a quality control measure, to ensure that the abnormal muscle response is really absent. Because of uncertainty as to which vessel was causing the hemifacial spasm, occasionally the spasm was not relieved by an MVD operation and re-operations were necessary. Monitoring of the abnormal muscle response has increased the cure rate of hemifacial spasm as a result of MVD operations, and it has made re-operations rare.[9,31]

Monitoring of the abnormal muscle contraction during MVD operations for hemifacial spasm has led to the observations that the symptoms of hemifacial spasm are often caused by more than one blood vessel and that one of the vessels causing symptoms can be very small. Even veins can cause the symptoms of hemifacial spasm.

Anesthetic Needs in Monitoring of Electromyographic Potentials

Whenever neurophysiologic monitoring involves recording EMG potentials, the patient cannot be paralyzed. Because administration of a muscle relaxant is common practice in anesthesia today, it is important that the anesthesia team be made aware of this in every individual case in which EMG monitoring is to be performed. Inhalation anesthetics, on the other hand, are not known to have any suppressive effect on EMG potentials, nor do such agents have any suppressive effect on BAEPs. Inhalation anesthetics do, however, markedly suppress the cortical components of sensory evoked potentials such as the frequently used SSEP. Monitoring SSEPs is not generally regarded to be beneficial in skull base operations, but monitoring SSEPs elicited by median nerve stimulation can be useful when tumors located near the lower medulla or upper spinal cord are removed. In such cases, short-latency SSEPs,

generated in the cuneate nuclei and medial lemniscus, may be monitored because these potentials are not affected by inhalation anesthetics.

References

1. Chopp M, Chen H, Dereski MO, et al. Mild hypothermic intervention after graded ischemic stress in rats. *Stroke.* 1991;22:37-43.
2. Clifton GL, Jiang JY, Lyeth BG, et al. Marked protection by moderate hypothermia after experimental traumatic brain injury. *J Cereb Blood Flow Metab.* 1991;11:114-121.
3. Daspit CP, Raudzens PA, Shetter AG. Monitoring of intraoperative auditory brainstem responses. *Otolaryngol Head Neck Surg.* 1982;90:108-116.
4. Delgado TE, Buchheit WA, Rosenholtz HR, et al. Intraoperative monitoring of facial muscle evoked responses obtained by intracranial stimulation of the facial nerve: a more accurate technique for facial nerve dissection. *Neurosurgery.* 1979;4:418-421.
5. Friedman WA, Kaplan BJ, Gravenstein D, et al. Intraoperative brain-stem auditory evoked potentials during posterior fossa microvascular decompression. *J Neurosurg.* 1985;62:552-557.
6. Grundy BL. Intraoperative monitoring of sensory-evoked potentials. *Anesthesiology.* 1983;58:72-87.
7. Grundy BL. Evoked potentials monitoring. In: Blitt CD, ed. *Monitoring in Anesthesia and Critical Care Medicine.* New York, NY: Churchill-Livingstone; 1985: 345-411.
8. Grundy BL, Jannetta PJ, Procopio PT, et al. Intraoperative monitoring of brainstem auditory evoked potentials. *J Neurosurg.* 1982;57:674-681.
9. Haines SJ, Torres F. Intraoperative monitoring of the facial nerve during decompressive surgery for hemifacial spasm. *J Neurosurg.* 1991;74:254-257.
10. Hardy RW Jr, Kinney SE, Lueders H, et al. Preservation of cochlear nerve function with aid of brain stem auditory evoked potentials. *Neurosurgery.* 1982;11:16-19.
11. Hashimoto I, Ishiyama Y, Yoshimoto T, et al. Brain-stem auditory-evoked potentials recorded directly from human brain stem and thalamus. *Brain.* 1981; 104:841-859.
12. Lang J. Facial and vestibulocochlear nerve, topographic anatomy and variations. In: Samii M, Jannetta PJ, eds. *The Cranial Nerves: Anatomy, Pathology, Pathophysiology, Diagnosis, Treatment.* New York, NY: Springer-Verlag; 1981:363-377.
13. Lang J. *Clinical Anatomy of the Head, Neurocranium, Orbit, and Craniocervical Region.* New York, NY: Springer-Verlag; 1983.
14. Lorento de No, R. Analysis of the distribution of action currents of nerve in volume conductors. *Stud Rockefeller Inst Med Res.* 1947;132:384-482.
15. Markand ON, Lee BI, Warren C, et al. Effects of hypothermia on brain stem auditory evoked potentials in humans. *Ann Neurol.* 1987;22:507-513.
16. Møller AR. Electrophysiological monitoring of cranial nerves in operations in the skull base. In: Sekhar LN, Schramm VL Jr, eds. *Tumors of the*

17. Møller AR. *Evoked Potentials in Intraoperative Monitoring*. Baltimore, Md: Williams & Wilkins; 1988.

18. Møller AR. Use of zero-phase digital filters to enhance brain-stem auditory evoked potentials (BAEPs). *Electroenceph Clin Neurophysiol*. 1988; 71:226-232.

19. Møller AR. Intraoperative monitoring of evoked potentials: an update. In: Wilkins RH, Rengachary SS, eds. *Neurosurgery Update, I; Diagnosis, Operative Technique, and Neuro-oncology*. New York, NY: McGraw-Hill Inc; 1990:169-176.

20. Møller AR. Neural generators of auditory evoked potentials (BAEP). In: Jacobson JT, ed. *The Auditory Brain stem Response*. 2nd ed. San Diego, Calif: CollegeHill Press; 1992.

21. Møller AR, Burgess JE. Neural generators of the brain stem auditory evoked potentials (BAEPs) in the rhesus monkey. *Electroenceph Clin Neurophysiol*. 1986;65:361-372.

22. Møller AR, Jannetta PJ. Compound action potentials recorded intracranially from the auditory nerve in man. *J Exp Neurol*. 1981;74:862-874.

23. Møller AR, Jannetta PJ. Auditory evoked potentials recorded intracranially from the brain stem in man. *Exp Neurol*. 1982;78:144-157.

24. Møller AR, Jannetta PJ. Evoked potentials from the inferior colliculus in man. *Electroenceph Clin Neurophysiol*. 1982;53:612-620.

25. Møller AR, Jannetta PJ. Monitoring auditory functions during cranial nerve microvascular decompression operations by direct recording from the eighth nerve. *J Neurosurg*. 1983;59:493-499.

26. Møller AR, Jannetta PJ. Preservation of facial function during removal of acoustic neuromas: use of monopolar constant-voltage stimulation and EMG. *J Neurosurg*. 1984;61:757-760.

27. Møller AR, Jannetta PJ. Neural generators of the auditory brain stem response. In: Jacobson JT, ed. *The Auditory Brainstem Response*. San Diego, Calif. College-Hill Press; 1984:13-31.

28. Møller AR, Jannetta PJ. Microvascular decompression in hemifacial spasm: intraoperative electrophysiological observations. *Neurosurgery*. 1985; 16:612-618.

29. Møller AR, Jannetta PJ. Synkinesis in hemifacial spasm: results of recording intracranially from the facial nerve. *Experientia*. 1985;41:415-417.

30. Møller AR, Jannetta PJ. Physiological abnormalities in hemifacial spasm studied during microvascular decompression operations. *Exp Neurol*. 1986; 93:584-600.

31. Møller AR, Jannetta PJ. Monitoring facial EMG responses during microvascular decompression operations for hemifacial spasm. *J Neurosurg*. 1987; 66:681-685.

32. Møller AR, Jannetta PJ, Møller MB. Neural generators of brain stem evoked potentials: results from human intracranial recordings. *Ann Otol Rhinol Laryngol*. 1981;90:591-596.

33. Møller AR, Møller MB. Does intraoperative monitoring of auditory evoked potentials reduce incidence of hearing loss as a complication of microvascular decompression of cranial nerves? *Neurosurgery*. 1989;24:257-263.

34. Møller AR, Møller MB, Jannetta PJ, et al. Auditory nerve compound action potentials and brain stem auditory evoked potentials in patients with various degrees of hearing loss. *Ann Otol Rhinol Laryngol*. 1991;100:488-495.

35. Møller MB, Møller AR, Jannetta PJ, et al. Diagnosis and surgical treatment of disabling positional vertigo. *J Neurosurg*. 1986;64:21-28.

36. Prass RL, Lüders H. Acoustic (loudspeaker) facial electromyographic monitoring, I: evoked electromyographic activity during acoustic neuroma resection. *Neurosurgery*. 1986;19:392-400.

37. Raudzens PA. Intraoperative monitoring of evoked potentials. *Ann NY Acad Sci*. 1982;388:308-325.

38. Raudzens PA, Shetter AG. Intraoperative monitoring of brainstem auditory evoked potentials. *J Neurosurg*. 1982;57:341-348.

39. Schramm J, Mokrusch T, Fahlbusch R, et al. Detailed analysis of intraoperative changes monitoring brain stem acoustic evoked potentials. *Neurosurgery*. 1988;22:694-702.

40. Sekhar LN, Møller AR. Operative management of tumors involving the cavernous sinus. *J Neurosurg*. 1986;64:879-889.

41. Sekiya T, Hatayama T, Iwabuchi T, et al. Thermal effect of irrigation in the cerebellopontine angle on brain stem auditory evoked potentials: experimental and clinical study. *Neurosurgery*. 1993 (in press).

42. Silverstein H, Norrell H, Hyman SM. Simultaneous use of CO_2 laser with continuous monitoring of eighth cranial nerve action potential during acoustic neuroma surgery. *Otolaryngol Head Neck Surg*. 1984; 92:80-84.

43. Spoendlin H, Schrott A. Analysis of the human auditory nerve. *Hear Res*. 1989;43:25-38.

44. Sugita K, Kobayashi S. Technical and instrumental improvements in the surgical treatment of acoustic neurinomas. *J Neurosurg*. 1982;57:747-752.

45. Watanabe E, Schramm J, Strauss C, et al. Neurophysiologic monitoring in posterior fossa surgery, II: BAEP-waves I and V and preservation of hearing. *Acta Neurochir (Wien)*. 1989;98:118-128.

CHAPTER 7

Trigeminal Neuralgia and Other Trigeminal Dysfunction Syndromes

Daniel C. Rohrer, MD, and Kim J. Burchiel, MD

Diagnosis

Cephalalaea was a term used in the first century by Aretaeus to describe the condition now known as trigeminal neuralgia. Numerous other depictions were noted in England between the thirteenth and seventeenth centuries. By 1677, John Locke accurately described the clinical features of this disease that serve as the diagnostic format to this day.

Trigeminal neuralgia (tic douloureux) is typically described as fleeting, lancinating pain lasting seconds to minutes that occurs in the sensory distribution of the trigeminal (V) nerve. The pain commonly strikes the third (mandibular) division of the nerve along the jaw or lower teeth or tongue and less commonly affects second (maxillary) and first (ophthalmic) divisions. Frequently more than one distribution is affected and the pain seemingly radiates from one division to the other. The pain almost always is unilateral, although very rarely bilateral trigeminal neuralgia can be seen. The typical pains always are paroxysmal, often described as "electrical" in quality by patients. There is usually a perioral trigger zone in the second or even third division. Triggering stimuli often include talking, eating, oral hygiene such as toothbrushing, wind or cold temperatures on the face. Light tactile non-noxious stimulation of the trigger zone produces the typical neuralgic pains commonly seen. Frequently, the pain occurs spontaneously either from environ-

mental stimuli or without apparent trigger. Because of the triggerability of the pain, the patients frequently do not groom the side of the face during acute episodes, may not eat or even swallow oral secretions. This disorder affects predominantly the older age group (60+), but individuals from their teens to more than 90 years old can be affected. There is a slight predominance of females to males in this disorder, 5.9 and 3.4 per 100,000 population, respectively.[47] The right side of the face is slightly more frequently affected than the left. There is also an elevated relative risk associated with hypertension and multiple sclerosis. Occasionally, familial occurrences also are reported.[50]

Neurologic examination in the typical case reveals no neurologic deficit. Sensory loss, even minimal, in the area of the pain or of the trigger zone suggests structural pathology or severe compression of the nerve in the posterior fossa. The typical pains are alleviated by carbamazepine. This in itself is a diagnostic test, for no other orofacial pain responds to this anticonvulsant. The disorder also is characterized by painfree intervals that can last from months to even years. Following a painfree interval, the pain returns exactly as before the hiatus.

Atypical trigeminal neuralgia combines features of typical idiopathic trigeminal neuralgia, that is, brief, lancinating, unilateral electrical pains, with a constant background pain that usually is described as either aching or burning. These pains are likewise unilateral, and facial sensory loss is more common in these individuals.

Secondary trigeminal neuralgia represents approximately 2% of the cases of trigeminal neuralgia, and atypical pain is more common. There is always a sensory loss, and these patients may harbor tumors or vascular lesions with compression of the nerve. The trigeminal reflexes (corneal blink, jaw jerk, and masseter inhibitory periods) also are always abnormal, and far field scalp potentials evoked by percutaneous infraorbital stimulation are altered in 80% of those measured.[19] The age range usually is less than the older age group affected with typical idiopathic trigeminal neuralgia, and male and female incidence is about equal.

Symptomatic trigeminal neuralgia occurs in association with multiple sclerosis and may present either typical or atypical pains. Patients with multiple sclerosis-associated trigeminal neuralgia also are younger and more likely to have bilateral facial symptoms.[10,11] *Post-traumatic trigeminal neuralgia* occurs approximately 5% to 10% of the time after facial trauma or oral surgery. It is reported to be seen in 1% to 5% of patients after the removal of impacted teeth. The painful episodes are sharp and episodic and often are triggered as is the pain of typical trigeminal neuralgia. Superimposed is a background of dull, throbbing, or burning pain such as with atypical trigeminal neuralgia. Those post-traumatic pain problems may represent either trigeminal neuroma or deafferentation pain, that is, pain following the loss of nervous system input. The term *trigeminal neuropathic pain* also has been used to describe this entity and probably is more accurate. This diagnosis overlaps substantially with *atypical facial pain.*

Atypical facial pain may be included with a number of disorders that come under the rubric of "pain of psychological origin in the head and face." No known physical cause or pathophysiologic mechanism for this type of pain exists. Once other etiologies of the pain are ruled out, such as sinus disease, migrainous neuralgia, "cluster" headache, etc., the diagnosis of atypical facial pain should be considered. Usually, there also is proof of contributing psychologic factors, and the characteristics of this patient group overlap the American Psychiatric Association definition of "psychogenic pain disorder." The pain usually is described as diffuse and/or nonanatomic in the orofacial region. There is a steady, often burning or aching quality. Atypical facial pain may mimic other syndromes. There often is obvious psychopathology, including delusions, hallucinations, and multiple physical complaints. Conversion or pseudoneurotic symptoms and signs may also be found. Psychological evaluation will reveal signs of somatization, depression, and illness behaviors. Patients typically undergo excessive treatment or exhibit medication-seeking behavior. Neurologic examination invariably is normal, or there may be poorly localized tenderness and vague, nonreproducible sensory loss.

The diagnosis of typical trigeminal neuralgia usually is not difficult if it is considered. Again, a patient with unilateral, fleeting, lancinating, electric-shock-like facial pains in the trigeminal sensory distribution that respond to carbamazepine has trigeminal neuralgia. The diagnosis of the overlap syndrome, atypical trigeminal neuralgia, may be more problematic, but again, fleeting pains are the hallmark. Patients with constant pain alone (trigeminal neuropathic and atypical facial) should be approached with great trepidation and not without thorough diagnostic evaluation, specifically including psychological evaluation.

Etiology
Trigeminal Neuralgia

Although there is no known proven etiology of trigeminal neuralgia, some autopsy results in patients with trigeminal neuralgia and multiple sclerosis indicate that demyelination within the descending tract of the trigeminal nerve or within the nerve itself can be correlated with the disorder. The mechanism of the pain in non-multiple sclerosis patients still is being debated. Considerable surgical evidence, however, indicates that in many, if not most, cases of trigeminal neuralgia, the nerve is compressed by an artery or less commonly a vein in the posterior fossa. It is at this point of cross-compression that the demyelination may occur, and thus, the cross-compression may be the inciting event. At surgery, the cross-compression of the nerve is typically at the level of the entry of the nerve into the pons. This also corresponds with data obtained with far field scalp potentials,[19,55,56] implicating damage to the same anatomic region of the trigeminal system.

As mentioned previously, other structural lesions such as tumors, aneurysms, or arteriovenous malformations can rarely cross-compress the nerve and produce quite typical pain. Secondary trigeminal neuralgia is reported with intrinsic tumors, such as neuromas of the trigeminal root,[84] meningiomas, and other cerebellopontine angle (CPA) lesions. Cavernous malformations of the parapontine region[87] to the upper cervical spinal cord[76] also are implicated. Vascular anomalies, such as severe vertebrobasilar ectasia[33,59] and variants of primitive trigeminal arteries,[64] may distort the brain stem and surrounding structures significantly enough to precipitate trigeminal neuralgia. Recently, various lesions causing enough brain stem displacement to result in contralateral trigeminal neuralgia have been described. These lesions include meningiomas, acoustic neuromas, cholesteatomas, and arachnoid cysts.[2,25,29,79] These secondary neuralgias are reportedly resolved with either removal or decompression of the contralateral mass.

Trigeminal Neuropathic Pain

The etiology behind trigeminal neuropathic pain is even more elusive. This form of trigeminal pain could be defined as constant, variable, nontriggerable, and unremitting. Adjectives used to describe these atypical pains include "burning," "aching," "drawing," "tight," "crawling," and others. Patients with so-called atypical facial pain do not have an apparent etiology for the pain and are thought

to have a high incidence of psychopathology. However, other patients with clear pathology of the trigeminal system have sensory loss and atypical pains similar to those described previously. The leading theory of causation in typical trigeminal neuralgia points to compression and possibly demyelination at the root entry zone of the trigeminal nerve. In our experience, atypical pains result from lesions in the distal trigeminal nerve.

All inpatient charts at our institution with diagnoses related to facial pain from 1977-1987 were reviewed in detail. Atypical facial pain patients, without clear-cut organic pathology or sensory loss, were specifically eliminated from this analysis. From this review 122 patients were identified: 81 patients with typical trigeminal neuralgia, 7 with glossopharyngeal neuralgia, and 34 with atypical pains, as characterized previously. Of this latter group, 12 had dental/temporomandibular pathology, 10 had head and neck cancer, 5 had atypical pains without specific diagnosis (with sensory loss), 4 had sinus disease, 2 were post-traumatic, and 1 had a CPA tumor. These data are consistent with a peripheral etiology of these pains.[7]

We propose that peripheral lesions of the trigeminal nerve behave as do other peripheral nerve lesions in that they produce sensory loss, deafferentation, and nonticlike pains. This may be caused by the asynchronous spatial-temporal dispersion of abnormal centrally propagating axonal activity in nociceptive and nonnociceptive fibers (neuromas, demyelination, inflammation) from the region of pathology. This is opposed to the putative synchronous multifiber volleys that may emanate from the proximal trigeminal root entry zone in patients with typical trigeminal neuralgia.

Medical Management

The medical treatment of typical idiopathic trigeminal neuralgia usually is very rewarding. Carbamazepine is started in doses of 100 mg bid and then increased by 200 mg a day every 2-3 days until reaching a final daily dose in the range of 800-1,000 mg. Prior to starting the medication, a baseline white blood cell count is obtained because it is not uncommon for mild leukopenia to occur during medical treatment. Rarely, a nondose-dependent and idiosyncratic bone marrow suppression (aplastic anemia) can occur early in treatment and must be watched for diligently. The white blood cell count is typically repeated a week after beginning therapy and then approximately 3-4 weeks later and then every several months while the patient is on the drug. Most typical cases of trigeminal neuralgia will respond to this medication to some extent. In fact, as mentioned previously, this is a powerful and reliable diagnostic modality in determining whether the patient has trigeminal neuralgia. Limitations to carbamazepine treatment are hypersensitivity reactions that preclude utilization of the drug, or at higher doses, symptoms of drowsiness, mental dullness, subjective dizziness, and ataxia. These latter common symptoms can be very troublesome in the elderly. In cases of hypersensitivity reactions, baclofen may be substituted with good effect. This drug is started at 5 mg tid and then increased by 5-10 mg every two to three days to a maximum dose of 80 mg per day. Baclofen usually is not helpful in patients who are otherwise able to take carbamazepine, but who continue to have neuralgic pains at high doses of the drug and are intolerant of the side effects. The anticonvulsant, phenytoin, also can be used but is rarely of additional benefit when either carbamazepine or baclofen have failed.

Recently, carbamazepine analogues, especially the keto derivative oxcarbazepine are gaining some attention within the European community.[23,68,97,98] Although drug dosages twice as high as those for carbamazepine are required to achieve adequate symptomatic relief, the adverse side effects occur much less frequently. In addition, the onset of beneficial effects occurs within 48 hours for most patients, and even less than 24 hours in some.

In general, about 70% of patients will respond at least initially to medical management. As time goes on, however, in many of these patients, the drugs become ineffective

and the pain breaks through the pharmacologic therapy. In fact, the majority of the patients eventually will fail medical management if followed carefully over many years.

Surgical Management

The surgical approach to trigeminal neuralgia is likewise highly effective. The procedures generally can be considered in two groups: minor percutaneous procedures and major operative procedures, which include microvascular decompression (MVD), trigeminal rhizotomy, trigeminal tractotomy, and nucleus caudalis dorsal root entry zone (DREZ) lesions. Dozens of operations have been developed over the past 5-6 decades, but certain percutaneous procedures and MVD seem to hold most of the surgical attention and promise at present.

Minor Percutaneous Procedures

Percutaneous procedures generally are performed on an outpatient basis or with at most a brief stay in the hospital. In general, the risks of the procedures are minimal and for this reason they generally are thought to be more appropriate for the elderly (more than 65 years old) or debilitated patient. The risk of mortality from these operations is close to zero and morbidity usually is minimal or acceptable.

Currently, three main percutaneous procedures are performed: percutaneous radiofrequency trigeminal gangliolysis, percutaneous retrogasserian glycerol rhizotomy and percutaneous balloon microcompression. These will be discussed briefly to afford proper comparison of the minor with the major surgical procedures used in our treatment algorithm of trigeminal neuralgia. Other minor procedures such as alcohol block, alcohol gangliolysis, and peripheral neurectomy have become somewhat outdated and will not be further discussed here. The more recent endeavors of chronic neurostimulation of the gasserian ganglion,[54] and retrograde adriamycin sensory ganglionectomy[46] also fall outside the confines of this chapter.

In all of the main percutaneous procedures, a needle or trocar is inserted under local or brief general anesthesia from a point on the cheek just lateral to the corner of the mouth, and then, under fluoroscopy, the needle is introduced into the ipsilateral foramen ovale (Hertl technique). The position of the needle then is fluoroscopically verified in the lateral position and the gangliolysis is performed. The percutaneous radiofrequency trigeminal gangliolysis procedure uses radiofrequency heating of the tip of an electrode to produce a thermal lesion in the ganglion, using the production of appropriate facial numbness in the area of pain and/or the trigger zone as the endpoint. Radiofrequency lesions are produced under brief general anesthesia using short-acting barbiturates such as methohexital or Propofol [Stuart Pharmaceuticals, Wilmington, Delaware].

The percutaneous retrogasserian glycerol rhizotomy procedure likewise is performed using a spinal needle until cerebrospinal fluid (CSF) from the trigeminal cistern is encountered. In the sitting position, a trigeminal cisternogram then is obtained using radio-opaque water-soluble contrast material (Isovue [Squibb Diagnostics, Princeton, New Jersey] 300 mg %) and then after removing this, anhydrous glycerol (approximately 0.3 ml) is instilled into the cistern. The patient remains in the seated position with the neck flexed slightly forward for 2 hours to obtain the maximum neurolytic effect.

Finally, the percutaneous balloon microcompression procedure utilizes a 14-gauge trocar placed into the region of the trigeminal ganglion after which a 4 French Fogerty catheter is inserted into this region, inflated with radio-opaque contrast material to a volume of 0.5-0.7 ml and held in place for 1-2 minutes. The latter two procedures do not routinely produce facial numbness and this is not used as an endpoint for the procedures. Sporadically, considerable numbness can be produced by the glycerol procedure, although it is reportedly rare using the balloon compression technique.

The most recently reported large series of percutaneous retrogasserian glycerol rhizotomies show 80% to 91% initial success in relieving pain. Except for one study reviewed here,[74] this success appears to be highly associated with the production of facial numbness (45% to 72%). Recurrence of facial pain appears to be approximately 50% within 2 years and has a direct association to prior ablative surgical procedures. Percutaneous radiofrequency trigeminal gangliolysis also shows an approximate 82% to 95% initial success rate,[12,61] which is directly associated with the production of facial numbness. Recurrence rates range from 5% to 42% at approximately 2 years, while nearly 50% classically remain in remission at 4-5 years. Unfortunate complications with percutaneous radiofrequency trigeminal gangliolysis include masseter weakness in 7% to 23% of cases, troublesome dysesthesias in 11% to 42%, corneal hypesthesia in 3% to 27%, frank neuroparalytic keratitis in fewer than 5%, and anesthesia dolorosa in fewer than 4%.[14] Percutaneous balloon microcompression shows a high rate of initial (93% to 100%) and delayed (50% to 90%) efficacy with little production of significant dysesthesias in most cases[6,13,14,57,58,61,62] and very rare production of corneal sensory loss. Although the incidence of ipsilateral masseter weakness may be more common in percutaneous balloon microcompression than in other percutaneous procedures, it appears to be primarily transient in nature.

Major Surgical Procedures

This section reviews the most commonly utilized modes of surgical therapy for trigeminal neuralgia that require general anesthesia and entail some operative risk of mortality for the patient. Although numerous techniques have been used over the years, four procedures have emerged as tested and effective surgical approaches to this disorder: MVD, rhizotomy, medullary tractotomy, and nucleus caudalis DREZ lesions. These operative techniques as used in the management of trigeminal neuralgia and the risks, expected results, and respective roles associated with these techniques are discussed here.

Microvascular Decompression

Elaborating on an original suggestion of Dandy[21] and later Gardner,[72,73] Jannetta[39-43,45] has demonstrated that patients with trigeminal neuralgia frequently have an artery or vein (occasionally a tumor) compressing the trigeminal nerve at its junction with the pons. Subsequently, many reports have documented a remarkable amelioration of trigeminal neuralgia following MVD of the trigeminal root, and this procedure has become one of the most important surgical approaches in patients with idiopathic trigeminal neuralgia.

The surgical procedure of MVD involves separation of the offending vessel from its point of contact with the posterior trigeminal root, typically observed at the root entry zone on the brain stem, and interposition of an inert plastic sponge or Teflon felt prosthesis between the vessel and the nerve. Reported series have demonstrated that with the exception of patients with multiple sclerosis, 62% to 64% of patients with trigeminal neuralgia have an artery (usually the superior cerebellar or anterior inferior cerebellar), 12% to 24% a vein, 13% to 14% have a combination of artery and vein, and 8% have a tumor or vascular malformation impinging on the nerve.* In a more recent report on microsurgical anatomy by Matsushima et al,[60] the lateral mesencephalic segment of the superior cerebellar artery near its bifurcation often (70% of cases) compressed the trigeminal nerve at multiple points on the nerve's medial surface. Nevertheless, a high incidence of neurovascular contact with the trigeminal nerve has been observed in autopsy studies in individuals with no history of trigeminal neuralgia and has been cited as evidence both for[30] and against[32] the hypothesis that trigeminal neuralgia is caused by such contact.

Magnetic resonance imaging (MRI) has the ability to clearly demonstrate the relationship of the cisternal portion of the trigeminal nerve to surrounding vertebrobasilar structures. MRI has been used as a screening

test not only to rule out CPA tumors and multiple sclerosis plaques in patients with trigeminal neuralgia, but also to possibly confirm compression or indentation of the trigeminal nerve by vascular structures.[37,86,93] Reviews of radiologic evidence of vascular compression in symptomatic patients compared to controls are mixed[37,86] as with the autopsy studies noted earlier. Nevertheless, although neurovascular contact may be an asymptomatic event, preoperative MRI demonstration of this phenomenon in symptomatic patients may influence the surgical treatment of choice toward MVD. Future advances with a combination of modalities, including magnetic resonance angiography, may further characterize the significance of radiologic neurovascular compression.

Although a posterior fossa craniectomy is required for MVD of the nerve, this has been justified by the potential advantages of: (1) treating what is thought to be the primary etiology of idiopathic trigeminal neuralgia, and (2) preservation of the trigeminal nerve, because relief apparently does not depend on the production of a sensory deficit.

Technique

MVD is a major surgical procedure, and patients must undergo a thorough preoperative evaluation of their cardiopulmonary, hematologic, and coagulation status. Baseline brain stem auditory-evoked responses (BAERs) and somatosensory-evoked potentials (SSEPs) are obtained prior to surgery. General anesthesia is administered by endotracheal tube with continuous BAER, SSEP, and facial nerve monitoring, and the patient may be positioned either in the semisitting or lateral recumbent position with the head secured by skeletal fixation. The semisitting position requires the placement of a transesophageal echocardiogram probe or precordial Doppler probe, as well as a right atrial catheter for detection and treatment of air embolism. We prefer a supine position with an ipsilateral shoulder roll with the head in fixation turned about 45° away from the surgeon and flexed

---

*References 1, 3, 9, 18, 20, 24, 42-45, 51, 69, 81, 83, 85, 89, 92, 101

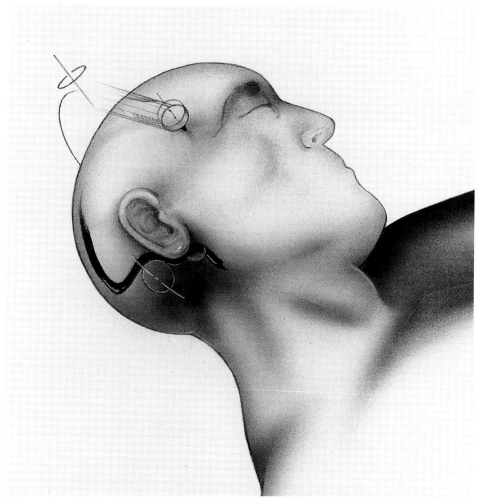

Figure 1. Patient positioning for MVD of the trigeminal nerve. The patient is placed in the supine position on an ipsilateral shoulder roll with the head in 3-point fixation, turned about 45° away from the surgeon, and flexed. The craniectomy is fashioned to expose the borders of the sigmoid sinus anteriorly and the lateral sinus superiorly.

(Figure 1). The patient is given 50 gm of mannitol and 40 mg of furosemide.

A 5-cm vertical retromastoid incision is made ipsilateral to the side of the facial pain four-fifths of the way from the inion to the mastoid tip, half above and half below a line that joins these landmarks. A 2.5-cm craniectomy then is made with a high-speed drill extending to the sigmoid sinus anteriorly and exposing the lateral sinus superiorly. The dura is opened in a semilunar fashion, roughly paralleling the transverse and sigmoid sinuses with the leaflet tacked up to the surrounding soft tissue. Small veins along the superior surface of the cerebellum joining the lateral sinus are coagulated and divided. The cerebellum is gently retracted medially with a self-retaining retractor, though almost no retraction is required in this position. The operating microscope is brought into position at this time. The petrosal vein usually is encountered along the superior petrous ridge and may be coagulated and divided, if necessary. The porus acusticus is identified with the facial, acoustic, and vestibular nerves, and these structures are carefully protected. The porus trigeminus then is identified, along with the nerve and its arachnoid investments. The latter are gently teased away from the nerve, exposing the arterial or other cross-compression source, which is typically at the junction of the nerve and brain stem at the root entry zone (Figure 2). Arteries can be mobilized easily, and, if necessary, a small pledget of Teflon felt interposed. Others have suggested the use of a Sundt clip-graft applied to the sensory root of the trigeminal nerve to protect it from recurrent vascular irritation.[53] Veins obviously indenting or deviating the nerve usually can be coagulated and divided. Final hemostasis is assured by a Valsalva maneuver, retractors are removed, and the dura, muscle, fascia, and skin are meticulously closed.

A somewhat different route is the infratentorial lateral supracerebellar approach described in detail elsewhere.[60] By dissecting over the tentorial cerebellar surface and exposing the anterolateral margin and anterior angle of the cerebellum, the superior cerebellar artery and its branches can be possibly better visualized and dissected away from the trigeminal nerve and its entry zone. Other regional cranial nerves can be avoided with this approach, but inspection of the inferior aspect of the trigeminal nerve may be more difficult.

Patients usually are observed postoperatively for 3-5 days and are maintained on their preoperative dosages of anticonvulsant medication, if any. Patients may continue to have tic pain for a few days postoperatively, particularly when the nerve has been manipulated slightly during decompression. This pain gradually subsides and disappears. Medication is withdrawn slowly at home after discharge. Early recurrences of pain often can be effectively treated by resumption of the previously ineffective drug doses.

Results and Complications

Initial success of MVD has been reported in 96% to 98% of cases and appears directly related to the presence of surgically relieved

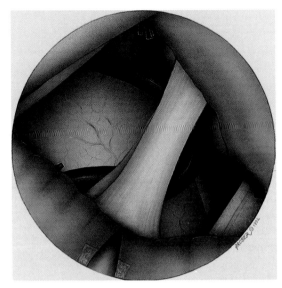

Figure 2. Operative view for MVD of the right trigeminal nerve. A retractor blade is only gently placed on the cerebellum. The cranial nerves IV-VIII usually are well visualized after dividing the petrosal vein and dissecting the arachnoid about the trigeminal nerve. A loop of the superior cerebellar artery is seen here compressing and deforming the trigeminal nerve at its REZ.

arterial cross-compression of the trigeminal nerve. Follow-up data suggest that patients followed for several years will experience a recurrence rate of severe pain in 12% to 29% of cases, or an average of approximately 22%. Moderate recurrences controlled with medication occur in 3% to 4% of cases, and minor and transient recurrences, usually not requiring medication, have been reported in up to 24% of cases.* Previously, it was implied that if patients remained painfree for more than 2 years, there would be a high likelihood of continued, lifelong, painfree existence. Contrary to that belief, a 1.5% per year recurrence of minor symptoms and a 3.5% per year recurrence of major symptoms exist for average long-term follow-ups greater than 8 years.[16] This may imply that MVD does not "cure" trigeminal neuralgia, but simply arrests its progress for a prolonged

---

*References 1, 3, 5, 9, 18, 20, 24, 42-45, 51, 63, 69, 81, 83, 85, 89, 92, 99-101.

period. If enough intrinsic damage to the system already has occurred, there remains a progressive erosion in the number of pain-free patients over time.

The nature of the clinical facial pain syndrome also appears to have prognostic implications for the long-term success rate of the procedure. Patients with paroxysmal pain may have as high as a 95% chance of remaining painfree postoperatively, while in those with both paroxysmal and constant pain, only approximately 58% may have long-term remission. In the latter group of patients, pain extending over two or three divisions also may indicate a worse prognosis for lasting postoperative remission than pain in a single division.[82]

Better results are obtained when there has been a shorter duration of symptoms prior to surgery.[5] If these symtoms have existed for longer than 8 years, intrinsic, nonreversible abnormalities may have developed. Patients whose painful symptoms later develop in more than one ipsilateral trigeminal distribution probably exemplify this theory.

Bilateral idiopathic trigeminal neuralgia, which is slightly more prominent in females and more familial in nature, may be successfully treated with MVD on both sides or just on the more symptomatic side. Pollack et al[71] have shown an initial 89%, 82%, 66%, and 60% success rate at 0, 1, 5, and 10 years, respectively. With repeat procedures included on patients with recurrent symptoms, an overall 74% maintained good or excellent pain relief.

As to the existence of previously placed surgical destructive lesions prior to MVD, the majority of reviews reveal a slightly lower success rate after MVD. This probably is true concerning minor recurrences of pain, but remains debated concerning long-term, major pain remission.[16]

Operative mortality for MVD is approximately 1%, and while immediate morbidity may be seen in as many as 33% to 60% of cases, significant persisting morbidity occurs in 10% to 23%. Morbidity is accounted for by an occurrence of trochlear (IV), trigeminal (V), abducens (VI), facial (VII), or vestibulo-cochlear (VIII) nerve dysfunction; gait ataxia or vertigo; supratentorial, cerebellar, or brain stem infarction; intracranial hematoma; seizures; CSF leak; or air embolism, Ipsilateral deafness, either partial or complete, has been a particularly troublesome complication and may occur in as many as 19% of cases. Pseudomeningocele, pulmonary embolism, pneumonia, and bacterial meningitis are rare complications. Minor transient complications, including postoperative herpes simplex outbreak, serous otitis media, aseptic meningitis, and superficial wound infection, can occur in 4% to 13%. Although trigeminal hypesthesia has been seen after MVD, interestingly, no cases of dysesthesias or anesthesia dolorosa have been reported.* Altogether, serious morbidity probably averages between 1% and 5% of cases.

Thus, while MVD entails a major operative procedure with the risks of mortality and significant morbidity, its success apparently does not depend on the production of a sensory deficit. It therefore avoids the risks, which are uncomfortable to both patient and physician, encountered in denervating procedures. Furthermore, MVD offers at least the potential for greater long-term pain relief without frequently repeated surgical procedures.

Rhizotomy

Trigeminal root section by the subtemporal extradural approach as described by Frazier has long been used in the treatment of trigeminal neuralgia. As newer procedures have been developed, reports of the outcome from subtemporal rhizotomy have all but vanished from the neurosurgical literature. One only can assume that younger neurosurgeons are not being exposed to this technique, and, as a result, it has fallen into disuse. Presently, a trigeminal rhizotomy is performed as an alternative to MVD when thorough exploration reveals no convincing vascular (or other) impingement. This has

---

*References 1, 3, 9, 18, 20, 24, 26, 31, 42-45, 51, 69, 81, 83, 85, 89, 92, 99-101.

been reported in 14% to 21%[18,69] of cases in which the original intent was to perform MVD. The subtemporal extradural and the posterior fossa approach will be reviewed and the relative risks of each compared.

Technique

The classic Frazier-Spiller procedure is performed under general anesthesia with the patient in skeletal fixation in the sitting position. An 8-cm vertical incision is made 2 cm in front of the external auditory meatus extending superiorly from the zygoma. The temporalis muscle is divided in the direction of its fibers, a burr hole is made in the temporal bone, and the burr hole then is enlarged to a 4-cm craniectomy. An extradural dissection is carried out medially and anteriorly to the foramen spinosum, which is plugged with wax or cotton, and the middle meningeal artery is coagulated and divided. Dissection proceeds medially to the foramen ovale where the third division of V is identified and the dura is carefully dissected from the dura propria of the ganglion and ganglion proper. First, the third and then the second divisions of the ganglion are exposed. The trigeminal root finally is visualized. Care must be taken not to put traction on the ganglion as this can result in indirect stretch of the greater superficial petrosal nerve and, occasionally, indirect injury of the facial nerve. An incision is made in the dura propria just posterior to the ganglion, and CSF of the cistern is encountered. The nerve rootlets then are cut or avulsed close to the lateral two-thirds of the ganglion, sparing the ophthalmic fibers, which often are separated from the mandibular division by a small interval. It is important to identify and spare the motor root as section of this results in atrophy of the temporalis muscle and ipsilateral jaw weakness. The dura is closed and the remaining wound is closed in layers.

Approach to the posterior root is performed as described for MVD. Upon visualization of the root, the lateral two-thirds are coagulated with the bipolar cautery and then

divided close to Meckel's cave. It is important to note that rhizotomy performed at the trigeminal root entry zone (REZ) must be of the inferior two-thirds of the root, due to the intrinsic somatotopic organization with the ophthalmic division most superior. Rhizotomy performed by these techniques usually spares ophthalmic sensation and, remarkably, touch sensation on the majority of the face as well. Postoperatively, these patients are treated in all respects like those patients having had MVD.

Results and Complications

Recurrence of pain following extradural rhizotomy occurs in approximately 15% of cases.[88] Operative mortality rates from large series of patients after subtemporal rhizotomy range from 0.8% to 1.6%. Facial weakness has been reported in from 7% to 8%. Paresthesias are a minor complaint in 56% and a severe complaint in 5%. Neuroparalytic keratitis occurs in 15% of cases.[88,91]

Section of the sensory root in the posterior fossa produces long-term pain relief in approximately 80% to 90% of cases, and there is a 1% to 2% incidence of mortality from the procedure. In about 28% of cases, the corneal reflex is impaired, but loss of corneal reflex and keratitis are distinctly unusual complications. Mild facial herpes develops in approximately one-half of the patients. Troublesome facial dysesthesias occur in about 8% of these patients, and another 20% may have mild paresthesias in the denervated area. Facial weakness can occur in 3% to 8%. Ten percent suffer hearing loss which remains permanent in about one-half of these patients. Complications of epidural and subdural hematoma, oculomotor paresis, infection, and thromboembolic events are rare but reported occurrences.[18,28,36,69,90,101]

Based on the available data, there is relatively little evidence favoring one of these approaches over the other for purposes of performing trigeminal rhizotomy. Both procedures have a remarkably similar efficacy, mortality, and morbidity. The possible exceptions are that keratitis appears to occur with some frequency after subtemporal rhizotomy, while it is virtually never seen after the posterior fossa approach, and that hearing loss is not a complication of the subtemporal procedure, but is not uncommon after posterior fossa surgery. Nevertheless, both procedures can yield good results, but should be reserved for patients in whom a minor procedure or MVD is not an option. When MVD is the primary goal of suboccipital craniectomy and no extrinsic vascular compression is found, partial sensory rhizotomy should be performed. In those with vascular contact, but no distortion of the trigeminal nerve root, some advocate both MVD and rhizotomy.

Trigeminal Tractotomy

Destruction of the descending tract of the trigeminal system in the dorsal medulla, the so-called Sjöqvist procedure,[78] produces analgesia and thermanalgesia in the distribution of the ipsilateral nerve with preservation of tactile sensation. This procedure can be used to treat intractable facial pain of both malignant and benign etiology, including that of refractory trigeminal neuralgia. Medullary tractotomy can be performed as either an open,[35,94] or percutaneous stereotaxic[66] procedure. Kunc[52] has previously stimulated the descending trigeminal tract mechanically under local anesthesia to define its anatomic limits. Here, the technique of open radiofrequency tractotomy with continuous peripheral trigeminal stimulation will be described.

Technique

Many of the reported complications of trigeminal tractotomy stem from poor anatomic localization of the descending tract and difficulty in correctly placing lesions within the medulla. The descending tract extends from the area of the second dorsal cervical nerve root medially to the line of emergence of the filaments of the spinal accessory nerve (XI). At the level of the obex, this tract becomes ventrolateral to the restiform body, and its identification becomes problematic. It is pref-

erable to perform the tractotomy after localization by evoked potentials recorded from the brain stem during continuous peripheral trigeminal stimulation.[35]

Under general endotracheal anesthesia, needle electrodes are inserted into the ipsilateral supraorbital, infraorbital, and mental foramina, and a second electrode is placed subcutaneously nearby each site for later bipolar stimulation of each division of the nerve. A similar pair of electrodes is applied to the ipsilateral wrist for median nerve stimulation. The patient is placed in the prone position in skeletal fixation, and through a vertical suboccipital incision, the arch of C1 and approximately 2-3 cm of the foramen magnum are opened. The dura is opened in the midline, exposing the medulla and upper cervical cord. Square-wave pulses (500 msec duration, 5-7 V, 2-3 Hz) are delivered to each facial electrode and the median electrode. The dorsolateral surface of the medulla is explored with a bipolar recording electrode connected to a bioamplifier and oscilloscope. The lateral "physiologic" border of the funiculus cuneatus is identified as the point at which stimulation of the median electrode produces no detectable evoked potential. Following this, the physiologic rostral-caudal and medial-lateral boundaries of the descending tract are delineated during stimulation of each of the facial electrodes individually. Each site is referenced to a common landmark, e.g. the obex or the most rostral cervical nerve rootlets. A radiofrequency electrode with a 2-mm bare tip then is inserted to a depth of 3 mm into the descending tract in the area that has shown the maximal evoked potential from stimulation of the trigeminal division(s) from which the pain originates, and a radiofrequency lesion (60 ma, 30 seconds) is made. The area then is surveyed again with the recording electrode during trigeminal stimulation, and radiofrequency lesions are repeated until evoked potentials are eliminated.

Results and Complications

Recent series of patients in which trigeminal tractotomy has been performed with physiologic monitoring are small. Virtually all patients have dense analgesia in the corresponding region of the face with gross preservation of the tactile sensation and only slight diminution of the corneal reflex. Some modifications in the topography and degree of sensory deficit and analgesia can be made post-tractotomy with various drugs. Levodopa will decrease the zone size of sensory deficit and thus potentially increase the amount of facial pain experienced. Conversely, methyldopa and the longer acting L-tryptophan will increase the sensory deficit zone size and thus decrease pain.[34,48]

Ipsilateral limb ataxia and contralateral limb sensory loss may be seen in 10% and 14% of patients, respectively.[35] This occurs secondary to extension of the lesion into adjacent structures such as the restiform body and the spinothalamic tract. Moreover, as there is difficulty in rendering the mandibular and oropharyngeal regions analgesic with tractotomy, more aggressive lesioning far dorsally may precipitate proprioceptive loss in the ipsilateral arm and leg. Although usually transient, these undesirable complications occasionally persist. No other morbidity and no other mortality have been reported in the more recent studies. However, prior to neurophysiologic monitoring, occasional deaths occurred in tractotomies for benign disease, more so in procedures for malignant disease.

This procedure has been classically more useful in the treatment of intractable pain associated with malignant disease of the head and neck, where 75% to 85% achieved substantial pain relief. When used in combination with appropriate rhizotomies, the beneficial yield may even improve.[49] However, advances in adjunctive cancer therapies, such as radiation and chemotherapy, as well as in improved delivery systems of analgesic medications may obviate the need for such an invasive procedure. As for chronic benign facial pain and that relating to trigeminal neuralgia, pain relief with trigeminal tractotomy has been variable, especially for mandibular division pain. Therefore, all other modalities should be exhausted prior to seriously considering this technique.

Nucleus Caudalis Lesions

This procedure differs from the pure trigeminal tractotomy in that the lesions are placed in such a manner that the secondary neurons carrying painful and thermal sensation are destroyed. These neurons reside within the pars caudalis of the spinal trigeminal nucleus. This region not only is associated with trigeminal pathways for pain and temperature, but also receives small somatosensory components of the facial, glossopharyngeal, and vagus nerves. Therefore, lesioning the pars caudalis, which extends from the lower aspect of the pars interpolaris to about the C2 spinal segment (where it becomes indistinguishable with the substantia gelatinosa), will theoretically result in ipsilateral hemifacial analgesia, including the ear, throat, and tongue. Within the nucleus caudalis, as within the trigeminal tract, topographic representation of trigeminal sensory input exists (Figure 3).

Technique

Nucleus caudalis lesioning has been performed both in an open and in a percutaneous fashion, with or without the use of a thermocouple DREZ electrode. The surgical procedure used in nucleus caudalis DREZ lesions derived from the work of Nashold et al[7,8,67] will be presented. The initial surgical exposure is similar to that for trigeminal tractotomy. A small suboccipital craniectomy and C1 to C2 laminectomies are performed, after which the dura is opened and the operating microscope positioned. The obex, entry zone for the dorsal C2 fiber, and the exit zone for the spinal accessory nerve then are identified. Again, intraoperative evoked potentials from each trigeminal division aid in lesion localization. Beginning inferiorly at the entry zone adjacent to the C2 dorsal root, the thermocouple DREZ electrode, with a 3-mm

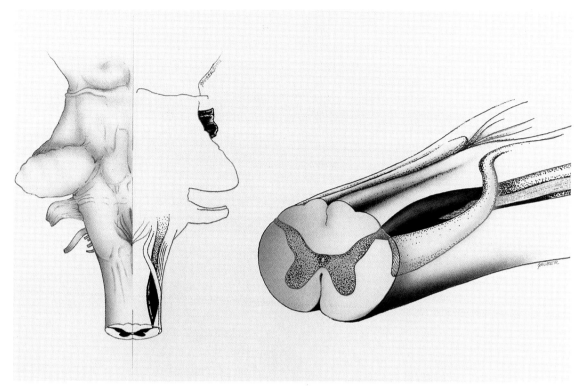

Figure 3. Dorsal and oblique lateral representations of the lower brain stem and cervicomedullary junction depicting the position of the pars caudalis of the spinal trigeminal nucleus. This "subnucleus" takes a position caudal to the other spinal trigeminal subnuclei, the pars oralis and the pars interpolaris. The nucleus caudalis remains medial to the trigeminal spinal tract throughout its entire rostrocaudal extent. Its relationship to the dorsal spinocerebellar tract is variable, however, as this pathway sweeps superiorly over the nucleus, from a medial to lateral direction, to eventually lie in a ventral position. At the first cervical level, the nucleus caudalis merges with the substantia gelatinosa and the trigeminal spinal tract merges with the dorsolateral tract of Lissauer. Note the location of the nucleus caudalis lateral and inferior to the obex.[80]

penetrating portion and a 2-mm uninsulated tip, is used to make multiple thermocoagulative caudalis lesions (at 75° C. for 15 seconds) at 1-mm intervals to a point approximately 2 mm above the obex. Spiegelmann et al[80] suggest using two different electrodes to lesion the full extent of the nucleus caudalis and trigeminal tract. For lesioning at the obex level to a few milimeters just below it, a laterally inserted, 90°-bent-tip Nashold electrode is used to spare the dorsal spinocerebellar tract. For the remainder of the inferior lesioning, a conventional DREZ electrode, with a 2-mm uninsulated tip, is used to coagulate the now superficial nucleus caudalis and trigeminal tract. After the lesions are completed, evoked potentials should not be elicitable.

Results and Complications

Relatively few, small clinical series of nucleus caudalis DREZ lesions[7,8,67,80] and other forms of nucleotomy procedures[38,70,77] are reported. Patients in these series have suffered from various etiologies of facial pain, including refractory postherpetic neuralgia, tic douloureux, dental extraction, glaucoma, anesthesia dolorosa, head and neck cancers, and post-traumatic facial pain. Certain generalizations still may be deduced. First, immediate postoperative pain relief can be seen in approximately 85% of cases, declining to 55% to 76% on a subsequent follow-up. In all the studies reviewed here, patients with postherpetic neuralgia have the best results in the long run, with good to excellent pain relief in 67% to 100% of cases. Patients with burning or sharp, lancinating pain have better results than those with dull, achy pain. In addition, patients with painful symptoms lasting less than 4 years fare better than those with more long-lasting symptoms. If these preoperative symptoms were associated with only minor or no sensory deficits, a better outcome also could be expected. Finally, the number of trigeminal dermatomes affected preoperatively has no bearing on the results, as all ipsilateral divisions are covered by unilateral nucleus caudalis DREZotomy.

As for patients with trigeminal neuralgia and other atypical facial pains, results were varied with good pain relief in only approximately 50% of cases. The encouraging results seen with refractory, postherpetic craniofacial neuralgia stem the notion that this entity may primarily involve the secondary afferent neurons in the nucleus caudalis. Therefore, this disease may represent an example of a "central" pain phenomenon,[67] that can be directly treated with this procedure.

Postoperative dysesthetic pain has not been reported thus far. Mild transient ipsilateral dysmetria affecting the upper more than the lower extremity has been observed in most patients.[8,38,80] This, however, did not cause a significant functional problem. Occasional mortality occurred, but usually was associated with other postoperative medical problems.

Summary and Conclusion

Concerning medical treatment in general, the more these pains resemble typical trigeminal neuralgia, the more likely patients will respond to anticonvulsant medications such as carbamazepine, baclofen, or phenytoin. If the pain has a constant or burning character, a tricyclic antidepressant such as amitriptyline in doses of 100-500 mg at bedtime in combination with fluphenazine 1-2.5 mg given orally, twice daily, represents a reasonable option. If a trigeminal neuroma or other mass lesion can be demonstrated, surgical excision can be recommended, but this is an

unusual occurrence. Further trigeminal deafferentation by neurectomy, gangliolysis, or rhizotomy is notably unsuccessful in the management of this condition and often worsens the pain state.

The best way to compare the outcomes for pain-relieving procedures such as these is to look at the point at which 50% of patients can be statistically expected to have return of pain. Initial efficacy for these surgical procedures is quite good. Most series report that more than 85% of patients will be painfree after any of the procedures described previously. If the patient continues to have pain after a percutaneous operation, the procedure simply can be repeated, and by that means almost all patients can be treated successfully. If MVD fails initially to relieve the pain, after an appropriate recovery interval a percutaneous procedure can be performed, which also is highly likely to result in a painfree state. For the percutaneous retrogasserian glycerol rhizotomy procedure, the expected painfree interval is approximately 1.5-2 years, and similar results have been seen with the balloon microcompression technique. The percutaneous radiofrequency trigeminal gangliolysis procedure produces about twice the painfree interval, or about 3-4 years, and out of the major operative procedures, pain relief can be expected to last an average of approximately 15 years after successful MVD.

Among the more major operative procedures, MVD is clearly the procedure of choice since it offers the potential benefits of greater long-term relief without sensory loss and its attendant complications. Rhizotomy should be used when peripheral procedures have been ineffective and/or when exploration of the trigeminal root does not reveal clear-cut vessels or other structures compressing the nerve. Trigeminal tractotomy should be reserved for those rare cases when all other surgical modalities have failed and the patient continues to have severe intractable trigeminal neuralgia. Similar reservations hold true for the use of nucleus caudalis DREZ lesions for the treatment of severe intractable trigeminal neuralgia. This procedure, however,

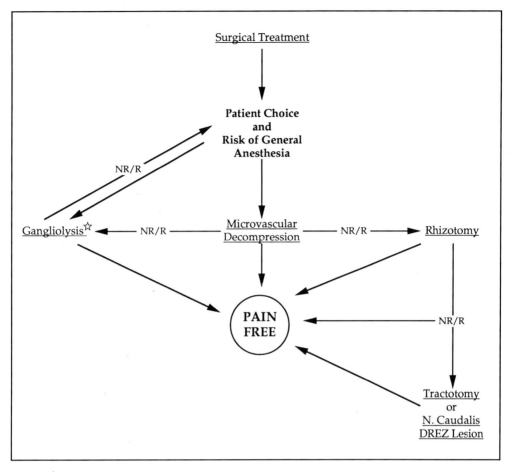

Figure 4. *Algorithm for the surgical management of trigeminal neuralgia. A decision is based on counseling with the patient and his or her overall risk for general anesthesia. NR/R = no relief or recurrence of pain, ☆ = glycerol, balloon, or radiofrequency gangliolysis.*

appears promising for the treatment of patients with the atypical pains of refractory postherpetic neuralgia or of burning or lancinating deafferentation pain of short duration and limited sensory loss.

In the future, other procedures not discussed earlier may prove useful in the treatment of typical and atypical trigeminal neuralgias. These include: high cervical epidural spinal-cord stimulation;[4] stereotaxic mesencephalotomy,[65] which may prove efficacious for treating the pain associated with head and neck cancer; and stereotactic lesions of the centrum medianum-parafascicularis complex of the thalamus.[95] These procedures are considered somewhat experimental at this time and should be offered only at those centers

conducting research into these potential modalities.

The choice between a major and a minor operative procedure in a patient with trigeminal neuralgia refractory to maximal medical therapy ultimately should be made between the patient and the physician. When presented with the expected outcome and morbidity and mortality data, most patients and families can make a reasonable, informed decision on the desired mode of surgery. In a younger, healthy patient, emphasis can be placed on the greater long-term success of MVD procedures, while in older patients, the decision process probably should be biased toward minor operative procedures of glycerol or radiofrequency gangliolysis, or peripheral neurectomy. If severe, refractory, atypical pain exists from either head and neck cancer or postherpetic neuralgia, trigeminal tractotomy or nucleus caudalis DREZ lesioning may have to be considered.

An analysis of the results of minor and major procedures for trigeminal neuralgia reveals a striking, and perhaps significant, fact. Most procedures that involve the ganglion or retrogasserian nerve appear to have a long-term efficacy of approximately 80%. Alcohol neurolysis and peripheral neurectomy have an initially similar response rate, but the recurrence rate increases after several years. This may derive from the regenerative capacity of the trigeminal nerve and the nature of the peripheral lesion.

In contrast, more "central" procedures seem to have an initial 6-12 month period where recurrences are greatest, followed by a relatively long interval during which recurrences are sporadic, but less frequent. Such procedures include glycerol and radiofrequency gangliolysis, percutaneous balloon microcompression, MVD, and trigeminal rhizotomy. This common response rate to such disparate techniques suggests that a common mechanism is operative.

It has been proposed that simply traumatizing the trigeminal nerve can alleviate or even eliminate the syndrome. Previous results with so-called "percussion" procedures certainly would support this, and data available on the results of the various surgical manipulations discussed in this chapter would be consistent with this as well.

Data have been presented that imply that spontaneous discharges within the nerve may, in part, be responsible for the clinical syndrome of trigeminal neuralgia.[83] Furthermore, abnormal neural activity in damaged axons may be eliminated by relatively minor (chemical) trauma to the nerve.[92] Thus, trauma to the nerve may irrevocably alter the pathophysiologic mechanism responsible for trigger or pain phenomena and might represent the basis for success of most procedures and their remarkably similar rates of success.

Where these surgical procedures seem to differ is in the realm of morbidity and mortality risk. Ideally, given their similar efficacies, the treating physician should elect the technique that has the least significant risk of complications. A dogmatic approach to the procedure of choice in the surgical treatment of trigeminal neuralgia is unwise because many excellent surgeons have obtained equally impressive results with widely varying methodologies. In the final analysis, a surgeon skilled in a few of the procedures discussed previously can deliver state-of-the-art quality patient care. Figure 4 depicts one algorithm out of many potential protocols for the surgical management of trigeminal neuralgia.

References

1. Apfelbaum RI. A comparison of percutaneous radiofrequency trigeminal neurolysis and microvascular decompression of the trigeminal nerve for the treatment of tic douloureux. *Neurosurgery.* 1977; 1:16-21.
2. Babu R, Murali R. Arachnoid cyst of the cerebellopontine angle manifesting as contralateral trigeminal neuralgia: case report. *Neurosurgery.* 1991; 28:886-887.
3. Barba D, Alksne JF. Success of microvascular decompression with and without prior surgical therapy for trigeminal neuralgia. *J Neurosurg.* 1984; 60:104-107.
4. Barolat G, Knobler RL, Lublin FD. Trigeminal neuralgia in a patient with multiple sclerosis treated with high cervical spinal cord stimulation: case report. *Appl Neurophysiol.* 1988;51:333-337.
5. Bederson JB, Wilson CB. Evaluation of microvascular decompression and partial sensory rhizotomy in 252 cases of trigeminal neuralgia. *J Neurosurg.* 1989; 71:359-367.
6. Belber CJ, Rak RA. Balloon compression rhizolysis in the surgical management of trigeminal neuralgia. *Neurosurgery.* 1987;20:908-913.
7. Bernard EJ Jr, Nashold BS Jr, Caputi F, et al. Nucleus caudalis DREZ lesions for facial pain. *Brit J Neurosurg.* 1987;1:81-91.
8. Bernard EJ Jr, Nashold BS Jr, Caputi F. Clinical review of nucleus caudalis dorsal root entry zone lesions for facial pain. *Appl Neurophysiol.* 1988; 51:218-224.
9. Breeze R, Ignelzi RJ. Microvascular decompression for trigeminal neuralgia: results with special reference to the late recurrence rate. *J Neurosurg.* 1982; 57:487-490.
10. Brisman R. Bilateral trigeminal neuralgia. *J Neurosurg.* 1987;67:44-48.
11. Brisman R. Trigeminal neuralgia and multiple sclerosis. *Arch Neurol.* 1987;44:379-381.
12. Broggi G, Franzini A, Lasio G, et al. Long-term results of percutaneous retrogasserian thermorhizotomy for "essential" trigeminal neuralgia: consid-

erations in 1000 consecutive patients. *Neurosurgery.* 1990;26:783-786.

13. Brown JA, Preul MC. Percutaneous trigeminal ganglion compression for trigeminal neuralgia: experience in 22 patients and review of the literature. *J Neurosurg.* 1989;70:900-904.

14. Burchiel KJ. Surgical treatment of trigeminal neuralgia: minor operative procedures. In: Fromm GH, ed. *Medical and Surgical Management of Trigeminal Neuralgia.* Mount Kisco, NY: Futura Publishing Co; 1987:71-99.

15. Burchiel KJ. Percutaneous retrogasserian glycerol rhizolysis in the management of trigeminal neuralgia. *J Neurosurg.* 1988;69:361-366.

16. Burchiel KJ, Clarke H, Haglund M, et al. Long-term efficacy of microvascular decompression in trigeminal neuralgia. *J Neurosurg.* 1988;69:35-38.

17. Burchiel KJ, Soldevilla FX, Loeser JD. Pathophysiology of atypical trigeminal neuralgia. Abstract presented at Congress of Neurological Surgeons meeting. 1991.

18. Burchiel KJ, Steege TD, Howe JF, et al. Comparison of percutaneous radiofrequency gangliolysis and microvascular decompression of the trigeminal nerve for the surgical management of tic douloureux. *Neurosurgery.* 1981;9:111-119.

19. Crucci G, Leandri M, Feliciani M, et al. Idiopathic and symptomatic trigeminal pain. *J Neurol Neurosurg Psychiatry.* 1990;53:1034-1042.

20. Cusick JF. Atypical trigeminal neuralgia. *JAMA.* 1981;245:2328-2329.

21. Dandy WE. Concerning the cause of trigeminal neuralgia. *Am J Surg.* 1934;24:447-455.

22. Dieckmann G, Bockermann V, Heyer C, et al. Five-and-a-half years' experience with percutaneous retrogasserian glycerol rhizotomy in treatment of trigeminal neuralgia. *Appl Neurophysiol.* 1987;50:401-413.

23. Farago F. Trigeminal neuralgia: its treatment with two new carbamazepine analogues. *Eur Neurol.* 1987;26:73-83.

24. Ferguson GG, Brett DC, Peerless SJ, et al. Trigeminal neuralgia: a comparison of the results of percutaneous rhizotomy and microvascular decompression. *Can J Neurol Sci.* 1981;8:207-214.

25. Florenza R, Llovet J, Pou A, et al. Contralateral trigeminal neuralgia as a false localizing sign in intracranial tumors. *Neurosurgery.* 1987;20:1-3.

26. Fritz W, Schäfer J, Klein HJ. Hearing loss after microvascular decompression for trigeminal neuralgia. *J Neurosurg.* 1988;69:367-370.

27. Fujimaki T, Fukushima T, Miyazaki S. Percutaneous retrogasserian glycerol injection in the management of trigeminal neuralgia: long-term follow up results. *J Neurosurg.* 1990;73:212-216.

28. Gelber BR, Gogela LJ, Pierson EW. Posterior fossa partial trigeminal rhizotomy: an alternative to microvascular decompression. *Nebr Med J.* 1989;74:105-108.

29. Haddad FS, Taha JM. An unusual cause for trigeminal neuralgia: contralateral meningioma of the posterior fossa. *Neurosurgery.* 1990;26:1033-1038.

30. Haines SJ, Jannetta PJ, Zorub DS. Microvascular relations of the trigeminal nerve: an anatomical study with clinical correlation. *J Neurosurg.* 1980;52:381-386.

31. Hanakita J, Kondo A. Serious complications of microvascular decompression operations for trigeminal neuralgia and hemifacial spasm. *Neurosurgery.* 1988;22:348-352.

32. Hardy DG, Rhoton AL Jr. Microsurgical relationship of the superior cerebellar artery and the trigeminal nerve. *J Neurosurg.* 1978;49:669-678.

33. Harsh GR IV, Wilson CB, Hieshema GB, et al. Magnetic resonance imaging of vertebrobasilar ectasia in tic convulsif: case report. *J Neurosurg.* 1991;74:999-1003.

34. Hodge CJ Jr, King RB. Medical modification of sensation. *J Neurosurg.* 1976;44:21-28.

35. Hosobuchi Y, Rutkin B. Descending trigeminal tractotomy: neurophysiological approach. *Arch Neurol.* 1971;25:115-125.

36. Hussein M, Wilson LA, Illingsworth R. Patterns of sensory loss following fractional posterior fossa Vth nerve section for trigeminal neuralgia. *J Neurol Neurosurg Psychiatry.* 1982;45:786-790.

37. Hutchins LG, Harnsberger HR, Jacobs JM, et al. Trigeminal neuralgia (tic douloureux): MR imaging assessment. *Radiology.* 1990;175:837-841.

38. Ishijima B, Shimoji K, Shimizu H, et al. Lesions of spinal and trigeminal dorsal root entry zone for deafferentation pain: experience of 35 cases. *Appl Neurophysiol.* 1988;51:175-187.

39. Jannetta PJ. Arterial compression of the trigeminal nerve at the pons in patients with trigeminal neuralgia. *J Neurosurg.* 1967;26(suppl):159-162.

40. Jannetta PJ. Microsurgical approach to the trigeminal nerve for tic douloureux. *Prog Neurol Surg.* 1976;7:180-200.

41. Jannetta PJ. Treatment of trigeminal neuralgia by suboccipital and transtentorial cranial operations. *Clin Neurosurg.* 1977;24:538-549.

42. Jannetta PJ. Treatment of trigeminal neuralgia by micro-operative decompression. In: Youmans JR, ed. *Neurological Surgery,* 2nd ed. Philadelphia, Pa: Saunders Company; 1982:3589-3603.

43. Jannetta PJ. Microsurgical management of trigeminal neuralgia. *Arch Neurol.* 1985;42:800.

44. Jannetta PJ, Tew JM. Treatment of trigeminal neuralgia. *Neurosurgery.* 1979;4:93.

45. Jannetta PJ, Zorub DS. Microvascular decompression for trigeminal neuralgia. In: Bucheit WA, Truex RC Jr, eds. *Surgery of the Posterior Fossa.* New York, NY: Raven Press; 1979:143.

46. Kato S, Otsuki T, Yamamoto T, et al. Retrograde adriamycin sensory ganglionectomy: novel approach for the treatment of intractable pain. *Stereotact Funct Neurosurg.* 1990;54-55:86-89.

47. Katusic S, Beard CM, Bergstralh E, et al. Incidence and clinical features of trigeminal neuralgia, Rochester, Minn., 1945-1984. *Ann Neurol.* 1990;27:89-95.

48. King RB. Pain and tryptophan. *J Neurosurg.* 1980;53:44-52.

49. King RB. Medullary tractotomy for pain relief. In: Wilkins RH, Rengachary SS, eds. *Neurosurgery.* New York, NY: McGraw-Hill; 1985:2452-2454.

50. Kirkpatrick DB. Familial trigeminal neuralgia: case report. *Neurosurgery.* 1989;24:758-761.

51. Kolluri S, Heros RC. Microvascular decompression for trigeminal neuralgia: a five-year follow-up study. *Surg Neurol.* 1984;22:235-240.

52. Kunc Z. Significant factors pertaining to the results of trigeminal tractotomy. In: Hassler R, Walker AE, eds. *Trigeminal Neuralgia: Pathogenesis and Pathophysiology.* Philadelphia, Pa: WB Saunders Co; 1970:90-100.

53. Laws ER Jr, Kelly PJ, Sundt TM, Jr. Clip-grafts in microvascular decompression of the posterior fossa: technical note. *J Neurosurg.* 1986;64:679-681.

54. Lazorthes Y, Armengaud JP, Da Motta M. Chronic stimulation of the Gasserian ganglion for treatment of atypical facial neuralgia. *Pacing and Clinical Electrophysiology.* 1987;10:257-265.

55. Leandri M, Favale E. Diagnostic relevance of trigeminal evoked potentials following infraorbital nerve stimulation. *J Neurosurg.* 1991;75:244-250.

56. Leandri M, Parodi CI, Favale E. Early trigeminal evoked potentials in tumours of the base of the skull and trigeminal neuralgia. *Electroencephalogr Clin Neurophysiol.* 1988;71:114-124.

57. Lichtor T, Mullan JF. A 10-year follow-up review of percutaneous microcompression of the trigeminal ganglion. *J Neurosurg.* 1990;72:49-54.

58. Lobato RD, Rivas JJ, Sarabia R, et al. Percutaneous microcompression of the gasserian ganglion for trigeminal neuralgia. *J Neurosurg.* 1990;72:546-553.

59. Lye RH. Basilar artery ectasia: an unusual cause of trigeminal neuralgia. *J Neurol Neurosurg Psychiatry.* 1986;49:22-28.

60. Matsushima T, Fukui M, Suzuki S, et al. The microsurgical anatomy of the infratentorial lateral supracerebellar approach to the trigeminal nerve for tic douloureux. *Neurosurgery.* 1989;24:890-895.

61. Meglio M, Cioni B. Percutaneous procedures for trigeminal neuralgia: microcompression versus radiofrequency thermocoagulation. Personal experience. *Pain.* 1989;38:9-16.

62. Meglio M, Cioni B, d'Annunzio V. Percutaneous microcompression of the gasserian ganglion: personal experience. *Acta Neurochir (Wien).* 1987; 39(suppl):142-143.

63. Meglio M, Cioni B, Moles A, et al. Microvascular decompression versus percutaneous procedures for typical trigeminal neuralgia: personal experience. *Stereotact Funct Neurosurg.* 1990;54-55:76-79.

64. Morita A, Fukushima T, Miyazaki S, et al. Tic douloureux caused by primitive trigeminal artery or its variant. *J Neurosurg.* 1989;70:415-419.

65. Nashold BS Jr. Brainstem sterotaxic procedures. In: Schaltenbrand G, Walker AE, eds. *Stereotaxy of the Human Brain: Anatomical Physiological and Clinical Applications.* New York, NY: Georg Thieme. 1982:475-483.

66. Nashold BS Jr, Crue BL. Stereotaxic mesencephalotomy and trigeminal tractotomy. In: Youmans JR, ed. *Neurological Surgery.* 2nd ed. Philadelphia, Pa: WB Saunders Co; 1982:3702-3716.

67. Nashold BS Jr, Lopes H, Chodakiewitz J, et al. Trigeminal DREZ for craniofacial pain. In: Samii M, ed. *Surgery in and around the Brain Stem and Third Ventricle: Anatomy, Pathology, Neurophysiology, Diagnosis, Treatment.* New York, NY: Springer-Verlag; 1986:54-59.

68. Patsalos PN, Elyas AA, Zakrzewska JM. Protein binding of oxcarbazepine and its primary active metabolite, 10-hydroxycarbazepine, in patients with trigeminal neuralgia. *Eur J Clin Pharmacol.* 1990; 39:413-415.

69. Piatt JH, Wilkins RH. Treatment of tic douloureux and hemifacial spasm by posterior fossa exploration: therapeutic implications of various neurovascular relationships. *Neurosurgery.* 1984;14:462-471.

70. Plangger CA, Fischer J, Grunert V, et al. Tractotomy and partial vertical nucleotomy: for treatment of special forms of trigeminal neuralgia and cancer pain of face and neck. *Acta Neurochir (Wien).* 1987; 39(suppl):147-150.

71. Pollack IF, Jannetta PJ, Bissonette DJ. Bilateral trigeminal neuralgia: a 14-year experience with microvascular decompression. *J Neurosurg.* 1988;68: 559-565.

72. Rand RW. Gardner neurovascular decompression of the trigeminal and facial nerves for tic douloureux and hemifacial spasm. *Surg Neurol.* 1981;16: 329-332.

73. Rand RW. The Gardner neurovascular decompression operation for trigeminal neuralgia. *Acta Neurochir (Wien).* 1981;58:161-166.

74. Sahni KS, Pieper DR, Anderson R, et al. Relation of hypesthesia to the outcome of glycerol rhizolysis for trigeminal neuralgia. *J Neurosurg.* 1990;72:55-58.

75. Saini SS. Retrogasserian anhydrous glycerol injection therapy in trigeminal neuralgia: observation in 552 patients. *J Neurol Neurosurg Psychiatry.* 1987; 50:1536-1538.

76. Saito N, Yamakawa K, Sasaki T, et al. Intramedullary cavernous angioma with trigeminal neuralgia: a case report and review of the literature. *Neurosurgery.* 1989;25:97-101.

77. Schvarcz JR. Craniofacial postherpetic neuralgia managed by stereotactic spinal trigeminal nucleotomy. *Acta Neurochir (Wien).* 1989;46(suppl):62-64.

78. Sjöqvist O. Studies on pain conduction in trigeminal nerve: a contribution to the surgical treatment of facial pain. *Acta Psychiatr Scand* 1938;17(suppl): 1-139.

79. Snow RB, Fraser RAR. Cerebellopontine angle tumor causing contralateral trigeminal neuralgia: a case report. *Neurosurgery.* 1987;21:84-86.

80. Spiegelmann R, Friedman WA, Ballinger WE, et al. Anatomic examination of a case of open trigeminal nucleotomy (nucleus caudalis dorsal root entry zone lesions) for facial pain. *Stereotact Funct Neurosurg.* 1991;56:166-178.

81. Swanson SE, Farhat SM. Neurovascular decompression with selective partial rhizotomy of the trigeminal nerve for tic douloureux. *Surg Neurol.* 1982; 18:3-6.

82. Szapiro J, Sindou M, Szapiro J. Prognostic factors in microvascular decompression for trigeminal neuralgia. *Neurosurgery.* 1985;17:920-929.

83. Taarnhøj P. Decompression of the posterior trigeminal root in trigeminal neuralgia: a 30-year follow-up review. *J Neurosurg.* 1982;57:14-17.

84. Tanaka A, Takaki T, Maruta Y. Neurinoma of the trigeminal root presenting as atypical trigeminal neuralgia: diagnostic values of orbicularis oculi reflex and magnetic resonance imaging: a case report. *Neurosurgery.* 1987;21:733-736.

85. Tarlov E. Percutaneous and open microsurgical techniques for relief of refractory tic douloureux. *Surg Clin North Am.* 1980;60:593-607.

86. Tash RR, Sze G, Leslie DR. Trigeminal neuralgia: MR imaging features. *Radiology.* 1989;172:767-770.

87. Tsubaki S, Fukushima T, Tamagawa T, et al. Parapontine trigeminal cryptic angiomas presenting as trigeminal neuralgia. *J Neurosurg.* 1989;71:368-374.

88. Tytus JS. Treatment of trigeminal neuralgia through temporal craniotomy. In: Youmans JR, ed. *Neurological Surgery 2nd ed.* Philadelphia, Pa: WB Saunders Co; 1982:3580-3585.

89. Van Loveren H, Tew JM Jr, Keller JT, et al. A

10-year experience in the treatment of trigeminal neuralgia: comparison of percutaneous stereotaxic rhizotomy and posterior fossa exploration. *J Neurosurg.* 1982;57:757-764.

90. Welch K. Treatment of trigeminal neuralgia by section of the sensory root in the posterior fossa. In: Youmans JR, ed. *Neurological Surgery. 2nd ed.* Philadelphia, Pa: WB Saunders Co; 1982:3586-3588.

91. White JC, Sweet WH. *Pain and the Neurosurgeon: A Forty Year Experience.* Springfield, Ill: Charles C. Thomas; 1969:179.

92. Wilson CB, Yorke C, Prioleau G. Microsurgical vascular decompression for trigeminal neuralgia and hemifacial spasm. *West J Med.* 1980;132:481-484.

93. Wong BY, Steinberg GK, Rosen L. Magnetic resonance imaging of vascular compression in trigeminal neuralgia: case report. *J Neurosurg.* 1989;70:132-134.

94. Young RF, Oleson TD, Perryman KM. Effect of trigeminal tractotomy on behavioral response to dental pulp stimulation in the monkey. *J Neurosurg.* 1981;55:420-430.

95. Young RF, Modesti LM. Stereotactic ablative procedures for pain relief. In: Wilkins RH, Rengachary SS, eds. *Neurosurgery.* New York, NY: McGraw-Hill Book Co; 1985:2454-2457.

96. Young RF. Glycerol rhizolysis for treatment of trigeminal neuralgia. *J Neurosurg.* 1988;69:39-45.

97. Zakrzewska JM, Patsalos PN. Oxcarbazepine: a new drug in the management of intractable trigeminal neuralgia. *J Neurol Neurosurg Psychiatry.* 1989; 52:472-476.

98. Zakrzewska JM. Medical management of trigeminal neuralgia. *Br Dent J.* 1990;168:399-401.

99. Zakrzewska JM. Cryotherapy for trigeminal neuralgia: a 10 year audit. *Br J Oral Maxillofac Surg.* 1991; 29:1-4.

100. Zhang KW, Zhao YH, Shun ZT, et al. Microvascular decompression by retrosigmoid approach for trigeminal neuralgia: experience in 200 patients. *Ann Otol Rhinol Laryngol.* 1990;99:129-130.

101. Zorman G, Wilson CB. Outcome following microsurgical vascular decompression of partial sensory rhizotomy in 125 cases of trigeminal neuralgia. *Neurology.* 1984;34:1362-1365.

CHAPTER 8

Hemifacial Spasm and Other Facial Nerve Dysfunction Syndromes

Robert H. Wilkins, MD

The dysfunction syndromes of the facial (VII) nerve include those involving hyperfunction and those involving hypofunction. The former category includes hemifacial spasm, Hunt's neuralgia, and, perhaps, cluster headaches. The latter group is composed of facial palsy of spontaneous onset (Bell's palsy). The emphasis in this chapter is on the aspects of these conditions that are dealt with surgically within the posterior fossa.

Hemifacial Spasm

Diagnosis

Hemifacial spasm is a syndrome of spontaneous and gradual onset that ordinarily makes its appearance in mid-life.[8,9,24,25,52,54,56,57] It affects women more often than men, with the reported ratios varying from 3:1 to 3:2. Its hallmark is intermittent twitching of the muscles of facial expression on one side of the face, the left side being favored at a ratio between 3:2 and 4:3.

As with tic douloureux, the patient may enjoy asymptomatic periods early in its course. Eventually, however, the problem occurs on a daily basis and the facial muscular contractions become stronger. Typically, the syndrome begins as a mild intermittent twitching of the muscles about one eye. As it progresses, more of the muscles supplied by the ipsilateral facial nerve become involved, including the platysma at times. In some patients, the stapedius muscle also will contract spasmodically, which the individual experiences as a peculiar tinnitus in the ipsilateral ear.[7,28] With time, tonic facial muscular contractions occur in addition to the rapid twitching; mild paresis eventually may develop in some of the involved muscles.

Jannetta has described an atypical form of hemifacial spasm that begins in the buccal muscles and spreads upward.[24,25] He encountered this form in 7.4% of 366 patients, and noted that the vascular compression of the facial nerve as found at operation in these patients tended to be on the postero-rostral aspect rather than the antero-caudal aspect of the nerve as most commonly encountered in patients with typical hemifacial spasm.

With either type of hemifacial spasm, the paroxysms of facial contraction are not accompanied by lacrimation or rhinorrhea, and they are not followed by a refractory period. Although the facial muscular contractions are involuntary and may occur during sleep, they may be modified to some extent by other events. Voluntary facial movements such as elevating the eyebrows may trigger the involuntary movements of hemifacial spasm. An effort to relax the face may result in momentary diminution of spasm. Hemifacial spasm frequently is intensified by fatigue, stress, anxiety, or self-consciousness, and occasionally its severity may be altered by a change in head position.

Hemifacial spasm is not a life-threatening disorder, but it alters the patient's facial appearance and may present a significant cosmetic problem. After repetitive contraction, the facial muscles may ache and feel tired. Any tinnitus caused by contractions of the stapedius muscle may annoy the patient. Of more importance, repetitive closure of the eyelids on one side will interfere with vision and may hamper reading, driving, and other important activities.

The key to the diagnosis of hemifacial spasm is the clinical observation of the abnormal facial movements. Typically, the physician will see evidence of frequent spontaneous spasms and occasional tonic contractions in the facial muscles on one side; slight ipsilateral facial weakness also may be noted, especially if the condition has been present for several years. Electromyography of the facial muscles may provide useful information if the diagnosis is unclear by clinical examination.[57]

Other studies ordinarily are not of help in establishing the diagnosis of hemifacial spasm, but may be valuable in disclosing the etiology in those relatively few patients with gross structural abnormalities such as an ectatic, elongated vertebrobasilar arterial system (megadolichovertebrobasilar anomaly); neoplasm; arteriovenous malformation; or arterial aneurysm. As a general rule, before treatment is undertaken, computed tomography (CT) scanning or magnetic resonance imaging (MRI) should be performed on all patients with hemifacial spasm to identify such lesions because the presence of one of these processes probably will influence the type of treatment chosen and might indicate the need for additional diagnostic studies such as angiography prior to treatment.

Associated Conditions

At times, hemifacial spasm is accompanied by ipsilateral dysfunction of another cranial nerve, probably because of an identical or similar etiology—for instance, nerve compression adjacent to the brain stem by the same epidermoid tumor or a similar artery. The acoustic nerve may be involved. As examples of this, 15 (14%) of the 106 patients reported by Ehni and Woltman had impaired hearing on the side involved by spasm,[9] and 56 (41%) of the 137 patients reported by Møller and Møller had an abnormal acoustic middle ear reflex.[35] The ipsilateral trigeminal (V) nerve may be involved by tic douloureux, and rarely nervus intermedius involvement may be manifest as geniculate neuralgia. The combination of hemifacial spasm and ipsilateral tic douloureux was termed *painful tic convulsif* in 1920 by Harvey Cushing,[6] and more than 50 patients with this condition have been reported since that time.[5,57] Yeh and Tew recently have used the term *tic convulsif* to denote the combination of hemifacial spasm and geniculate neuralgia.[59] At least four individuals with this combination have been described in the medical literature since 1963.[57]

Jannetta has postulated that vascular compression of the left side of the medulla between the entry or exit zones of the glossopharyngeal (IX) and vagus (X) nerves and the inferior olive is a cause of arterial hypertension.[22,23,27] Because of the close proximity of this area to the exit zone of the facial nerve, one might expect that patients with left hemifacial spasm are more likely to be hypertensive than those with right hemifacial spasm. While operating on 27 hypertensive patients for a vascular compression syndrome such as hemifacial spasm or trigeminal neuralgia, Jannetta also inspected the lateral aspect of the medulla. In 20 of 22 patients whose operations were on the left side, he noted arterial compression of the medulla in the area mentioned previously. Yet in 5 patients with right-sided operations, Jannetta saw no such vascular compression. Among 30 of my own patients, 8 of 19 (42%) with left hemifacial spasm were hypertensive, compared with 3 of 11 (27%) with right hemifacial spasm; this difference is not statistically significant (Chi-square test: $p = 0.70$).[57]

TABLE 1*
Clinical Differentiation of HFS from Other Facial Movements[a]

	Sex	Age	Side	Voluntary control	Sleep	Clinical characteristics	Association	Electrophysiologic testing
Hemifacial spasm	F > M	50-70	Unilateral	No	May be present	Tonic/clonic movement of facial muscles innervated by cranial nerve VII	Vessel compressing on cranial nerve VII root at entry zone (dolichoectatic vessel) Tumor AVM	Blink reflex latency normal; usually synkinetic movement with appearance of response in muscles other than orbicularis oculi on the affected side. EMG: Arrhythmic discharge, 20-40 sec
Blepharospasm	M = F	50-70	Bilateral	Yes (somewhat)	Absent	Bilateral synchronous spasms of the orbicularis oculi	Midbrain and thalamic infarcts Progressive supranuclear palsy Meige's syndrome	Blink reflex latency normal. May see increased amplitude; no synkinesis EMG: facial muscles normal voluntary motor units
Orofacial dystonia (Meige's syndrome)	M = F	Any age	Bilateral	No	Absent	Writhing movements often involving the tongue and respiration	Drugs Basal ganglia disease	Blink reflex normal EMG: normal
Facial synkinesis after Bell's palsy	M = F	Any age	Unilateral	No	Present	Unilateral facial weakness; may see "crocodile tears," gustatory lacrimation	Prior history of facial paralysis	Blink reflex: increased latencies of R1 and R2 on the affected side EMG: evidence of synkinesis and fibrillation potentials and reduced motor units
Spastic paretic facial contracture	M = F	Any age	Unilateral	No	Present	Hemifacial smile present at all times but paretic on voluntary movement	Brain stem glioma Multiple sclerosis	Blink reflex: may see increased latencies of R1 and R2 on the affected side EMG: fibrillation potential and reduced number of motor units. Myokymia may be seen.
Facial myokymia	M = F	Any age	Unilateral (rarely bilateral)	No	Present	Constant, rapid undulation and flickering muscles ("bag of worms appearance")	Multiple sclerosis Intramedullary tumor	Blink reflex latency normal EMG: myokymic discharge (grouped fasciculations)
Facial tic	M = F	Children	Bilateral or unilateral	Yes	Present	Stereotypic movements: brief, repetitive, suppressible	Gille de la Tourette's syndrome	Blink reflex latency normal EMG: normal (usually)
Focal seizure of the face	M = F	Any age	Unilateral	No	—	Movements occurring with head and eye deviation	Focal cortical lesion	Blink reflex latency normal EMG: normal EEG: abnormal

[a]AVM, arteriovenous malformation; EEG, electroencephalogram; EMG, electromyogram.
*From Reference 8.

Differential Diagnosis

Various conditions can cause abnormal facial movements, and hemifacial spasm must be differentiated from them (Table 1). Ordinarily, this is not difficult. At times, postparalytic hemifacial spasm can resemble spontaneous hemifacial spasm, but with the former there should be a history of previous facial palsy. Blepharospasm[16,21] often is confused with hemifacial spasm by physicians and others who do not understand the difference between the two. Of interest, a single support group exists for both of these conditions—the Benign Essential Blepharospasm Research Foundation.

The condition that most closely mimics spontaneous hemifacial spasm is postparalytic hemifacial spasm, which follows facial paresis such as that caused by Bell's palsy or trauma to the facial nerve. Each has one or more of four features involving the muscles supplied by the affected facial nerve: spontaneous spasms, contractures, intrafacial associated movements (facial synkinesis), and weakness. With spontaneous hemifacial spasm, the spasms are the dominant feature, whereas the contractures and synkinesis are the most noticeable aspects of postparalytic hemifacial spasm.

Spastic paretic facial contracture and facial myokymia are conditions that ordinarily arise from a lesion within the brainstem such as a glioma, multiple sclerosis, or a tuberculoma. The spastic facial contracture and weakness may resemble the contractures and weakness of long-standing hemifacial spasm but the myokymia can be differentiated from the twitching of hemifacial spasm. Such myokymia has been described as a continuous, undulating, wormlike, spreading movement.

Essential blepharospasm is a condition manifested by involuntary bilateral repetitive and symmetrical blinking of the eyes. At times it may be accompanied by bilateral dystonic spasms of the lower facial or oromandibular muscles as Meige's syndrome. These disorders are easily differentiated from hemifacial spasm because they are bilateral.

Other conditions may also superficially resemble hemifacial spasm, such as habit spasms (idiopathic tics), focal cortical seizures, tardive dyskinesia, and the wincing that occurs in response to the pain of tic douloureux. However, these are sufficiently different that they should not be confused with hemifacial spasm.[56]

Etiology and Pathogenesis

Over the years following the original recognition of hemifacial spasm as a clinical entity, there has been debate about the etiology and pathogenesis of this condition. It is now known that various pathologic processes occasionally can cause hemifacial spasm, primarily by involving the ipsilateral facial nerve.[57] The association usually is one of compression or distortion of the nerve in the cerebellopontine angle by an ectatic, elongated, and tortuous vertebrobasilar arterial system; a neoplasm; an arteriovenous malformation; or an arterial aneurysm. During the past two decades, evidence has accumulated that in most patients, the condition seems to be caused by compression, by an adjacent blood vessel, of the zone of exit of the facial nerve from the brain stem.[18,22,24,25,37,57]

How these factors result in hemifacial spasm still is being investigated and argued. There currently are three main theories about the pathogenesis of hemifacial spasm.[8,57]

Some investigators have proposed that communication occurs between adjacent axons within the facial nerve, perhaps because focal compression and demyelination permit the formation of a false synapse (ephapse).[12-14,38-40] Such ectopic excitation and ephaptic transmission then results in an abnormal conduction of impulses through the peripheral portion of the facial nerve.

Other investigators, however, have postulated that the important pathophysiologic changes in hemifacial spasm occur within the facial motor nucleus, perhaps in response to a peripheral stimulus.[11] Møller has been a strong advocate of this idea.[31,32]

The third theory is that aberrant regeneration occurs within the facial nerve, perhaps from a point of nerve compression, such that some of the axons originally supplying one facial muscle become misdirected to another.[8,57] This idea seems to have more relevance to the development of postparalytic hemifacial spasm than it does to the development of spontaneous hemifacial spasm.

Treatment

Various approaches have been taken to the treatment of hemifacial spasm.[57] In those few patients with a structural abnormality along the course of the facial nerve that can be detected by CT or MRI, such as a neoplasm in the cerebellopontine angle, the treatment of choice is to remove the lesion and decompress the facial nerve. Most patients, however, do not fall into this category and must be treated in other ways.

Some forms of nonoperative treatment have been tried.[57] Most of these, involving approaches such as psychotherapy, electrical stimulation, massage, and radiotherapy, have not been beneficial. And, in general, medication has not proved effective, although some patients have been helped by haloperidol, clonazepam, carbamazepine, orphenadrine, or baclofen.

In recent years, Type A botulinum exotoxin has been injected in small doses into various facial muscles to reduce their contractions.[57] Complete or nearly complete relief of the symptoms is achieved in 90% to 100% of the patients, but muscle weakness is substituted for hyperactivity. Relief is temporary—lasting an average of 3-4 months—so injections have to be repeated periodically for an indefinite time.

Operative treatment of hemifacial spasm has been of two main types.[57] The first is designed to injure or interrupt the facial nerve at some point along its course, and the second is aimed at removing the presumed cause of the condition but leaving the facial nerve intact.

Various ingenious techniques have been used to injure or interrupt the facial nerve.[57] Some surgeons have compressed or otherwise traumatized the facial nerve in the cerebellopontine angle, and others have divided it partially or totally just after its exit from the stylomastoid foramen. As a rule, these approaches substitute facial paralysis or paresis for the abnormal muscular contractions. Furthermore, as the facial nerve regenerates or otherwise recovers from the injury, the hemifacial spasm returns along with the ability to contract the facial muscles voluntarily. In addition, it has been shown that the simultaneous performance of a nerve anastomosis using the hypoglossal or spinal accessory nerve to restore facial function and to prevent regrowth of the facial nerve into its distal channels has not been a guarantee against the recurrence of the hemifacial spasm.

An alternative to the operative exposure of the facial nerve trunk has been the percutaneous injection of alcohol or phenol into the nerve trunk to injure it chemically, or the percutaneous insertion of a needle into the nerve trunk to injure it mechanically or with a radiofrequency current. Other surgical approaches have included the division or injection of peripheral facial nerve branches. All of these alternatives have the disadvantages

of replacing the abnormal movements with weakness and of not producing a permanent cessation of the hemifacial spasm.

Microvascular Decompression

The most successful form of treatment to date has been microvascular decompression (MVD) of the facial nerve at the brain stem.* I discussed the historic aspects of the development of this approach in Chapter 4 of this book.

This procedure usually is performed with the patient in a lateral recumbent or in a sitting position. The facial nerve is exposed through a retromastoid craniectomy, and the existence of vascular compression is sought at the brain stem. If one or more arteries or arterial branches are discovered, these are dissected away from the area(s) of compression and this displacement is maintained by the insertion of an inert material such as polyvinyl alcohol foam or shredded Teflon® (E.I. du Pont de Nemours & Co., Wilmington, Delaware) felt. The most commonly encountered arteries are the vertebral artery, the posterior inferior cerebellar artery (PICA), and the anterior inferior cerebellar artery (AICA), with the relative frequencies of involvement varying among the authors who have reported series of patients treated for hemifacial spasm by MVD.[57] If one or more veins are discovered, these usually are coagulated with bipolar current and divided to prevent recanalization. During the operation, brain stem auditory evoked potentials (BAEPs) are monitored as a way of detecting early and potentially reversible changes in auditory function.[33-35,41,44,57,58]

Among Jannetta's 366 patients with hemifacial spasm (HFS),

. . . the etiology was thought to be arterial in 323 (multiple arteries in 96), venous in 7, and both arterial and venous in 33; of the other three patients, one had a tumor, one had an aneurysm, and one had an arteriovenous malformation. [25]

---

*References 18, 22, 24, 25, 28, 29, 37, 43, 54, 56, 57

Furthermore, Jannetta noted that of the patients with vascular compression, those with typical HFS had this vascular effect on the anterocaudal aspect of the facial nerve exit zone, whereas those with atypical HFS almost always had the effect on the posterorostral aspect. . . . In Jannetta's series, [24] the most common artery involved in typical HFS was the posterior inferior cerebellar artery. This was also the experience of Loeser and Chen. [29]57

In a personal series of 74 patients, 1 had a meningioma in the ipsilateral cerebellopontine angle. Among the first 48, whose operative findings were analyzed, [43] arterial contact with the facial nerve was noted in 46 (96%) patients, in 15 of whom there was visible anatomical distortion of the nerve. As in Jannetta's experience, [24] it was not uncommon that more than one vessel seemed to contribute to the vascular compression in a single patient. In 22 instances the nerve was contacted by the PICA; in 17, by the AICA; and in 11, by the vertebral artery. In 10 other instances, an artery contacting the nerve could not be named because of insufficient exposure. One patient had osseous contact with the nerve, and one patient had no perceptible abnormality.[57]

In 1990, Jannetta reported the outcome of 366 patients.[25] "Initially, 215 (58%) had a complete response, 141 (39%) had a partial response, and 10 (3%) had no response. The long-term results among 334 patients followed for 12 to 189 months (mean, 68 months) with a 10% reoperation rate, showed that 298 (89%) had a complete response, 17 (5%) had a partial response, and 19 (6%) had no response."[57]

In 1983, Loeser and Chen assessed the results of 20 personal patients and 15 series of patients from the medical literature.[29] "The 433 patients from the 16 series had 450 operations: 366 (84%) were 'cured' initially and 17 (4%) were 'cured' by a second operation. The incidence of relapse after complete cessation of spasm was less than 10%. However, the length of follow-up in the 16 series was as short as 1 month."[57]

In 1984, we reported the results of MVD for the first 48 of a personal series of patients with hemifacial spasm.[43]

After an average follow-up period of 42.5 months, 30 (62.5%) had complete relief (excellent result)

and 12 (25%) had only infrequent and mild periorbital twitching (good result). Six patients either noted no significant improvement or sustained a recurrence after initial relief. A later assessment of 41 of these patients who were followed from 5 to 12 years (average, 8.1 years) postoperatively showed that initially 32 had an excellent result and 6 had a good result. This favorable immediate outcome tended to persist with time. Of the 32 with an excellent result, only 3 experienced recurrence, at 1, 6, and 54 months after operation, respectively. Three of the 41 patients underwent a second operation. At the time of last follow-up, 30 had an excellent result, 6 had a good result, and 5 had significant residual or recurrent HFS.[57]

Among a larger group of 74 personal patients treated for hemifacial spasm, 7 have had a re-exploration.[57]

The complications of MVD for hemifacial spasm center around inadvertent injury to the cranial nerves and vessels in the lower cerebellopontine angle.[57] In 1983, Loeser and Chen summarized the complications of 450 MVD operations from 16 patient series.[29]

There were 341 (76%) operations with no complications, 38 (8%) with temporary complications, and 71 (16%) with permanent complications. Among the complications were 58 (13%) instances of auditory nerve dysfunction and 26 (6%) instances of facial nerve dysfunction. There was one (0.2%) reported death.[57]

. . . . In a personal series of 74 patients, the complication rate tended to diminish as the experience of the surgeon grew, with the exception of the incidence of significant ipsilateral hearing loss, which did not improve until the institution of intraoperative monitoring of auditory evoked potentials. . . . Prior to the institution of intraoperative auditory evoked potential monitoring at our hospital in 1984, 10 (6.6%) of 152 primary microvascular decompression operations for HFS or tic douloureux were followed by a profound ipsilateral hearing loss or deafness. Subsequently, however, none of the 109 primary operations (assessed through June 1989) caused profound hearing loss or deafness. [44,59]57

. . . . However, evoked potential monitoring is not an absolute safeguard against deafness. Even with direct intraoperative monitoring of auditory compound action potentials from the eighth nerve.

. . . ,Møller and Møller [35] noted that 1 of 39 patients undergoing a first microvascular decompression operation for HFS 'lost his hearing instantaneously during decompression of the facial nerve.' Likewise, Nishihara et al. [41] encountered a severe reduction in hearing in 2 of 94 patients having microvascular decompression as treatment of HFS or tic douloureux, despite both BAEP and direct auditory compound action potential monitoring. Furthermore, . . . the dissection involved in reexploration of the cerebellopontine angle in a patient with persistent or recurrent HFS is especially hazardous. Two (29%) of seven such patients in the author's practice sustained ipsilateral deafness despite intraoperative BAEP monitoring; in both cases, the evoked potentials were lost abruptly and did not recover despite immediate cessation of retraction and operative manipulation.[57]

Hunt's Geniculate Neuralgia; Cluster Headache

The nervus intermedius is part of the facial nerve complex. It consists of a series of filaments that lie between, and communicate with, the facial and vestibular nerves in the cerebellopontine angle. Its fibers subserve the autonomic and sensory aspects of facial nerve function.

The greater superficial petrosal nerve leaves the nervus intermedius within the temporal bone at the geniculate ganglion and enters the cranial cavity through the hiatus of the facial canal. It runs forward on the floor of the middle fossa, passing under the gasserian ganglion and lateral to the internal carotid artery. It is joined by the deep petrosal nerve from the sympathetic plexus around the internal carotid artery to form the vidian nerve, which passes forward through the pterygoid canal to the sphenopalatine ganglion.

Preganglionic parasympathetic fibers from the lacrimal nucleus travel through the nervus intermedius and greater superficial petrosal nerve to reach the sphenopalatine ganglion. . . . Postganglionic fibers mediate secretory impulses to the lacrimal gland via the zygomatic nerve and its anastomosis with the lacrimal nerve. Other postganglionic fibers carry secretory and vasodilatory impulses to the mucous glands and vessels of the nasal epithelium. . . . Additional preganglionic parasympathetic fibers, leaving the medulla with the fibers mentioned above, pass through the nervus intermedius but leave the greater superficial petrosal nerve to join the internal carotid artery plexus. Within this plexus are neurons that give

rise to vasodilatory postganglionic fibers that pass to the cerebral arteries. . . .[36]

The sensory functions of the facial nerve have been examined by many investigators, but especially by J. Ramsay Hunt, who was a Professor of Neurology at Columbia University College of Physicians and Surgeons. For more than 30 years, he studied the sensory system of the facial nerve and various pain syndromes that he related to this system— forms of geniculate neuralgia. He concluded in 1937 that the sensory system of the facial nerve has four separate pathways for the transmission of sensory impulses.[20] The first involves sensory filaments from the geniculate ganglion that supply the tympanic membrane, a cutaneous area on the external ear, and (along with cranial nerve VIII) the internal ear. The second includes sensory fibers of the greater superficial petrosal and vidian nerves passing from the geniculate ganglion through the sphenopalatine ganglion and distributed with its orbital, posterior nasal, and palatal branches. The third pathway consists of nerve fibers of deep sensibility of the face that originate in the geniculate ganglion and pass with the peripheral motor branches to the facial musculature. The fourth pathway is essentially gustatory, involving the chorda tympani nerve, but also contains fibers that transmit common sensation from the ipsilateral anterior two-thirds of the tongue.

Hunt classified geniculate neuralgia into primary, secondary, and reflex forms, and thought that the most common secondary form is that following herpetic inflammation of the geniculate ganglion (postherpetic form). Concerning the location of the pain, he classified geniculate neuralgia into otalgic and prosopalgic forms consistent with the sensory distributions of the facial nerve as described previously.[20]

He concluded his 1937 paper as follows:

To summarize, the neuralgic affections of the various cranial nerves are:

1. True trigeminal neuralgia, which is distributed in one or more branches of the trifacial nerve

and in which the pain is localized in the more superficial structures of the face and intra-oral region. . . . In cases of neuralgia of the third division of the fifth nerve there is often associated otalgia.

2. Geniculate neuralgia, which involves the deeper structures of the face. This is characterized by pain in the deep posterior orbital, palatal and nasal regions, with painful pressure sensation in the face. This is geniculate deep prosopalgia, and with it there is associated geniculate otalgia.

3. Glossopharyngeal neuralgia, which is characterized by neuralgic pains in the distribution of the glossopharyngeal nerve at the base of the tongue and the adjacent regions of the throat and by associated otalgia.

4. Superior laryngeal neuralgia, of vagal origin, in which the pains are localized in the region of the larynx, with associated otalgia.

All these various forms are accessible to surgical intervention by the cranial method of approach through the posterior fossa, which exposes the fifth, seventh, ninth, and tenth cranial nerves. If this procedure is carried out with the use of local anesthesia, it is possible by touching any one of the nerves to reproduce the neuralgic pain, thus confirming the clinical diagnosis, which is often involved and difficult.[20]

In 1909, Alfred Taylor operated on a patient with otalgia that was thought to represent "tic douloureux of the sensory filaments of the facial nerve."[4] He exposed the cerebellopontine angle and divided the facial nerve, nervus intermedius, and upper fasciculus of the acoustic nerve. At follow-up evaluation 5 months postoperatively, the patient reported having been relieved of her ear pain.

White and Sweet summarized the surgical treatment of that patient and 8 more in 1969.[53] In these cases and some others,[2,3,17,42,46,59] the nervus intermedius has been shown to be important in the mechanism of aural pain, either because cutting it stopped the pain, stimulating it provoked the pain, or some other suggestive circumstance existed.

In 1980, Ouaknine and coworkers reported on a 48-year-old woman who had a 21-year history of left geniculate neuralgia associated with left

tinnitus and reduced auditory acuity and occasional dizziness. [42] She died from the rupture of an arteriovenous malformation of the temporal lobe. At autopsy, a redundant loop of the left posterior inferior cerebellar artery was found to be cross-compressing the facial, intermediate, and cochleovestibular nerves. . . . However, as discussed by Ouaknine and colleagues, in relatively few cases of cranial neuralgia have the exact neurovascular relationships of the nervus intermedius been studied. . . .[55]

Therefore, the relative importance of vascular compression as an etiologic factor in otalgic geniculate neuralgia has not yet been determined.

Rupa and associates treated 18 patients with primary otalgia by a total of 31 surgical procedures.[46] Seventeen patients had sequential rhizotomies and 1 patient had MVD alone. The nerves sectioned, singly or in combination, were the nervus intermedius (14 patients), geniculate ganglion (10 patients), glossopharyngeal nerve (14 patients), vagus nerve (11 patients), tympanic nerve (4 patients), and chorda tympani nerve (1 patient). MVD was performed in 9 patients in whom vascular loops were discovered. By this inclusive and repetitive approach, the authors were able to provide pain relief to 72% of their patients for a mean follow-up period of 3.3 years.

As implied by the previous discussion, there are many causes of otalgia other than geniculate neuralgia, and several sources of sensory innervation of the external, middle, and inner ear, and the tonsillar area.[51] Except for the postherpetic variety, otalgic geniculate neuralgia has proved difficult to diagnose with certainty.[2,3,17]

Likewise, the diagnosis of prosopalgic geniculate neuralgia is also difficult to substantiate. As Bronson Ray stated, "there is a variety of syndromes of face pain. . . . Included in this group are: sphenopalatine neuralgia or Sluder's headache, vidian neuralgia, buccal neuralgia, Horton's cephalalgia, lower-half headache, atypical facial neuralgia, and carotidynia. There are others with less commonly mentioned names. Each of these syndromes has some special feature which supposedly sets it apart from the other, but each borders on the other and distinguishing features are frequently spurious."[45]

Of these forms of facial pain, one seems to be fairly common—cluster headache.* "Cluster headache (also called migrainous neuralgia, Horton's syndrome, and histamine cephalalgia among other terms) is a typical form of cranial pain syndrome that can occur episodically or chronically. . . . It is predominantly a disorder of adult men, with reported male to female ratios ranging between 4.5:1 and 6.7:1. The pain is typically unilateral and retro-orbital, oculotemporal or oculofrontal in location, excruciating in severity, and boring and non-throbbing in character. In association with the pain, the patient may exhibit ipsilateral signs of autonomic dysfunction such as rhinorrhea or nasal congestion, increased lacrimation, ptosis, and miosis."[36]

Various medical regimens have been and are used to prevent or treat episodic or chronic cluster headache.[10,17,36,48,49,53] But the headaches of some patients are or become refractory to such management, which has led to the development of various surgical strategies designed to interrupt the transmission of nociceptive and autonomic impulses, including those transmitted through the facial nerve.[36]

Beginning in 1940, Gardner and his associates [15] treated cluster headache by resecting the greater superficial petrosal nerve in an attempt to interrupt abnormal parasympathetic discharges responsible for dilation of the cerebral, meningeal, and nasal mucosal blood vessels, the pain resulting from which was being transmitted over the trigeminal nerve. However, they also thought it possible that the operation interrupted painful impulses coming over the geniculate somatic afferent fibers from the dura mater, internal carotid artery, and vidian nerve. By the time of their report in 1947, Gardner, et al., had performed this procedure on 13 patients. The results were excellent in 25% and fair to good in 50%; 25% of the patients experienced no relief.

*References 10, 15, 17, 19, 30, 36, 48-50, 53

Other surgeons subsequently performed this same procedure for cluster headache. . . . In 1970, Stowell [50] reported 36 patients so treated for cluster headache over a 20-year period. Of these, 32 had complete relief, but 15 subsequently experienced recurrence of headache (eight by 1 year, three more by 2 years, and four more by 3 years). . . .

. . . it seems that the main drawback to the treatment of cluster headache by greater superficial petrosal neurectomy is the incidence of headache recurrence, which in some cases may result from nerve regeneration. Because of the relatively high failure and recurrence rates associated with this type of surgical treatment, other approaches have been tried.

Two of these approaches involve interruption of the same neural system, either peripheral to the greater superficial petrosal nerve (the sphenopalatine ganglion) or central to it (the nervus intermedius). In 1962, Brown [1] reported that the injection of alcohol into the sphenopalatine ganglion of 28 patients with cluster headache did not reliably stop the headache. Meyer, et al., [30] in 1970, presented 13 patients with intractable cluster headache who were treated by sphenopalatine ganglionectomy; seven obtained little relief, four were improved, and only two had complete relief (for more than 1 year).[36]

In contrast, Salar et al reported the successful relief of pain in each of 7 patients treated by percutaneous radiofrequency thermocoagulation of the sphenopalatine ganglion, with follow-up periods of 6 to 28 months.[47] Although the diagnosis in the 7 patients was sphenopalatine ganglion neuralgia, the description of the syndrome given by the authors blends with that of cluster headache.

Surgical interruption of the nervus intermedius has been used by various surgeons to treat cluster headache, either as the sole procedure or in combination with injury to some portion of the trigeminal system.[17,36,53] Likewise, surgical injury to some portion of the trigeminal system has been used as the primary treatment, either alone or in combination with division of the nervus intermedius.[10,17,19,36,53] Finally, MVD of the trigeminal and facial nerves at the brain stem, solely or in combination, has been tried.[36] The problems with all of these approaches have been the inconsistency of pain relief and the high probability of recurrence of the cluster headache. A reliable surgical method for curing cluster headache has not yet been developed.

Bell's Palsy

Jannetta and Bissonette noted in 1978 that "the etiology of Bell's palsy, like a number of other cranial nerve afflictions which consist of rapid or sudden loss of function, has never been satisfactorily explained despite extensive analysis by a number of investigators over the years. These entities may have a simple mechanical explanation in some patients. This consists of the sudden shift of an arterial loop in the cerebellopontine angle stretching the appropriate nerve."[26]

In support of their thesis, Jannetta and Bissonette presented 5 patients with Bell's palsy who were found at operation to have the facial-acoustic nerve bundle stretched and compressed from the anterior aspect. The first patient was a 57-year-old woman who underwent sectioning of the right nervus intermedius for intractable nervus intermedius neuralgia in April of 1972. She had had right-sided Bell's palsy 7 years previously, with complete resolution of the facial weakness. "At operation, the facial nerve was noted to be stretched by an arterial loop about 1 cm. from the brain stem. . . . The artery was left undisturbed."[26] The other four patients were operated upon between July 1973 and November 1975 for Bell's palsy. All were found to have vascular compression of the facial nerve at a point between the brain stem and the porus acusticus, and all improved after surgical decompression of the nerve.

In 1981, Jannetta reported the operative findings of 11 patients with intractable Bell's palsy.[23] There were 8 males and 3 females, varying in age from 29 to 73 years. The palsy was on the right in 3 and on the left in 8. It had been present between 11 days and 8 years. In 10 patients, the facial nerve was noted to be stretched by an arterial loop; the nerve also was swollen in 2 patients, who were operated on at 11 and 41 days after the onset, respectively. One patient had no treatment. Of the 10 treated patients, 7 improved, although 6 had residual weakness and 5 had synkinesis.

Summary

Hemifacial spasm can be diagnosed by observation and clinical history. It is thought to arise primarily from compression of the facial nerve at the brain stem, usually by an adjacent artery. Although many approaches to treatment have been tried, the most effective is MVD of the facial nerve at the brain stem. This operation has well-recognized risks, including ipsilateral deafness. The latter complication ordinarily can be avoided by the use of intraoperative monitoring of auditory evoked potentials.

Hunt's geniculate neuralgia of either the nonherpetic otalgic or prosopalgic type is difficult to diagnose. Experience with the surgical treatment of either type has been so limited that no meaningful conclusions can be drawn. In contrast, cluster headache of either the episodic or chronic type is a commonly recognized condition for which a number of surgical treatments have been tried. Unfortunately, no surgical approach thus far has provided satisfactory long-term relief for the majority of patients treated.

The etiology of Bell's palsy remains a matter for conjecture. Jannetta has postulated that in some patients, Bell's palsy may be caused by vascular compression of the facial nerve in the cerebellopontine angle, but the evidence in support of this idea is limited so far.

References

1. Brown LA. Mythical sphenopalatine ganglion neuralgia. *South Med J.* 1962;55:670-672.
2. Bruyn GW. Nervus intermedius neuralgia (Hunt). *Cephalalgia.* 1984;4:71-78.
3. Bruyn GW. Nervus intermedius neuralgia (Hunt). *Handbook Clin Neurol.* 1986;48:487-494.
4. Clark LP, Taylor AS. True tic douloureux of the sensory filaments of the facial nerve. *JAMA.* 1909; 53:2144-2146.
5. Cook BR, Jannetta PJ. Tic convulsif: results of 11 cases treated with microvascular decompression of the fifth and seventh cranial nerves. *J Neurosurg.* 1984;61:949-951.

6. Cushing H. The major trigeminal neuralgias and their surgical treatment based on experiences with 332 gasserian operations. *Am J Med Sci.*1920;160: 157-184.

7. Diamant H, Enfors B, Wiberg A. Facial spasm: with special reference to the chorda tympani function and operative treatment. *Laryngoscope.* 1967; 77:350-358.

8. Digre K, Corbett JJ. Hemifacial spasm: differential diagnosis, mechanism, and treatment. *Adv Neurol.* 1988;49:151-176.

9. Ehni G, Woltman HW. Hemifacial spasm: review of one hundred and six cases. *Arch Neurol Psychiatry.* 1945;53:205-211.

10. Ekbom K. Chronic migrainous neuralgia. *Handbook Clin Neurol.* 1986;48:247-255.

11. Ferguson JH. Hemifacial spasm and the facial nucleus. *Ann Neurol.* 1978;4:97-103.

12. Gardner WJ. Concerning the mechanism of trigeminal neuralgia and hemifacial spasm. *J Neurosurg.* 1962;19:947-958.

13. Gardner WJ. Cross talk—the paradoxical transmission of a nerve impulse. *Arch Neurol.* 1966;14: 149-156.

14. Gardner WJ, Sava GA. Hemifacial spasm: a reversible pathophysiologic state. *J Neurosurg.* 1962;19: 240-247.

15. Gardner WJ, Stowell A, Dutlinger R. Resection of the greater superficial petrosal nerve in the treatment of unilateral headache. *J Neurosurg.* 1947; 4:105-114.

16. Grandas F, Elston J, Quinn N, et al. Blepharospasm: a review of 264 patients. *J Neurol Neurosurg Psychiatry.* 1988;51:767-772.

17. Gybels JM, Sweet WH. *Neurosurgical Treatment of Persistent Pain: Physiological and Pathological Mechanisms of Human Pain.* Basel, Switzerland: S Karger; 1989:70-91.

18. Haines SJ, Torres F. Intraoperative monitoring of the facial nerve during decompressive surgery for hemifacial spasm. *J Neurosurg.* 1991;74:254-257.

19. Hassenbusch SJ, Kunkel RS, Kosmorsky GS, et al. Trigeminal cisternal injection of glycerol for treatment of chronic intractable cluster headaches. *Neurosurgery.* 1991;29:504-508.

20. Hunt JR. Geniculate neuralgia (neuralgia of the nervus facialis): a further contribution to the sensory system of the facial nerve and its neuralgic conditions. *Arch Neurol Psychiatry.* 1937;37:253-285.

21. Jankovic J, Orman J. Blepharospasm: demographic and clinical survey of 250 patients. *Ann Ophthalmol.* 1984;16:371-376.

22. Jannetta PJ. Neurovascular compression in cranial nerve and systemic disease. *Ann Surg.* 1980;192: 518-524.

23. Jannetta PJ. Cranial nerve vascular compression syndromes (other than tic douloureux and hemifacial spasm). *Clin Neurosurg.* 1981;28:445-456.

24. Jannetta PJ: Hemifacial spasm. In: Samii M, Jannetta PJ, eds. *The Cranial Nerves: Anatomy, Pathology, Pathophysiology, Diagnosis, Treatment.* New York, NY: Springer-Verlag; 1981:484-493.

25. Jannetta PJ. Cranial rhizopathies. In: Youmans JR, ed. *Neurological Surgery: A Comprehensive Reference Guide to the Diagnosis and Management of Neurosurgical Problems.* 3rd ed. Philadelphia, Pa: WB Saunders Co; 1990:4169-4182.

26. Jannetta PJ, Bissonette DJ. Bell's palsy: a theory as to etiology. Observations in six patients. *Laryngo-*

27. Jannetta PJ, Segal R, Wolfson SK Jr. Neurogenic hypertension: etiology and surgical treatment, I: observations in 53 patients. *Ann Surg.* 1985;201: 391-398.

28. Kim P, Fukushima T. Observations on synkinesis in patients with hemifacial spasm: effect of microvascular decompression and etiological considerations. *J Neurosurg.* 1984;60:821-827.

29. Loeser JD, Chen J. Hemifacial spasm: treatment by microsurgical facial nerve decompression. *Neurosurgery.* 1983;13:141-146.

30. Meyer JS, Binns PM, Ericsson AD, et al. Sphenopalatine ganglionectomy for cluster headache. *Arch Otolaryngol.* 1970;92:475-484.

31. Møller AR. Hemifacial spasm: ephaptic transmission or hyperexcitability of the facial motor nucleus? *Exp Neurol.* 1987;98:110-119.

32. Møller AR. The cranial nerve vascular compression syndrome, II: a review of pathophysiology. *Acta Neurochir (Wien).* 1991;113:24-30.

33. Møller AR, Jannetta PJ. Monitoring auditory functions during cranial nerve microvascular decompression operations by direct recording from the eighth nerve. *J Neurosurg.* 1983;59:493-499.

34. Møller AR, Møller MB. Does intraoperative monitoring of auditory evoked potentials reduce incidence of hearing loss as a complication of microvascular decompression of cranial nerves? *Neurosurgery.* 1989;24:257-263.

35. Møller MB, Møller AR. Loss of auditory function in microvascular decompression for hemifacial spasm: results in 143 consecutive cases. *J Neurosurg.* 1985;63:17-20.

36. Morgenlander JC, Wilkins RH. Surgical treatment of cluster headache. *J Neurosurg.* 1990;72:866-871.

37. Nagahiro S, Takada A, Matsukado Y, et al. Microvascular decompression for hemifacial spasm: patterns of vascular compression in unsuccessfully operated patients. *J Neurosurg.* 1991;75:388-392.

38. Nielsen VK. Pathophysiology of hemifacial spasm. I: ephaptic transmission and ectopic excitation. *Neurology.* 1984;34:418-426.

39. Nielsen VK. Electrophysiology of the facial nerve in hemifacial spasm: ectopic/ephaptic excitation. *Muscle Nerve.* 1985;8:545-555.

40. Nielsen VK. Electrophysiology of hemifacial spasm. In: May M, ed. *The Facial Nerve.* New York, NY: Thieme; 1986:487-497.

41. Nishihara K, Hanakita J, Kinuta Y, et al. Importance of intraoperative monitoring of ABR and compound action potential of the eighth cranial nerve during microvascular decompression surgery. *No Shinkei Geka.* 1986;14:509-518. English abstract.

42. Ouaknine GE, Robert F, Molina-Negro P, et al. Geniculate neuralgia and audiovestibular disturbances due to compression of the intermediate and eighth nerves by the postero-inferior cerebellar artery. *Surg Neurol.* 1980;13:147-150.

43. Piatt JH Jr, Wilkins RH. Treatment of tic douloureux and hemifacial spasm by posterior fossa exploration: therapeutic implications of various neurovascular relationships. *Neurosurgery.* 1984;14: 462-471.

44. Radtke RA, Erwin CW, Wilkins RH. Intraoperative brainstem auditory evoked potentials: significant decrease in postoperative morbidity. *Neurology.* 1989;39:187-191.

45. Ray BS. The surgical treatment of headache and

scope. 1978;88:849-854.

atypical facial neuralgia. *J Neurosurg.* 1954;11: 596-606.

46. Rupa V, Saunders RL, Weider DJ. Geniculate neuralgia: the surgical management of primary otalgia. *J Neurosurg.* 1991;75:505-511.

47. Salar G, Ori C, Iob I, et al. Percutaneous thermocoagulation for sphenopalatine ganglion neuralgia. *Acta Neurochir (Wien).* 1987;84:24-28.

48. Sjaastad O. Cluster headache. *Handbook Clin Neurol.* 1986;48:217-246.

49. Sjaastad O. Chronic paroxysmal hemicrania (CPH). *Handbook Clin Neurol.* 1986;48:257-266.

50. Stowell A. Physiologic mechanisms and treatment of histaminic or petrosal neuralgia. *Headache.* 1970; 9:187-194.

51. Vinken PJ, Bruyn GW, Klawans HL, et al. Headache. *Handbook Clin Neurol.* 1986;48.

52. Wartenberg R. *Hemifacial Spasm: A Clinical and Pathophysiological Study.* New York, NY: Oxford University Press; 1952.

53. White JC, Sweet WH. *Pain and the Neurosurgeon:* *A Forty-Year Experience.* Springfield, IL: Charles C Thomas; 1969:257-265, 345-372, 622-627.

54. Wilkins RH. Hemifacial spasm: treatment by microvascular decompression of the facial nerve at the pons. *South Med J.* 1981;74:1471-1474.

55. Wilkins RH. Surgical therapy of neuralgia: vascular decompression procedures. *Semin Neurol.* 1988; 8:280-285.

56. Wilkins RH. Hemifacial spasm. *Contemp Neurosurg.* 1991;13(6):1-6.

57. Wilkins RH. Hemifacial spasm: a review. *Surg Neurol.* 1991;36:251-277.

58. Wilkins RH, Radtke RA, Erwin CW. The value of intraoperative brainstem auditory evoked potential monitoring in reducing the auditory morbidity associated with microvascular decompression of cranial nerves. *Skull Base Surg.* 1991;1:106-109.

59. Yeh H, Tew JM Jr. Tic convulsif, the combination of geniculate neuralgia and hemifacial spasm relieved by vascular decompression. *Neurology.* 1984; 34:682-684.

CHAPTER 9

Evaluation of Vestibulocochlear Dysfunction Syndromes, Selection of Patients, and Surgical Technique for Selective Microsurgical Vestibular Nerve Section for Intractable Meniere's Syndrome

Edward C. Tarlov, MD, and Dennis S. Poe, MD

Vestibulocochlear dysfunction syndromes encompass a small portion of neurosurgical practice. Patients with tinnitus, hearing loss, and dizziness are in the purview of otolaryngologists, neuro-otologists, and otoneurologists. In the United States, few of the latter two types of specialists exist and many patients must rely on the varied expertise of neurologists and otolaryngologists. Unfortunately, neurosurgical attention will grant beneficial outcomes to only a minority of these patients. This chapter outlines some of the background for determining which patients can reliably be helped by an otoneurosurgical approach and which patients with atypical and poorly understood conditions associated with vertigo should be cautioned against surgery. We begin with the caveat that a little empathy can go a long way. There is a danger of overdiagnosis and of overtreatment. For some patients, the answer to treatment lies in the elegant ancient aphorism of France's great Voltaire: "Amuse the patient until nature brings about a cure." Nevertheless, among the large population of patients with disorders of imbalance and dizziness is a small number with the episodic vertigo, unilateral tinnitus, and fluctuating hearing loss of Meniere's syndrome. Sodium restriction, diuretics, and vestibular sedatives are the initial treatment of choice. However, refractory patients who are symp-

tomatic and still have useful hearing may benefit from selective microsurgical section of the vestibular nerve in the posterior fossa. This operation uses the principles of the standard neurosurgical approaches to the cranial nerves in the cerebellopontine angle, and therefore, a careful judgment as to whether the symptoms are sufficiently severe to warrant an intracranial operation is imperative.

As with most procedures in functional neurosurgery, patient selection is all important and to this end the history is critical. Dizziness is a nonspecific term used by patients. The initial challenge is to determine what a patient really means by dizziness. An imbalance in visual, proprioceptive, and vestibular signals alters perception of orientation of the head and body in space. Only a small number of patients with complaints of dizziness actually have vertigo, the illusion of movement, which is not necessarily rotary. A clinical diagnosis by an experienced otologist is much more valuable than an exhaustive evaluation of nonspecific symptoms.

The precipitating factors and severity of vertigo are important in diagnosis. Benign positional vertigo results from head movement, lasts seconds, and usually is not disabling. Vertebrobasilar ischemia generally is associated with neurologic symptoms in addition to vertigo and referable to the posterior circulation; these may include visual symptoms and facial or other somatic sensory or motor symptoms. Occasionally, vertebrobasilar ischemia occurs when the head is turned and held in a position long enough to compromise blood flow to the brain stem. The classic vertigo of Meniere's syndrome is of sudden, spontaneous onset. Head movements exacerbate symptoms, but are not the precipitating event. The vertigo is typically severe, often completely disabling while active, lasting minutes or hours. Following a severe attack, disequilibrium or positional vertigo can last for hours, days, or weeks, and may be confused with benign positional vertigo.

Labyrinthitis or vestibular neuronitis can cause vertigo, which is identical to a Meniere's attack, but this is self-limited and not recurrent. The effects of these disorders should subside after several weeks. If severe symptoms recur, Meniere's syndrome should be suspected.

Migraines also can cause vertigo that is indistinguishable from Meniere's. The diagnosis of migraine depends on an additional history of associated headaches or other classic neurologic symptoms.

Controversy exists over the importance of perilymph fistulas as a cause of spontaneous vertigo. Symptoms are identical to Meniere's and can be differentiated only by direct visualization of the inner ear by endoscopy or by middle ear exploration. Changes of pressure in the middle ear with air travel, coughing, sneezing, or by pneumatic manipulation of the tympanic membrane are thought to be more commonly associated with fistulas. The symptoms caused by these maneuvers are not reliable in differentiating the patients with Meniere's syndrome.

The sensation of an impending faint is known as presyncopal light-headedness. It can result from orthostatic hypotension, vasovagal attack, hyperventilation, or decreased cardiac output. These syncopal episodes must be distinguished from psychological causes of dizziness, anxiety disorders, panic attacks, and dizziness that can follow ocular surgery.

An excellent discussion of the evaluation of dizziness in patients may be found in the recent work of Baloh and Honrubia.[2] In our practice at the Lahey Clinic, most patients with vestibulocochlear dysfunction syndromes are evaluated in the Department of Otolaryngology and sometimes in Neurology, and referred for joint neurosurgical otologic approaches if Meniere's syndrome is diagnosed.

Proper preoperative selection of patients is critical to the success of any operation. Regarding the treatment of tic douloureux, surgery is highly successful only in patients with typical symptoms. Operations on the trigeminal (V) nerve in patients with atypical facial pains are fraught with problems for the patient and surgeon (see Chapter 7). Similarly, sectioning the vestibular nerve for disorders other than typical Meniere's syndrome is not likely to be successful.

Preservation of hearing usually was not an issue in the era before microsurgery. Many of these patients were deaf before operation, but even those with some hearing could not expect to have preservation of cochlear nerve function postoperatively. Facial palsy also was an occasional consequence of the procedure. Up to a decade ago, the neurosurgical operation for intracranial vestibular nerve section was seldom performed in most neurosurgical units. The disorder was managed by otolaryngologic procedures, including labyrinthectomy, which was performed only on patients who already were deaf, and endolymphatic shunting, which has not produced encouraging results for relief of vertigo.[13,14]

With present microsurgical methods,[6,21-24] selective intracranial section of the vestibular nerve can be carried out safely with preservation of hearing and facial (VII) nerve function. In relieving the disabling vertigo of Meniere's syndrome, the operation can be performed with few lasting side effects. To ensure successful outcomes, however, accurate preoperative diagnosis of Meniere's syndrome is essential. Also, the operation is not likely to relieve vertigo from other causes.

The diagnosis of true Meniere's syndrome

is not common among the spectrum of patients with complaints of dizziness. The incidence of the disorder varies in different studies between estimates of 1/100,000 to 1/1,000 population.[19,23] In most instances, onset is between the ages of 30 and 60 years, with younger and older persons rarely affected.

Strict clinical criteria for diagnosis should be used. Vertigo is the first symptom in the majority of patients and it generally is the most disabling feature of the disease. Recurring attacks usually increase in frequency. Tinnitus is commonly present and sometimes may be the only reliable indicator of which labyrinth is involved. Tinnitus on the side of the affected ear is common. The stage of fluctuating hearing loss may last from a few weeks to several years before deafness occurs. Hearing fluctuations and deafness usually are associated with bouts of vertigo. Ultimately, hearing loss is almost always permanent in untreated patients, and vertigo may continue after deafness is complete. Drop attacks occasionally occur as the result of the loss of tonic influences of the otolith. In severe attacks, the patient may be thrown to the ground, or if seated, may suddenly become disoriented with respect to gravity. Nystagmus may accompany the attacks, but its direction is not of localizing value. Occasionally, spontaneous nystagmus to the side opposite the diseased labyrinth occurs. Electronystagmography with caloric testing usually is abnormal and may demonstrate canal paresis with diminished responses to warm and cold water or air on the affected side. On otologic testing, the majority of patients show low-frequency perceptive hearing loss with fairly good discrimination and negative tone decay on impedance audiometry. Brain stem auditory-evoked response (BAER) testing demonstrates normal latencies.

The most important differential diagnosis is between Meniere's disease and acoustic neuroma. The latter lesion does not cause vertigo as severe as does Meniere's syndrome. The loss of vestibular function usually is slow, producing mild ataxia rather than par-

oxysmal disturbances. Magnetic resonance imaging (MRI) with gadolinium enhancement is helpful in excluding other diagnoses. BAER testing is 96% accurate for acoustic neuroma-better than either computed tomography (CT) scanning with contrast or MRI without gadolinium. BAER testing can identify a vestibulocochlear (VIII) nerve lesion but is not specific for its nature.

Approximately 20% of patients with Meniere's syndrome will have bilateral involvement, and because of this relatively high incidence, attempts at preserving existing hearing have considerable importance. Nevertheless, destruction of the labyrinth, which results in a total loss of hearing, has continued as a standard otologic operation. It is not a desirable form of treatment in patients with unilateral Meniere's syndrome if there is useful hearing in the affected ear or if there is loss of hearing on the other side from other causes. Neither is it desirable in bilateral Meniere's syndrome if both ears are affected early in the disease, if one labyrinth has been destroyed before disease appears in the other ear, or if hearing is poor in one ear and rapidly failing in the other. In these cases, microsurgical vestibular nerve section is appropriate.

On the basis that malabsorption of the endolymph may be the pathology,[12]—a matter of some controversy[18,19]—a variety of operations to relieve excess pressure of the endolymph have been carried out, principally aimed at preserving or improving hearing and relieving tinnitus. Shunting operations, creating fistulas from the endolymphatic sac to the mastoid cavity or the subarachnoid space, have been carried out for many years. The endolymphatic sac-to-subarachnoid shunt has been described by House,[13] and the endolymphatic sac-to-mastoid shunt by Shea.[20] The value of shunting procedures for Meniere's syndrome is unproven, however, and the controversy about the efficacy of these procedures remains. Glasscock et al,[8-10] reviewed the results of these shunting procedures and found that among 112 patients, 66% were relieved of further vertigo and 47% were relieved of tinnitus; 35% had decreased hearing and 45% had stable hearing after shunting. The natural course of the illness is characterized by remissions; and because the hearing loss fluctuates, lengthy and careful followup is required to determine the effect of the therapy on hearing.

The pioneer neurosurgeons had a great deal of experience with vestibular nerve section in Meniere's syndrome and the operation proved to be reliable in their hands. Dandy[3,4,11] refined the operation to the extent that only 2 deaths occurred among his 587 patients. Vertigo was relieved entirely in 90%, was unchanged in 5%, and was worse in 5%. In the majority of these 587 patients, the entire vestibulocochlear nerve bundle was sectioned, with total loss of auditory as well as vestibular function. Fifty-four of the patients had facial paralysis, which was permanent in 17. Of 95 patients in whom only the vestibular portion of the nerve was sectioned, 9 had improved hearing, 27 had unchanged hearing, 46 had loss of hearing, and 13 were totally deaf. In Falconer's[5] experience during the 1960s, 8 patients had some degree of hearing on the operated side.

Jannetta,[15] who did much to develop the surgical treatment of tic douloureux, expanded his theory of vascular compression in cranial rhizopathies to include some patients with complaints of dizziness.[16] These patients did not have Meniere's syndrome, but rather a new syndrome, "disabling positional vertigo," was described.[16] The nine patients who Jannetta et al described experienced constant positional vertigo or disequilibrium severe enough to cause constant and disabling nausea. These patients had no hearing disturbance and no loss of vestibular function. Typically, they had been seen by a number of physicians. The vertigo, although described as constant, was precipitated by changes in head position. In two of the nine patients, vertigo was post-traumatic. All but one patient had specific changes in BAER, resembling those in patients with acoustic nerve tumors, and consisting of a latency shift of wave II and an abnormal amplitude and shape of wave III.

To relieve the condition, Jannetta et al[15] used microvascular decompression (MVD) of one vestibular nerve.

Neurosurgeons agree on the criteria for diagnosing typical trigeminal neuralgia and hemifacial spasm, but positional vertigo can occur from peripheral causes (vestibular neuronitis), from central diseases (brain stem and cerebellar demyelinating diseases, trauma, and arteriosclerosis), and from functional disturbances.

In other related conditions, operation is seldom seriously considered. Benign paroxysmal positional vertigo is a self-limited clinical entity rarely lasting a year. The patient experiences vertigo on tilting the head back to look up or in lying on or rolling over onto the affected ear. Finding calcium concretions in the semicircular canal at postmortem examination has led to naming this condition "cupulolithiasis." The patient is advised to avoid the provocative position. If the condition persists longer than a year, the branch of the vestibular nerve to the posterior canal can be divided through the tympanic membrane via the internal auditory canal with relief of symptoms,[7] but at considerable risk of hearing loss. A newer procedure, in which the posterior canal is opened and the membranous labyrinth is compressed to ablate its function, may prove as effective.

Jannetta et al[16] recommended MVD for patients who had constant disabling positional vertigo in the upright position. The description may stretch and confuse the term "positional vertigo." Their concept of neural hyperactivity because of vascular compression of the cranial nerves at their root entry zone requires further attention and evaluation. Yet, in tic douloureux, even when the strongest case for a vascular compressive mechanism can be made, several phenomena are unexplained. (See Chapter 3.)

Post-traumatic syndromes with dizziness and vestibular disorders involving litigation are almost never helped significantly by surgery. The dizziness of postinfectious syndromes, vascular disease, demyelination, and brain stem tumors is similarly not likely to be helped by vestibular nerve surgery. BAER testing can identify a vestibulocochlear nerve lesion, but does not provide etiologic specificity.

Autopsy studies of temporal bones in patients who died following operation have shown dilatation of the endolymph spaces at the expense of the perilymph spaces. This pathologic finding is thought to cause symptoms because perilymph and endolymph pressures must be equal for normal cochlear and vestibular function. Similar to hydrocephalus or glaucoma, accumulation of endolymph most likely is caused by deficient reabsorption.

Operative Indications

When hearing on the affected side is absent and the patient is disabled by severe vertigo, labyrinthectomy is indicated, and is effective in eliminating these attacks. The imbalance following labyrinthectomy ordinarily is short-lived, and good compensation usually occurs without significant residual imbalance. Labyrinthectomy may be carried out via a transmastoid or transcanal approach.

We recommend selective microsurgical vestibular nerve section when hearing preservation is a consideration and the vertiginous attacks are severe and refractory to medical management. Hearing preservation is an important consideration when hearing is normal or nearly normal in the affected ear, or when there is any evidence of bilateral involvement, in effect, whenever hearing has not already been lost. The morbidity of the operation has been quite low, and it has proven thus far to be very effective for lasting control of disabling vertigo.

The vestibular nerve can be safely exposed via three routes. In an extradural approach along the floor of the middle fossa, the vestibular nerve may be sectioned in the internal auditory canal. The second route, the extradural transmastoid exposure of the endolymphatic sac, is familiar to otologists. The mastoid is drilled away, exposing the sigmoid sinus. The dural opening is bounded anteriorly by the internal auditory meatus and posteriorly by the sigmoid sinus. The exposure of the vestibulocochlear nerve bundle, although adequate to section the vestibular nerve, is quite limited.

The posterior fossa approach provides positive identification of the vestibulocochlear nerve complex by confirmation of its proximity to the flocculus, visualization of the trigeminal nerve rostrally and the glossopharyngeal, vagus, and spinal accessory nerves below, and identification of the bony internal auditory meatus. We have performed this operation as a combined neurosurgical-otologic procedure, and prefer it because closure of the very thin, tangentially exposed dura anterior to the sigmoid sinus is difficult. With the patient in the supine position, the head turned contralaterally, little cerebellar retraction is necessary once cerebrospinal fluid (CSF) has been aspirated. The structures behind the endolymphatic sac are well seen from within the dura when the procedure is carried out in this manner.

Patient Positioning

In developing microsurgical approaches for trigeminal neuralgia, particularly in the elderly, it became clear that the supine position offered a safe and wide exposure to the cerebellopontine angle. Once the surgeon becomes familiar with the use of this position, the view obtained is virtually identical to that obtained in the sitting position except that the surgical field is rotated 90°. Although we consider the sitting position safe, we use the supine position more often for all cerebellopontine angle surgery. The principal hazards of the sitting position (i.e. hypotension and air embolism) are eliminated without losing most of the technical advantages. The head of the operating table is slightly elevated, a step that markedly reduces venous pressure. The neck is rotated contralaterally and moderately flexed (Figure 1). When CSF has been aspirated from the cisterna magna, almost no cerebellar retraction is necessary. The surgeon is seated behind the patient's head.

We use BAER monitoring during the

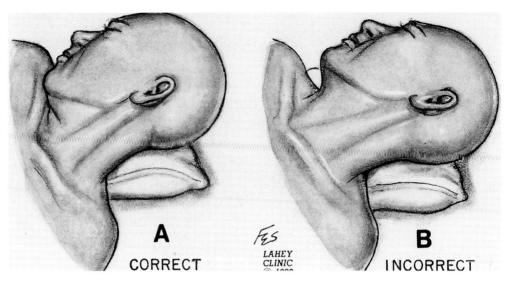

Figure 1. The ipsilateral shoulder is elevated on a roll. (A) The neck is slightly flexed to gain proper trajectory. (B) The head is supported in three-point pin fixation. The bony exposure may be higher than optimal as shown in Figure 2; if the bony exposure is in the proper location, the corresponding intracranial exposure may be too low. This is especially important in short-necked or large-shouldered individuals, where the effects of slight imperfections of position can be exaggerated.

procedure, which may help to preserve hearing. Electrodes are placed on the vertex, on each ear lobe, and over the chest wall. A small microphone is inserted in each ear. The monitoring provides early warning of stretching or direct injury to the cochlear nerve during the course of the operation.

Surgical Technique

Overall orientation in the supine position from the surgeon's viewpoint is shown in Figure 1. The chin should be flexed as in Figure 1A. If the neck is not properly flexed (Figure 1B), the craniotomy may be improperly positioned (Figure 2, dotted line). A Mayfield three-point head fixation unit allows the use of the Leyla-Yasargil self-retaining retractor system. Hair shaving is minimal. A paramedian incision 1 cm posterior to the mastoid prominence is used. A piece of pericranium is harvested for later dural closure. A small laterally placed craniotomy centered just below the junction of the transverse and sigmoid sinuses is performed (Figure 2). We use a small bone flap (Figures 3 and 4), which is replaced at the end of the procedure.

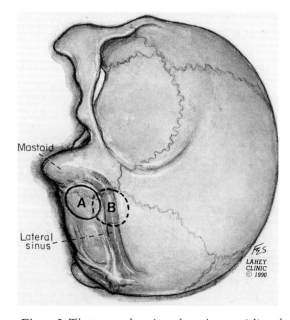

Figure 2. The proper location of craniotomy (A) and the improper location of craniotomy (dotted lines at B), if head is not sufficiently flexed.

We use the high-speed drill to enter the skull over and just below the junction of the lateral and sigmoid sinuses. A #3 Penfield dissector is used to strip the dura below the transverse sinus and medial to the sigmoid

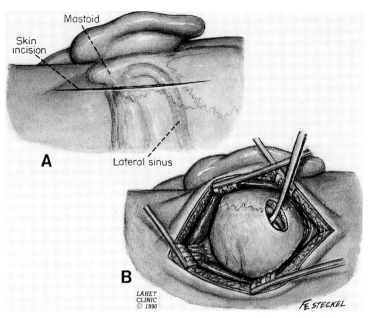

Figure 3. *Craniotomy technique, medial to mastoid* ***(A)***. *An opening is drilled* ***(B)*** *through the mastoid area to expose the dura just below the junction of the transverse and sigmoid sinuses. This opening may be enlarged slightly with a curet or small Kerrison rongeur to admit a #3 Penfield dissector to strip the dura as shown.*

Figure 4. *A craniotome* ***(A)*** *is used to cut a small flap. The bone edges are thoroughly waxed to prevent CSF leak. Holes are drilled in the medial and inferior edges of the craniotomy defect to secure the bone flap. The dura is opened as shown* ***(B)***. *If the cranial defect is too medial, excessive brain retraction may be required.*

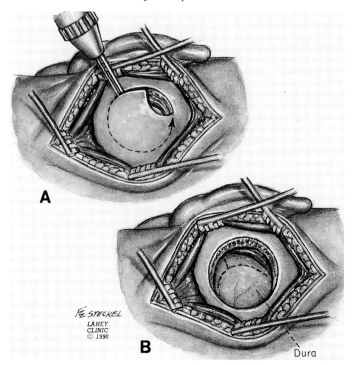

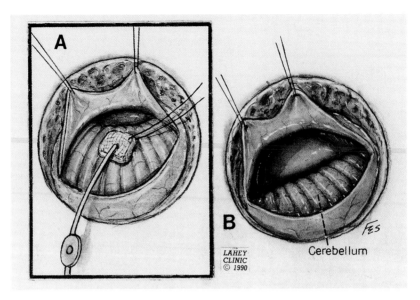

Figure 5. *The CSF is aspirated from over the cerebellar hemisphere once the dura has been opened (**A**) and tented laterally. This is less traumatic than exposing the cisterna magna. Slow, careful aspiration at this step will greatly reduce the necessity for retraction. (**B**) The slack exposure obtained after the CSF has been drained is visible.*

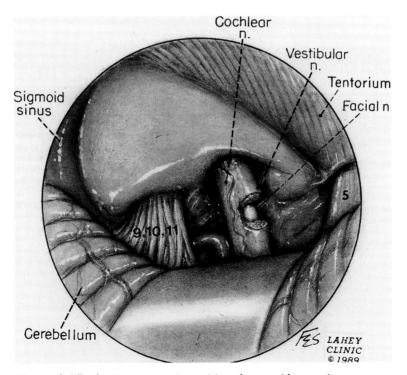

Figure 6. *The brain retractor is positioned to avoid excessive pressure which would indent the cerebellum and cause cerebellar injury or contusion. Correct pressure may be obtained by aspirating copious amounts of CSF after the initial dural opening.*

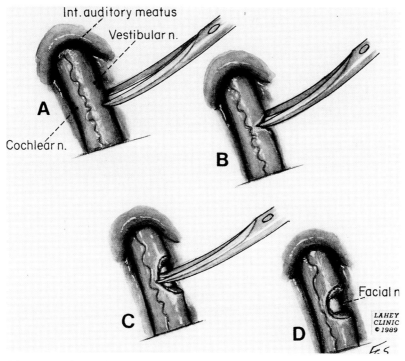

Figure 7. (A) Arachnoid has been reflected medially off the vestibular complex. (B) Cochlear and vestibular nerves are exposed. (C) Microscissors divide the vestibular nerves, and (D) edges of the nerve are retracted as division is continued, exposing the facial nerve.

sinus (Figure 3B). The craniotome then is used to turn a small flap (Figure 4). The edges are drilled for stay sutures to secure it at the end of the operation.

The dura is opened laterally and sutured to the muscles. CSF is aspirated from the subarachnoid space over the cerebellar convexity (Figure 5). A considerable quantity of fluid may be aspirated to create a slack cerebellar exposure, reducing or eliminating the need for cerebellar retraction. Further CSF is aspirated from the cerebellopontine cisterns to gain a slack exposure of the angle and the region of the internal auditory meatus (Figure 6). It is advantageous to take extra time at this stage for adequate aspiration of CSF. The petrosal vein must be carefully avoided. For operations on nerve VIII, often it is not necessary to disturb the petrosal vein, but if it is stretched, it should be coagulated and divided.

Once the retractor has been positioned correctly, a wide view of the vestibulocochlear nerve complex from the internal auditory meatus to the brain stem is obtained. The vestibular portion of the vestibulocochlear nerve occupies the superior 50% of the combined bundle (Figure 7). It is a darker gray in appearance than the more inferiorly lying cochlear division. At the level of the internal auditory meatus, a plane of cleavage between the vestibular and cochlear division may be visible. Gently depressing the vestibular portion of the nerve inferiorly allows visualization of the whiter facial nerve lying anterosuperiorly. Significant vessels coursing along the vestibulocochlear nerve bundle should be spared to preserve hearing.

A clear plane of cleavage between the vestibular and cochlear portions cannot always be visualized. When this is the case, the superior 50% of the combined cochlear and vestibular bundle is sectioned. Following such sections, most patients tested have no vestibular function. We have found residual function in some patients using maximal ice

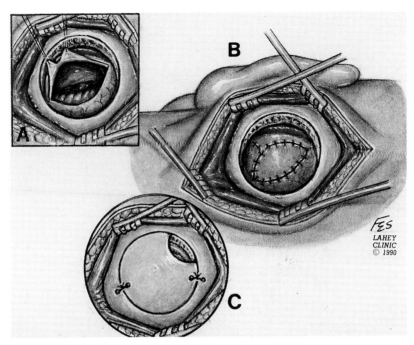

Figure 8. (A) Slack exposure seen at the end of operation. (B) Dural graft sutured in place. (C) Bone flap replaced.

water stimulation. Because the cochlear nerve and its blood supply are delicate, manipulation of the cochlear nerve is avoided. The surgeon's view of the sectioned vestibular and preserved cochlear and vestibular is depicted in Figure 6.

A pericranial graft obtained during the exposure is used to provide a patulous dural closure (Figure 8). The muscles, subcutaneous tissues, and skin then are closed in layers, and a small dressing is applied. Steroid preparation and postoperative treatment for several days can reduce the side effects of the procedure, but steroids tend to obscure the recognition of meningeal inflammation, thus should be reserved only if meningeal symptoms develop and are proven not to be septic in origin.

This procedure can be carried out without producing loss of hearing in most instances. All of the patients in our series have had relief of their disabling attacks of dizziness. Postoperative vertigo appears to be proportional to preoperative vestibular function as determined by electronystagmography. CSF leak has not been a problem. No facial weakness or other effects outside the vestibulocochlear nerve system have occurred. The procedure is extremely effective in the surgical treatment of intractable Meniere's syndrome when relief of vertigo with hearing preservation is desired.

References

1. Adams CBT, Chir M. Microvascular compression: an alternative view and hypothesis. *J Neurosurg.* 1989;70:1-12.
2. Baloh RW, Honrubia V. *Clinical Neurophysiology of the Vestibular System.* 2nd ed. Philadelphia, Pa: FA Davis; 1990:91-111, 214-219.
3. Dandy, WE. Meniere's disease: its diagnosis and a method of treatment. *Arch Surg.* 1928;16:1127-1152.
4. Dandy WE. Treatment of Meniere's disease by section of only the vestibular portion of the acoustic nerve. *Bull Johns Hopkins Hosp.* 1933;53:52-55.
5. Falconer MA. Treatment of Meniere's disease. *Br Med.* 1963;2:179.
6. Fluur E, Tovi D. Microscopic intracranial section of the vestibular nerve in Meniere's disease: a preliminary report. *Acta Otolaryngol (Stockh).* 1965; 59:604-606.
7. Gacek RR. Singular neurectomy update. *Ann Otol Rhinol Laryngol.* 1982;91:469.
8. Glasscock ME III, Miller GW. Middle fossa vestibular nerve section in the management of Meniere's disease. *Laryngoscope.* 1977;87:529-541.
9. Glasscock ME III, Davis WE, Hughes GB, et al.

Labyrinthectomy versus middle fossa vestibular nerve section in Meniere's disease: a critical evaluation of relief of vertigo. *Ann Otol Rhinol Laryngol.* 1980;89:318-324.

10. Glasscock ME III, Miller GW, Drake FD, et al. Surgical management of Ménière's disease with the endolymphatic subarachnoid shunt: a five-year study. *Laryngoscope.* 1977;87:1668-1675.

11. Green RE. Surgical treatment of vertigo, with follow-up on Walter Dandy's cases: neurological aspects. *Clin Neurosurg.* 1959;6:141-151.

12. Hallpike CS, Cairns H. Observations on the pathology of Meniere's syndrome. *J Laryngol & Otol.* 1938;53:625-654.

13. House WF. Subarachnoid shunt for drainage of hydrops: a report of 63 cases. *Arch Otolaryngol.* 1964;79:338-354.

14. House WF, Fraysse B. Revision of the endolymphatic subarachnoid shunt for Meniere's disease: review of 59 cases. *Arch Otolaryngol.* 1979;105:559-600.

15. Jannetta PJ. Microsurgical approach to the trigeminal nerve for tic douloureux. *Prog Neurol Surg.* 1976;7:180-200.

16. Jannetta PJ. Møller MB, Møller AR. Disabling positional vertigo. *N Engl J Med.* 1984;310:1700-1705.

17. McKenzie KG. Intracranial division of the vestibular portion of the auditory nerve for Ménière's disease. *Can Med Assoc J.* 1936;34:369-381.

18. Schuknecht HF. Meniere's disease: a correlation of symptomatology and pathology. *Laryngoscope.* 1963;73:651-665.

19. Schuknect, HF. Meniere's disease. In: *Otolaryngology, I.* Philadelphia, Pa: JB Lippincott Co; 1991

20. Shea JJ. Teflon film drainage of the endolymphatic sac. *Arch Otolaryngol.* 1966;83:316-319.

21. Tarlov EC. Microsurgical vestibular nerve section for intractable Meniere's syndrome—technique and results. *Clin Neurosurg.* 1986;33:667-684.

22. Tarlov EC. Selective microsurgical vestibular nerve section for intractable Meniere's syndrome. In: Rengachary SS, Wilkins RH, eds. *Neurosurgical Operative Atlas.* Baltimore, Md: Williams and Wilkins; 1991;1:51-58.

23. Tarlov EC, Oliver P. Selective vestibular nerve section combined with endolymphatic sac to subarachnoid shunt for intractable Meniere's syndrome: surgical technique. *Contemporary Neurosurgery.* 1983;4:1.

24. Tarlov EC, Poe D. Selective microsurgical vestibular nerve section for intractable Meniere's syndrome. *Contemporary Neurosurgery.* 1991;13:1-6.

CHAPTER 10

Glossopharyngeal (Vagoglossopharyngeal) Neuralgia

Robert H. Wilkins, MD

Clinical Syndrome

Glossopharyngeal neuralgia is a pain syndrome that was so named because the pain is perceived primarily in the distribution of the glossopharyngeal (IX) nerve. It has many similarities to trigeminal neuralgia. Like trigeminal neuralgia, it is ordinarily a sharp, lancinating, unilateral pain that lasts for a few seconds to a minute before it wanes, only to be followed a short time later by another paroxysm of pain. Such paroxyms usually occur in clusters, and the clusters may recur in an irregular fashion over a period of days, weeks, or months before the episode stops spontaneously. Early in the course of the disorder, there may be long painfree intervals between episodes,[15] but the episodes of recurring neuralgia ordinarily become more frequent and more distressing with time.[2,19] The individual paroxyms of pain tend to be severe and they typically will cause the patient to interrupt all voluntary activity until the pain subsides. These paroxyms may occur without any obvious precipitating event or may be triggered by a non-noxious stimulus such as the act of swallowing.

As is true with trigeminal neuralgia, glossopharyngeal neuralgia almost always occurs in adults, with the peak age of onset between 40 and 60 years.[2,19] Among 217 patients with glossopharyngeal neuralgia reported by Rushton et al,[15] the pain began when the patient was 50 years of age or older in 57% of the cases.

About 5% to 8% of patients with trigeminal neuralgia will be found to have a benign tumor (e.g. epidermoid tumor, meningioma, acoustic neuroma) in the cerebellopontine angle (CPA), and about 2% to 3% will be discovered to have multiple sclerosis.[20] A small percentage will be found to have some other condition affecting the ipsilateral trigeminal (V) nerve. Many of the patients with such structural lesions will have appropriate neurologic deficits, at times beyond the trigeminal nerve distribution, that should alert the physician to the existence of the underlying problem. The remainder of the patients with trigeminal neuralgia, if explored surgically, can be shown to have vascular compression of the trigeminal sensory root adjacent to the pons.[14]

In like fashion, glossopharyngeal neuralgia may arise because of a structural lesion affecting the glossopharyngeal nerve (secondary glossopharyngeal neuralgia) or in the absence of such a lesion (idiopathic glossopharyngeal neuralgia). Among the patients with idiopathic glossopharyngeal neuralgia, some seem to have vascular compression of the glossopharyngeal and vagus nerves at the medulla oblongata, a topic that will be discussed in more detail later in this chapter. Among the patients with secondary glossopharyngeal neuralgia, the etiologic lesion may affect adjacent cranial nerves such as the vagus (X) and spinal accessory (XI) nerves, and it often produces appropriate neurologic deficits.

However, the spectrum of structural abnormalities is somewhat different from the spectrum associated with trigeminal neuralgia.[2,4] The neoplasms found in patients with glossopharyngeal neuralgia often are malignant and often affect the nerve extracranially. Infections or inflammations have been implicated etiologically in some cases of glossopharyngeal neuralgia but seldom in patients with trigeminal neuralgia. An elongated styloid process may rarely be the cause of glossopharyngeal neuralgia, but not of trigeminal neuralgia. And, finally, multiple sclerosis is almost never encountered in patients with glossopharyngeal neuralgia.[15]

Other differences between glossopharyngeal neuralgia and trigeminal neuralgia also exist.[2,15,19] Trigeminal neuralgia is about 70 to 100 times more common than glossopharyngeal neuralgia. Glossopharyngeal neuralgia affects men as frequently as women, while trigeminal neuralgia favors women in about a 3:2 ratio. Glossopharyngeal neuralgia is more common on the left side of the head (3:2), whereas trigeminal neuralgia is more common on the right side of the head (5:3). Bilateral involvement, ordinarily in sequence rather than simultaneous, occurs in less than 2% of patients with glossopharyngeal neuralgia, but it occurs in about 4% of patients with trigeminal neuralgia.

Glossopharyngeal neuralgia has more variability of expression than does trigeminal neuralgia.[2,19] With glossopharyngeal neuralgia, atypical features are so common that they are almost the rule rather than the exception. For example, the pain may be constant; may be perceived as an aching, burning, or pressure sensation; may last for periods up to days or weeks; or may have its onset or radiation outside the distribution of the glossopharyngeal nerve.[19]

Trigeminal neuralgia is experienced in some part of the area innervated by the ipsilateral trigeminal nerve, frequently in the mandibular (V_3) division. Despite its previously mentioned variability, glossopharyngeal neuralgia typically occurs within the distribution of the ipsilateral glossopharyngeal nerve. Through its branches, the glossopharyngeal nerve receives sensory input from two main areas: the external and middle ear, and the pharynx and posterior third of the tongue.[13] On this basis, the pain of glossopharyngeal neuralgia can be experienced primarily in the ear (otalgic type), primarily in the throat (pharyngeal type), or in both locations.

In either location, glossopharyngeal neuralgia can be confused with geniculate neuralgia or even with mandibular division trigeminal neuralgia.[5,16,19] Further confusion in diagnosis may occur because of the fact that glossopharyngeal neuralgia is accompanied by trigeminal neuralgia in approximately 10% of patients with the former disorder.[2,15] The application of a 10% cocaine solution or some other surface anesthetic to the region of the tonsil and pharynx will help to establish the diagnosis of glossopharyngeal neuralgia if the patient is relieved of pain for 1-2 hours afterward, even during swallowing and the probing of a trigger zone.[15]

The glossopharyngeal nerve shares certain brain stem nuclei with the vagus nerve and also shares some areas of peripheral innervation.[13] In about 10% to 15% of patients, paroxysms of pain are accompanied by bradycardia or asystole, which, in turn, may cause syncope and even convulsions.[2,5,10,18,19] This phenomenon does not seem to result from a hypersensitive carotid sinus; the vagus system has been implicated, as will be discussed below.

In 1969, White and Sweet stated: "The disorder was originally called *glossopharyngeal neuralgia* by Harris (1921), but it has been clear for over twenty years that vagal fibers are often implicated. In our previous volume we adhered to the customary term initiated by Harris for the sake of brevity, but now have decided this should be changed to *vagoglossopharyngeal neuralgia*. The original term is in our opinion lulling too many surgeons into inadequacies both in analysis and in surgery of these patients."[19]

Etiology and Pathogenesis

As stated previously, an etiologic factor other than vascular compression may be encountered in some patients with glossopharyngeal neuralgia. Chief among the structural lesions causing glossopharyngeal neuralgia are neoplasms, infections, and inflammations. For this reason, and especially if the patient has a neurologic deficit, thin-slice high-resolution computed tomography (CT) and/or magnetic resonance imaging (MRI) is recommended before decisions are made about treatment.[17]

Jannetta has championed the idea that vascular compression of the glosspharyngeal and vagus nerves at the medulla oblongata is the etiology in most cases of "idiopathic" glossopharyngeal neuralgia. In 1980, he reported that 15 of 17 patients who underwent surgical exploration of the glossopharyngeal and vagus nerves at the medulla were found to have such vascular compression (in 9 cases by the posterior inferior cerebellar artery and in 6 cases by other vessels).[7] Normally, however, there are close associations between these nerves and vessels,[21] and the etiologic significance of such associations still is not entirely clear.

The pathogenesis of glossopharyngeal neuralgia is not well understood. Little has been written on this subject except in relation to the possible role of vascular compression, and in relation to the cardiovascular responses that sometimes occur during paroxysms of glossopharyngeal neuralgia. Hypotheses to explain how vascular compression causes neural dysfunction have been discussed in Chapters 2 and 3 in this book, and also by Bruyn.[2]

Concerning the cardiovascular responses, White and Sweet postulated: "Bradycardia, and much less often, hypotension and direct cerebral effects, occur from impulses induced in the sinus nerve of Hering by especially severe paroxysms of pain in the glossopharyngeal domain. The afferent impulses related to the pain jump the insulation firing cardiovascular regulatory fibers at an artificial synapse somewhere in the peripheral nerve or rootlets."[19]

In addition to the mechanism of ephaptic transmission between the somatic afferent fibers and the visceral afferent fibers (carotid sinus nerve of Hering) in the glossopharyngeal nerve proposed by White and Sweet, van Loveren et al[17] have implicated central collateral pathways between the nucleus tractus solitarius and the dorsal motor nucleus of the vagus nerve to explain some of the cardiovascular phenomena of glossopharyngeal neuralgia. They stated: "Transvenous cardiac pacing will prevent bradycardia but may not affect the hypotension because of vasodilatation produced by increased vagal outflow."[17]

Furthermore, Wallin et al[18] have provided evidence that inhibition of peripheral sympathetic activity also may contribute to the hypotension. Their patient regularly developed asystole and fainted during paroxysms of glossopharyngeal neuralgia. Although the patient had documented bradycardia and sometimes asystole of up to 8 seconds in duration during his attacks, a cardiac pacemaker did not prevent syncope. The authors documented that spontaneous sympathetic activity in muscle nerves disappeared during the attacks, and blood pressure fell despite a functioning pacemaker.

In 1986, Bruyn[2] reviewed the available evidence bearing on the pathogenesis of glossopharyngeal neuralgia, including information about the cardiovascular responses. Although he noted that a case could be made for either a central or a peripheral mechanism, he strongly favored the former. After presenting the clinical features of glossopharyngeal neuralgia in detail, Bruyn stated: "The clinical data reviewed . . . seem to allow only one interpretation: undue afferent loading (trigger factors!) through the IXth nerve fibres causes an abrupt discharge of solitary tract neurons (consciously perceived as neuralgia pain after the impulses have been relayed to thalamus and cortex) as well as spill over to, and discharge of, the ambiguous and vagal dorsal motor nuclei, including bradycardia, sinus arrest, asystole, arterial hypotension and, in a sporadic case, diminution of respiratory rate."[2]

Surgical Treatment

Glossopharyngeal neuralgia usually is responsive initially to the medications that are effective in controlling trigeminal neuralgia, such as carbamazepine (Tegretol; Basel Pharmaceuticals, Summit, New Jersey) and phenytoin (Dilantin; Parke-Davis, Morris Plains, New Jersey).[5,15,17,19] If such therapy is, or becomes, ineffective, or if significant side effects occur, surgical treatment should be considered.

Historically, several approaches to surgical therapy have been taken, including removal of the styloid process, superior laryngeal neurectomy or injection, extracranial section of the glossopharyngeal nerve and pharyngeal branch of the vagus nerve, and bulbar tractotomy.[19] At present, surgeons usually choose one of three approaches: intracranial section of the glossopharyngeal and upper vagal rootlets, microvascular decompression (MVD) of these rootlets, or percutaneous destruction of the glossopharyngeal nerve.

Intracranial Section of the Glossopharyngeal and Upper Vagal Rootlets

This operation dates back to the 1920s. According to White and Sweet:

When the pain recurred following his extracranial section of the glossopharyngeal nerve, Adson after careful cadaver dissections proceeded in 1925 to the first intracranial (preganglionic) root section. Serious bleeding during operation led to death four hours later. . . . It remained for Dandy to carry out the first 2 successful glossopharyngeal rhizotomies for this disorder. . . . Dandy's superb report of relief of pain in 2 severely afflicted patients by a glossopharyngeal rhizotomy coupled with his usual excellent illustrations . . . have led to the general belief that idiopathic neuralgia of the throat can be cured in this way.[19]

In 1927, Dandy stated: "An operation by which the ninth nerve is sectioned intracran-

ially was carried out. . . . The superiority of this operation over section of the glossopharyngeal nerve in the neck is due to the fact that other nerves are not injured and the nerve is cut above the ganglion, thereby precluding return of the malady. The operation is practically without danger to life and leaves no subjective or objective disturbance in its wake.[5]

Since 1927, however, it has become apparent that to increase the likelihood of permanent relief, the surgeon also should cut the upper vagal rootlets.[5,19] This procedure rarely yields extensive anesthesia in the oropharyngeal and aural regions.[5,19]

In 1981, Rushton et al[15] reported 217 cases of glossopharyngeal neuralgia seen at the Mayo Clinic between 1922 and 1977. They summarized their experience with surgical treatment as follows:

In 1923, intracranial section of the glossopharyngeal nerve at the jugular foramen was undertaken. A total of 71 patients have been treated in this manner. When some patients failed to gain relief of pain, it was decided that sectioning of the upper three or four rootlets of the vagus nerve should be included in the procedure . . . . a total of 44 patients have undergone this procedure. In addition, ten patients also underwent section of the fifth cranial nerve for an associated trigeminal neuralgia. . . .

A total of 129 patients have had surgical procedures for glossopharyngeal neuralgia: 110 patients obtained good relief of pain and 13 patients did not. Occasionally, the pain was initially relieved but returned two to six weeks postoperatively. Six patients underwent further operation. . . .

The most common postoperative disability was related to swallowing. Twenty-five patients had difficulty swallowing, and many complained of a feeling of having a foreign body in the throat and a "tickling" or drawing sensation in the pharynx. . . .

Patients who have the classic symptoms of glossopharyngeal neuralgia and who obtain relief by cocainization of the throat are candidates for surgical section of the glossopharyngeal nerve and probably of the upper two to three rootlets of the vagus nerve. When the patient's pain is in the inner ear and is unaffected by cocaine treatment, one should consider sectioning of the nervus intermedius of the seventh nerve at the time of operation. . . .

It is not uncommon at the time of manipulation of the ninth and tenth nerves to note a decrease in blood pressure or a sudden tachycardia. Several patients had a pronounced drop in blood pressure, and this necessitated emergency supportive measures by the anesthesiologist. . . .

Interest has been renewed in the possibility that trigeminal neuralgia and glossopharyngeal neuralgia may be caused by compression of the nerves by arterial or venous loops. . . . Review of our operative reports revealed that in 19 patients a specific comment was made about compression of the ninth or tenth nerve by an arterial loop. . . . it is interesting that the surgeons who commented specifically about the arterial loop also mentioned that the nerve was enlarged and congested in five patients.

A few patients with bilateral glossopharyngeal neuralgia have been seen. Patients with this rare condition may be helped by microvascular decompression. Bilateral sectioning of the ninth cranial nerve may result in loss of the ability to swallow.[15]

Rushton et al, as noted previously, commented on the hypotension and tachycardia that may occur during manipulation of the glossopharyngeal and vagus nerves at operation. Of equal or greater significance is the temporary hypertension that may occur when the glossopharyngeal nerve is cut, interrupting the afferent vasodepressor impulses from the ipsilateral carotid sinus.[5,19] Depending on the severity of this response, appropriate medical management may be necessary to prevent the complications of acute hypertension such as intracerebral hemorrhage.

Microvascular Decompression of the Glossopharyngeal and Vagus Nerves at the Medulla Oblongata

As stated previously, Jannetta reported in 1980 that vascular compression of the glossopharyngeal and vagus nerves at the medulla was identified at operation in 15 of 17 patients with glossopharyngeal neuralgia. Of the 2 patients without documented vascular compression, 1 had undergone prior surgery and the postoperative scar prevented inspection of the nerve root entry and exit zone, and the other was operated on by another

surgeon and Jannetta was not present at the operation to confirm the findings.[8] Among the 15 patients with documented vascular compression, the posterior inferior cerebellar artery was the vessel involved in 9 patients, and various other vessels were the compressive agents in the other 6 patients. In 1990, Jannetta reported 28 patients with glossopharyngeal neuralgia, all of whom had cross-compression of the glossopharyneal and vagus nerve fascicles at the brain stem.[9]

Based on these and related observations, Jannetta and others have performed MVD of the glossopharyngeal and vagus nerves to treat glossopharyngeal neuralgia. Among six patients reported in 1977 by Laha and Jannetta,[11] five were found to have neural compression by a tortuous vertebral artery or posterior inferior cerebellar artery. MVD was performed in four patients, in one of whom the glossopharyngeal and upper vagal rootlets also were cut. Of the three patients who were treated by MVD alone, one had relief of pain for a follow-up period of 6 months, one had incomplete relief of pain, and one died in the immediate postoperative period from an intracerebral hemorrhage related to severe postoperative hypertension.

In 1980 and 1981, Jannetta reported on an enlarged personal series of 11 patients with glossopharyngeal neuralgia, 9 of whom were treated by MVD.[7,8] Recurrences were experienced by 2 patients in whom small fragments of muscle were used to keep the offending vessel separated from the neural structures; Jannetta subsequently switched to using shredded Teflon (E. I. du Pont de Nemours & Co., Wilmington, Delaware) for this purpose, to prevent resorption of the implanted padding. At the time of the reports, six of the nine patients treated by MVD were painfree, but the lengths of follow-up were not specified. In addition to the death from the hypertensive crisis mentioned previously, the surgical complications included one instance of temporary hypertension and four of decreased palatal function and gag reflex (two temporary after MVD and two permanent after nerve section).[7]

A few other surgeons also have reported

individual cases or small series of patients treated for glossopharyngeal neuralgia by MVD.[5,6] In general, their findings and results have been similar to those of Jannetta.

Percutaneous Glossopharyngeal Rhizotomy

As an alternative to an open operation such as those just described, various surgeons have used percutaneous methods to injure the glossopharyngeal nerve in order to treat glossopharyngeal neuralgia. The most widely used form of this treatment at present is percutaneous radiofrequency rhizotomy at the pars nervosa of the jugular foramen,[5,17] a procedure that has been made easier by the use of CT for guidance of the inserted electrode.[1]

Gybels and Sweet listed some of the advantages of the technique as follows: "It is impossible from the anterior approach to enter the intracranial cavity via the jugular foramen. Consequently, no intracranial hemorrhages from needle puncture can occur. The lower or petrous ganglion of IX and the lower or nodose ganglion of X lie below the jugular foramen. Hence one's lesion is central to the cells of origin of nearly all of the primary afferent fibers in both nerves. This may explain the low recurrence rate in the idiopathic group. A further attractive feature in contrast to trigeminal rhizotomy is that denervation dysesthesias probably do not occur."[5]

Gybels and Sweet summarized the results of eight series of patients treated in this way.[5] These 21 patients, who had been reported between 1977 and 1988, generally did well. The complications encountered included intraoperative bradycardia and hypotension, and postoperative vocal cord paralysis and dysphagia.

Conclusions

Glossopharyngeal neuralgia, better termed

vagoglossopharyngeal neuralgia because of the involvement of the vagus system in addition to the glossopharyngeal system in the manifestations of the disorder, occurs infrequently but has been well described. Although some clinical features may be confusing, glossopharyngeal neuralgia ordinarily can be diagnosed without difficulty. Appropriate radiologic studies (e.g., CT and MRI) should be conducted to identify a structural lesion such as a neoplasm. If this is found, it is dealt with directly, and carbamazepine or phenytoin are used to treat the pain if this is necessary.

When no structural lesion is found on the radiologic studies, the patient usually is treated medically. If the medication is or becomes ineffective or if significant side effects occur, one of several forms of surgical treatment can be considered.

Gybels and Sweet prefer to begin with a percutaneous radiofrequency rhizotomy at the jugular foramen. "In the patients in whom this fails, open posterior fossa operations should lead to IX and partial X rhizotomies regardless of neurovascular relationships because of the absence of dysesthesias after rhizotomy of these roots and the greater likelihood of recurrence of pain after MVD."[5]

Onofrio has a somewhat different opinion, favoring the open rhizotomy approach over the other two methods: "Section of the ninth and upper fibers of the tenth cranial nerves causes little or no defineable neurologic deficit. Microvascular decompression . . . invites recurrence of pain postoperatively and seems unwarranted. . . . Radiofrequency procedures for extracranial destruction of the ninth nerve are unacceptable in that, like extracranial alcohol blocks of the jugular foramen, they invite unacceptable tenth nerve dysfunction."[12]

At the present time, I also prefer the open rhizotomy form of surgical treatment, for the reasons just given.

Experience with this operation has accumulated over many years and it has been shown to be easily performed, effective, and safe, especially in the current era of neurosurgical technique.

References

1. Arbit E, Krol G. Percutaneous radiofrequency neu-rolysis guided by computed tomography for the treatment of glossopharyngeal neuralgia. *Neuro-surgery.* 1991;29:580-582.

2. Bruyn GW. Glossopharyngeal neuralgia. In: Vinken PJ, Bruyn GW, Klawans HL, et al, eds. *Handbook of Clinical Neurology.* Volume 48. 1986:459-473.

3. Dandy WE. Glossopharyngeal neuralgia (tic dou-loureux): its diagnosis and treatment. *Arch Surg.* 1927;15:198-214.

4. Deparis M. Glossopharyngeal neuralgia. In: Vinken PJ, Bruyn GW, eds. *Handbook of Clinical Neurol-ogy.* Volume 5. Amsterdam: North-Holland; 1968:350-361.

5. Gybels JM, Sweet WH. *Neurosurgical Treatment of Persistent Pain: Physiological and Pathological Mechanisms of Human Pain.* Basel, Switzerland: S Karger; 1989:91-103.

6. Hamer J. Microneurosurgical findings of glosso-pharyngeal neuralgia. In: Samii M, ed. *Surgery in and around the Brain Stem and the Third Ventricle.* New York, NY: Springer-Verlag; 1986:285-289.

7. Jannetta PJ. Neurovascular compression in cranial nerve and systemic disease. *Ann Surg.* 1980;192: 518-524.

8. Jannetta PJ. Cranial nerve vascular compression syndromes (other than tic douloureux and hemifa-cial spasm). *Clin Neurosurg.* 1981;28:445-456.

9. Jannetta PJ. Cranial rhizopathies. In: Youmans JR, ed. *Neurological Surgery: a Comprehensive Refer-ence Guide to the Diagnosis and Management of Neurosurgical Problems.* 3rd ed. Philadelphia, Pa: WB Saunders Co; 1990:4169-4182.

10. Kong Y, Heyman A, Entman ML, et al. Glossopha-ryngeal neuralgia associated with bradycardia, syn-cope, and seizures. *Circulation.* 1964;30:109-113.

11. Laha RK, Jannetta PJ. Glossopharyngeal neuralgia. *J Neurosurg.* 1977;47:316-320.

12. Onofrio BM. Glossopharyngeal rhizotomy. In: Rengachary SS, Wilkins RH, eds. *Neurosurgical Operative Atlas.* Volume 12. Baltimore, Md: Wil-liams & Wilkins; 1991:323-326.

13. Peele TL. *The Neuroanatomic Basis for Clinical Neurology.* 3rd ed. New York, NY: McGraw-Hill; 1977:216-219.

14. Piatt JH Jr, Wilkins RH. Treatment of tic doulou-reux and hemifacial spasm by posterior fossa explo-ration: therapeutic implications of various neuro-vascular relationships. *Neurosurgery.* 1984;14: 462-471.

15. Rushton JG, Stevens JC, Miller RH. Glossopharyn-geal (vagoglossopharyngeal) neuralgia: a study of 217 cases. *Arch Neurol.* 1981;38:201-205.

16. Stookey B, Ransohoff J. *Trigeminal Neuralgia: Its History and Treatment.* Springfield, Ill: Charles C Thomas; 1959:103-111.

17. van Loveren HR, Tew JM Jr, Thomas GM. Vago-glossopharyngeal and geniculate neuralgias. In: Youmans JR, ed. *Neurological Surgery: a Compre-hensive Reference Guide to the Diagnosis and Management of Neurosurgical Problems.* Volume 6. 3rd ed. Philadelphia, Pa: WB Saunders Co; 1990: 3943-3949.

18. Wallin BG, Westerberg CE, Sundlöf G. Syncope induced by glossopharyngeal neuralgia: sympathetic outflow to muscle. *Neurology.* 1984;34:522-524.

19. White JC, Sweet WH. *Pain and the Neurosurgeon: A Forty-Year Experience.* Springfield, Ill: Charles C Thomas; 1969:128, 265-302.

20. Wilkins RH. Trigeminal neuralgia: introduction. In: Wilkins RH, Rengachary SS, eds. *Neurosurgery.* New York, NY: McGraw-Hill; 1985:2337-2344.

CHAPTER 11

Neoplasms and the Cranial Nerves of the Posterior Fossa

Franco DeMonte, MD, FRCS(C), and Ossama Al-Mefty, MD

Because of the remarkable density of vital neurovascular structures contained within the posterior fossa, surgery in this region always has intrigued the neurosurgeon. In the premicrosurgical era, the morbidity and mortality associated with surgery in the posterior fossa were daunting and many lesions were considered unapproachable. But with the advent of the operating microscope and microsurgical techniques, surgical barriers have begun to fall. Neoplasms of the posterior fossa, however, still present some of the greatest tests of surgical problem solving and skill. Operative mortality rates for petroclival meningiomas, for example, still ranged from 10% to 20% as recently as the mid-1980s.[22,41,65] An increased understanding of the anatomy of the skull base has allowed surgeons to design approaches that maximize visibility and minimize operating distance and brain retraction.[2] These surgical routes have increased the incidence of total tumor removal, while decreasing rates of morbidity and mortality.[6,56,57]

Demographics of Posterior Fossa Neoplasms

As a group, intraparenchymal tumors of neuroectodermal origin comprise the most common neoplasms found in the posterior fossa[10] (Table 1). Cranial nerve symptoma-tology usually results from increased intracranial pressure secondary to obstructive hydrocephalus, and is a late event. An exception to this process would be glial tumors of the brain stem, which usually have direct nuclear or fascicular involvement and subsequent dysfunction of the cranial nerves early in the course of the disease. Discussion of these tumors, however, is beyond the scope and intent of this chapter.

Acoustic neuromas (schwannomas of the vestibulocochlear [VIII] nerve) account for 80% to 90% of tumors at the cerebellopontine angle (CPA),[14] and are the next most common tumors of the posterior fossa.[10] They typically result in sensorineural hearing loss with a predominant deficit in speech discrimination, tinnitus, and disequilibrium. These neoplasms are discussed in Chapter 12. This chapter focuses on meningiomas, nonacoustic schwannomas, paragangliomas, epidermoid tumors, and chordomas, and how these tumors

TABLE 1
Incidence of Posterior Fossa Tumors*

Tumor Type	Incidence
Gliomas	42.8%
Vestibular schwannomas	36.5%
Meningiomas	7.1%
Epidermoid tumors	0.73%
Chordomas	0.31%

*Modified from Olivecrona's series of 954 posterior fossa tumors, as reported by Castellano and Ruggiero.[10]

TABLE 2
Clinical Syndromes of the Basal Posterior Fossa

A. CPA Syndrome

Early   1. CN VIII signs only
       2. CN VIII signs,
          early CN V and VII, and cerebellar
          signs

Late   3. CN VIII signs,
          established CN V, VII, and
          cerebellar signs,
          CN IX, X, XI signs,
          brain stem signs
       4. Increased intracranial pressure,
          papilledema

B. Jugular Foramen Syndromes

- Palsies of CN IX, X, XI—Vernet's syndrome
- Palsies of CN IX, X, XI, XII—Collet-Sicard syndrome
- Palsies of CN IX, X, XI, XII, and sympathetics—Villaret's syndrome

C. Clival Syndrome

- Stage 1—Unilateral CN VI palsy
- Stage 2—Bilateral cranial nerve palsies
- Stage 3—Brain stem signs

D. Foramen Magnum Syndrome

- Suboccipital neck pain (C2 dermatome)
- Ipsilateral dysesthesia
- Contralateral dissociated sensory loss
- Progressive weakness—ipsilateral upper extremity, counterclockwise to lower extremity involvement, and finally contralateral upper extremity
- Wasting of intrinsic hand muscles

TABLE 3
Basal Posterior Fossa Syndromes and Their Common Neoplastic Causes

Clival Syndrome
Chordomas
Petroclival meningiomas
Paragangliomas
Nasopharyngeal carcinomas
Intrinsic brain stem tumors

Jugular Foramen Syndrome
Paragangliomas
Schwannomas
Metastatic tumors
Meningiomas

CPA Syndrome
Acoustic schwannomas
Meningiomas—CPA or petroclival
Epidermoid tumors
Trigeminal schwannomas
Cholesterol granulomas

Foramen Magnum Syndrome
Meningiomas
Schwannomas
Chordomas
Intramedullary tumors

the various clinical syndromes of the cranial nerves in the posterior fossa and of the relative incidence of different pathologic processes encountered in this area, they can formulate an intelligent and concise differential diagnosis. Table 2 lists the clinical syndromes encountered; Table 3 lists the most common neoplastic processes that produce them. With these lists in mind, a well-directed and intelligent choice of investigations can be made. The results of these investigations will help the clinician-surgeon formulate an appropriate treatment plan.

Meningiomas

Petroclival meningiomas and those of the CPA (posterior surface of the petrous bone lateral to the trigeminal nerve) result in cranial nerve signs and symptoms much more frequently than other meningiomas located within the posterior fossa.[3,10,20,40,53]

Meningiomas arising from the upper two-thirds of the clivus medial to the trigeminal root are classified as clival or petroclival

affect the cranial nerves in the posterior fossa. Management of each of these lesions is discussed briefly.

The distance from Meckel's cave to the hypoglossal canal ranges from 13.5-34.0 mm.[34] Within that space are the trigeminal, facial, vestibulocochlear, glossopharyngeal, vagus, spinal accessory, and hypoglossal (V, VII, VIII, IX, X, XI, and XII) nerves. The oculomotor (III) and trochlear (IV) nerves are only slightly superior and anterior to the trigeminal nerve, and the abducens (VI) nerve lies just medial to the facial and vestibulocochlear nerves.

A pathologic process affecting any part of the posterior fossa skull base can impinge on one or more of the cranial nerves, resulting in their dysfunction. If surgeons are aware of

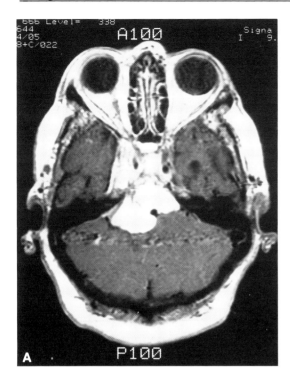

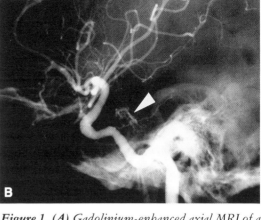

Figure 1. (A) Gadolinium-enhanced axial MRI of a large petroclival meningioma that also involves the cavernous sinus bilaterally and encases the basilar artery. The patient was troubled with significant ataxia, numbness of the right face, and weakness of the left leg. (B) Left lateral carotid angiogram. The typical supply from the internal carotid artery to this petroclival meningioma is seen (arrowhead). This vessel rarely can be entered for embolization.

tumors (Figure 1). In a review of 32 cases, Cherington and Schneck found headache to be the most frequent symptom of a petroclival meningioma, occurring in two-thirds of patients.[11] Headache was the initial complaint in 50%. Eighty percent of patients had either diminution or loss of sensation in the ipsilateral distribution of the trigeminal nerve. A similar percentage had papilledema and ataxia or disequilibrium. Half of the patients had evidence of ipsilateral hearing loss and involvement of the pyramidal tract. Forty percent had ipsilateral facial palsy, and just under a third had evidence of glossopharyngeal and vagus nerve dysfunction. Diplopia occurred in a third as well, 60% of which was the result of an abducens palsy.

More recent series of clival tumors also show a high incidence of involvement of the trigeminal nerve (35% to 85%),[6,56,65] evidenced usually by a decreased corneal reflex or hypesthesia but at times by facial pain.[56] Vestibulocochlear nerve dysfunction is also common, occurring in 30% to 70% of modern series.

Meningiomas arising from the posterior surface of the petrous bone lateral to the tri-

geminal nerve are classified as CPA meningiomas. In Yasargil and Mortara's series, the initial symptom or manifestation of the tumor was headache in 37%, decreased hearing or vertigo in 30%, facial pain in 27%, and facial numbness or paresthesias in 13% of patients.[65] Castellano and Ruggiero found a higher incidence of unilateral hearing loss as the primary manifestation (57% of patients) in their series.[10]

By the time the patient comes for medical treatment, however, the incidence of cranial nerve involvement had risen. Facial pain was present in 23% to 64%, while numbness or paresthesias occurred in 9% to 60% of patients. Unilateral hearing loss was present in 14% to 80%. Half of the patients have facial weakness or hemifacial spasm. Evidence of cerebellar dysfunction includes nystagmus in 45% to 75% and dys-synergia in 50% to 70%.[10,54,65]

Historically, surgical removal of basal posterior fossa meningiomas has been plagued by high rates of operative morbidity and mortality. In the review by Castellano and Ruggiero, there was a 43% mortality rate for patients with CPA tumors and a greater than

TABLE 4
**Relationships of the Cranial Nerves
to Petroclival and CPA Meningiomas**

Cranial Nerve	Petroclival	Cerebellopontine Angle
IV		Superior and lateral
V		Superior and anterior
VI	Anterior and inferior	Anterior
VII–VIII		Posterior
IX–X–XI		Inferior

60% mortality rate for patients with tumors arising from the clivus.[10] Pioneers of petroclival meningioma surgery in the microsurgical age still reported mortality rates ranging from 9% to 17%.[22,41,65] More recently, in series reported by experienced skull-base surgeons, the operative mortality has dropped (0% to 2%).[6,51,56] Recent series of surgery of CPA meningiomas also have reported 0% mortality rates.[50,54] Surgical morbidity, however, still is a concern (8% to 35% for patients with petroclival tumors) and is, to a large extent, related to new deficits in cranial nerves (20% to 45% for petroclival tumors, 23% for CPA tumors) and vascular injury (possibly 8% to 17%).[6,51,54,56]

The cranial nerves of the posterior fossa have a relatively constant anatomic relationship to petroclival and CPA meningiomas[54,55] (Table 4). The trochlear nerve usually is superior and lateral to these tumors. In one-sixth of petroclival tumors (17%), it may be superior and anterior. The trigeminal nerve is superior and anterior in most cases, but occasionally is directed anterior to the tumor. The abducens nerve is almost universally anterior and inferior to petroclival tumors and directly anterior to CPA meningiomas. The facial and vestibulocochlear nerve complex generally is posterior, although a tongue of tissue may grow posterior to the complex, displacing it anteriorly or inferiorly. For the most part, the lower cranial nerves are inferior to the tumor.

Surgical approaches to these basal meningiomas are myriad and include retrosigmoid, subtemporal-transtentorial, combined subtemporal-transtentorial and retrosigmoid, petrosal, preauricular-infratemporal fossa, transtem-

poral, and transcondylar approaches, which will be discussed later in this chapter.

Nonacoustic Schwannomas

Schwann cell tumors may arise from any of the cranial nerves of the posterior fossa. The vestibular nerves are by far the most frequent sites of schwannoma origin. After acoustic neuromas, most common are trigeminal nerve schwannomas, and those Schwann cell tumors arising from the facial nerve and the nerves exiting the jugular foramen. Nerve sheath tumors of nerves subserving ocular movement and those originating from the hypoglossal nerve are exceedingly rare; information about them is confined to only a few case reports.[37,61,62]

Trigeminal schwannomas account for 0.07% to 0.36% of intracranial tumors and 0.8% to 8% of intracranial Schwann cell tumors.[42,47] Fifty percent are located primarily in the middle fossa arising from the ganglionic segment of the trigeminal nerve (Figure 2).

Facial hypesthesia or pain, and corneal hypesthesia are the initial complaints in about 60% of patients with schwannomas of the trigeminal nerve arising from the ganglionic segment. At presentation, a full 80% to 90% of patients experience these complaints. Some patients (10% to 20%), however, never develop evidence of trigeminal dysfunction. A higher frequency of facial pain (52%) is encountered in patients with tumors of the ganglionic segment as opposed to tumors involving the trigeminal root (28%).[42] By the time of diagnosis, diplopia is present in 50%, and is the initial symptom in about 15% of patients. This usually results from

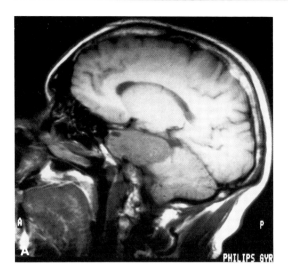

Figure 2. (A) Sagittal MRI. A large, well-defined lesion of decreased signal intensity is centered in the middle fossa and extends into the upper posterior fossa. (B) Gadolinium-enhanced axial MRI. The axial image of the same patient demonstrates intense contrast-enhancement of the tumor. This trigeminal schwannoma manifested itself with a palsy of the right abducens nerve and trigeminal neuralgia. Note the involvement of the cavernous sinus, encasement of the carotid, and the degree of brain stem compression.

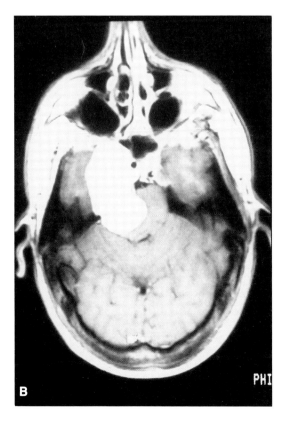

involvement of the abducens nerve as it courses medial to the tumor in its cavernous portion. Facial weakness and hearing loss occur rarely and are thought to result from involvement of the greater superficial petrosal nerve, the facial nerve, and the eustachian tube or cochlea in the temporal bone.[43]

Schwannomas arising from the trigeminal root tend to remain confined to the posterior fossa and account for 20% to 30% of total cases. They typically present as a CPA syndrome with a combination of hearing loss, tinnitus, and facial nerve and cerebellar dysfunction. Early involvement of the trigeminal nerve tends to imply the diagnosis; however, up to 10% of patients with acoustic schwannomas initially present with symptoms of trigeminal nerve dysfunction. As a corollary, 6% of patients with trigeminal schwannomas initially complain of hearing loss.

Dysfunction of the lower cranial nerves or long tract signs are not uncommon, and are identified in 30% to 50% of patients at diagnosis.

Dumbbell or hourglass tumors occupying both the middle and posterior fossae make up 15% to 25% of trigeminal schwannomas. They present with a composite of the symptoms and findings of tumors occurring in the middle and posterior fossae.

As with basal meningiomas, the relationships of the cranial nerves to trigeminal schwannomas are relatively constant[47] (Table 5). The trochlear nerve is identified on the superior pole of the tumor, while the oculomotor nerve and the abducens nerve are seen medial. The facial and vestibulocochlear nerve complex is displaced posteroinferiorly.

TABLE 5
Relationships of the Cranial Nerves to Trigeminal Schwannomas

Cranial Nerve	Relationship to Tumor
III	Medial
IV	Superior
VI	Medial
VII-VIII	Posteroinferior

Complete excision of a schwannoma results in cure and is the goal of any surgical procedure. In a recent series of 16 patients, total removal was accomplished in 12 initially and subsequently in 2 others (including 5 of 6 with cavernous sinus involvement).[47] Tumors within the posterior fossa usually are approached through a retrosigmoid craniectomy. Combined approaches, such as supratentorial and infratentorial or subtemporal and infratemporal fossa approaches, have been carried out successfully.[42,47]

Before 1970, a mortality rate of 25% had been reported for patients with these tumors.[42] In 2 recent reports encompassing 30 patients,[42,47] 2 deaths occurred: 1 operative and 1 related to a recurrence 4 years after surgery. Morbidity consisted of new or worsened deficits of the trigeminal nerve in 16 patients (53%), abducens nerve palsy in 2, and facial nerve palsy in 1. Cerebrospinal fluid (CSF) leaks occurred in 2 patients, hydrocephalus in 1, temporal lobe contusion with a subdural hematoma in 1, and meningitis in 1. With careful dissection, function of the trigeminal nerve can be preserved, or at times improved, through tumor removal.

A tumor of the facial nerve sheath produces slowly progressive facial weakness as the typical clinical syndrome. Sudden facial weakness, however, occurs in about 11% of cases, and a full 27% of patients with facial nerve schwannomas never manifest facial weakness.[38] Facial spasm has been reported in up to 17% of patients. Hearing loss occurs in about 50% of patients and may be conductive, sensorineural, or mixed. Tinnitus and vertigo, or dizziness, occur in 13% and 10%, respectively. External manifestations of the tumor, such as a mass, pain, or otorrhea, occur in 30% or more of patients. Schwann cell tumors of the facial nerve involve the tympanic or vertical segments in most patients (58% and 48%, respectively). Multiple segments are almost always affected. Treatment consists of resecting the tumor and grafting the facial nerve with the greater auricular or sural nerves.

In most patients, it is difficult, if not impossible, to identify the specific nerve of origin of a schwannoma of the jugular foramen.[46] The origin, however, is of minor importance; the clinical presentation and the surgical management are more a function of anatomic location than specific nerve origin.[17,25,29] Kaye and colleagues classified tumor locations into three types (A to C).[29] Type A tumors primarily are intracranial with only a small extension into the bone. Tumors having their main mass within the temporal and occipital bones with or without an intracranial component are classified as Type B. Type C tumors primarily are extracranial with only a minor extension into the bone or the posterior fossa.

Patients with Type A tumors may not have dysfunction of the lower cranial nerves. Their clinical syndrome may be indistinguishable from that of an acoustic neuroma, with deafness, vertigo, and ataxia being common. Types B and C tend to present with various forms of the jugular foramen syndrome. In these patients, hoarseness usually is the initial symptom.

The surgical approach to these lesions depends on the anatomic location of the tumor. Tumors primarily contained in the posterior fossa can be dealt with through a standard retrosigmoid craniectomy. Types B and C, however, require combined approaches for optimal exposure and complete removal. We have found the combined infratemporal-posterior fossa approach quite useful in this instance.[2,5] It allows both intracranial and extracranial exposure of the jugular foramen and all of the neurovascular structures in and around it.

The postoperative management of the dysfunction of cranial nerves IX, X, XI, and XII is by far the most important aspect of managing tumors of the jugular foramen. If extensive dissection around the jugular foramen is necessary, it has been our practice to perform a tracheostomy to avoid the complications of aspiration. Patients must be kept *nil per os* until definite objective evidence of an adequate swallowing mechanism without aspiration is obtained. Direct pharyngoscopy, esophagoscopy, and laryngoscopy are performed, followed by a modified barium swallow.

These investigations will reveal pooling of secretions, dysfunction of the swallowing mechanism, and any aspirations that may occur.

Paragangliomas

Paragangliomas are the most common tumors of the middle ear and, after acoustic neuromas, are the most common tumors of the temporal bone.[28] Even more so than meningiomas, these tumors have a predilection for females. Women make up more than 80% of patients in series of tympanic, jugular, and vagal paragangliomas. Most of these tumors occur in the sixth decade of life.

Paragangliomas are slow-growing tumors that extend along planes of least resistance (that is, along blood vessels and mastoid aircell tracts, and through cranial nerve foramina). Malignancy occurs in 10% of these patients, and catecholamine secretion is detected in 5%.[1,15]

Hearing loss occurs in 90% of patients with glomus tympanicum tumors and 70% of patients with glomus jugulare tumors, but occurs only rarely in patients with glomus vagale tumors.[60] Hearing loss is more often conductive than sensorineural. Sensorineural hearing loss implies that the tumor involves the inner ear or cochlear nerve and occurs in 4% to 18% of glomus tympanicum or jugulare tumors and in 14% of glomus vagale tumors. Pulsatile tinnitus, an audible bruit, or spontaneous aural bleeding can be seen in 60% to 70% of patients with tympanicum or jugulare tumors and in 30% of those with vagale paragangliomas (Figure 3).

Involvement of the facial nerve is the next most common symptom or sign, occurring in 18% of patients with tympanicum tumors and 21% of those with glomus jugulare tumors.[60] The facial nerve is most commonly affected in its vertical mastoid segment, but occasionally can be compressed in the soft tissue of the stylomastoid foramen.[28]

In a series of 100 tumors of the jugular foramen, Jackson and colleagues reported 59 glomus jugulare tumors and 18 glomus vagale tumors.[26] It is not surprising, then, that the various nerves passing through the jugular

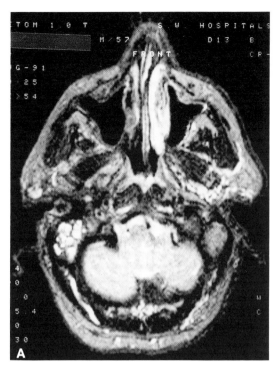

Figure 3. (A) Axial MRI. The "salt and pepper" appearance of this tumor on the T2-weighted image is typical of glomus tumors. The patient had a history of tinnitus, hearing loss, and ear pain. (B) Coronal CT scan showing irregular destruction of the bone of the jugular foramen just inferolateral to the cochlea, which is clearly seen.

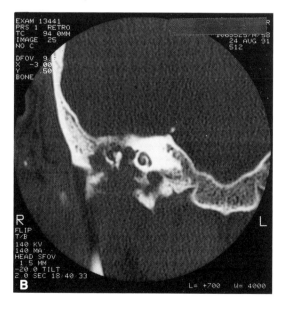

foramen are dysfunctional in 13% of patients with glomus jugulare tumors and in 70% of those with glomus vagale tumors. A change

TABLE 6
Fisch's Classification of Paragangliomas*

Class A	Tumors limited to middle ear cleft.
B	Tumors limited to the tympanomastoid area without destruction of bone in the infralabyrinthine compartment.
C	Tumors extending into and destroying bone of the infralabyrinthine and apical compartments of the vertical portion of the carotid canal.
C_1	Tumors destroying the bone of the jugular foramen and jugular bulb with limited involvement of the vertical portion of the carotid canal.
C_2	Tumors destroying the infralabyrinthine compartment of the temporal bone and invading the vertical portion of the carotid canal.
C_3	Tumors involving the infralabyrinthine and apical compartments of the temporal bone with invasion of the horizontal portion of the carotid canal.
D	Tumors with intracranial-intradural extension.
D_1	Tumors with an intracranial-intradural extension up to 2 cm in diameter.
D_2	Tumors with an intracranial-intradural extension greater than 2 cm in diameter that require a combined two-stage otologic and neurosurgical removal.
D_3	Tumors with inoperable intracranial-intradural extension.

*Data from Fisch[16]

of voice may precede other symptoms by 2-3 years in patients with glomus vagale tumors. Vocal cord paralysis is the usual finding on examination.[36] If it occurs, hypoglossal paresis denotes tumor extension into the hypoglossal canal or high in the neck.

Although still advocated by some, radiation therapy for paragangliomas probably should be reserved for palliative treatment only.[2] It has been shown to result in fibrous and vascular sclerosis, but to have little effect on the neoplastic cells themselves,[9] including their secretory potential.[52]

Surgical resection is the treatment of choice for paragangliomas of the head and neck, and the surgical approach selected should be based on the size and extension of the tumor[1] (Tables 6 and 7). Small glomus tympanicum or jugulare tumors limited to the promontory, middle ear, and jugular bulb can be approached and removed through the external ear canal using standard otologic approaches. Larger lesions (i.e. Class B [Fisch and colleagues] or Class II [Jackson and colleagues]) may be removed through a transmastoid approach. Fisch Class C or D or Jackson Class III or IV tumors, however, require an infratemporal fossa approach (as described by Fisch) or a combined approach.

The senior author's combined infratemporal-posterior fossa approach provides superb exposure and allows total removal of both intradural and extradural tumors in one stage.[5]

Chordomas

Chordomas are rare neoplasms accounting for 0.1% to 0.2% of all intracranial tumors.[33] About 35% of chordomas involve the cranium; two-thirds of these lie in the clivus.[39] Tumors arising from the rostral clivus have been classified as basi-sphenoidal chordomas, while those arising caudal to the spheno-occipital synchondrosis have been classified as basi-occipital (Figure 4). These tumors usually grow extradurally (one-third extend ventrally into the nasal cavities, the paranasal sinuses, and the pharynx), but may penetrate the dura as they become large or recur.[33,58]

By virtue of their relation to the upper brain stem and sella, basi-sphenoidal chordomas tend to cause dysfunction of the upper cranial nerves (that is, visual loss and cavernous sinus syndrome) and pituitary endocrinopathy. Basi-occipital chordomas are more likely to result in palsy of lower cranial nerves and long tract signs. Lateral exten-

TABLE 7
Jackson's Classification of Glomus Tumors*

Glomus Tympanicum Tumors

Class I	Small mass limited to the promontory.
II	Tumor completely filling middle ear space.
III	Tumor filling the middle ear and extending into the mastoid.
IV	Tumor filling the middle ear and extending into the mastoid or through the tympanic membrane to fill the external ear canal. May also extend anterior to the internal carotid artery.

Glomus Jugulare Tumors

Class I	Small tumor involving the jugular bulb, middle ear, and mastoid.
II	Tumor extending under the internal auditory canal. May have intracranial extension.
III	Tumor extending into the petrous apex. May have intracranial extension.
IV	Tumor extending beyond the petrous apex into the clivus or infratemporal fossa. May have intracranial extension.

*Data from Jackson.[27]

sions of these lesions give rise to unilateral symptoms.[48]

In 1945, Givner reviewed the 100 cases of spheno-occipital chordomas reported at that time and found that paresis of the abducens nerve was the most frequent symptom and occurred in 34 patients.[19] This paresis tended to precede the onset of paralysis of other ocular nerves. The paresis initially was unilateral, but became bilateral in the later

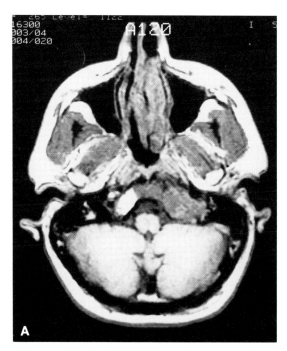
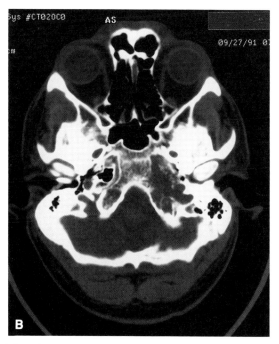

Figure 4. (*A*) *Axial MRI. This patient developed a palsy of the left abducens nerve. The MRI shows a loss of the normal high signal intensity of the clival bone marrow and a mass lesion of the left petroclival region.* (*B*) *Axial CT scan. A large irregular area of bony destruction and expansion is seen in the left petroclival area. These findings are typical of a chordoma.*

stages of the disease. He also noted that, in every instance of facial nerve dysfunction, the abducens nerve also was involved. In their series of 44 patients, Kendall and Lee reported an 84% incidence of cranial nerve palsies.[30] Half of these were bilateral. In a series of 26 cranial chordomas reported by Raffel and colleagues, diplopia was the most common symptom, occurring in 21 patients.[48] On examination, there were 15 instances of abducens nerve palsy and 5 cases of oculomotor nerve palsy. In 12 patients, diplopia was the initial symptom of their disease process. Dysfunction of the trigeminal nerve occurred in 5 patients and cranial nerves VII-XII were affected in 9. In the recent series of Sen and colleagues, 9 of their 17 patients were diagnosed after investigation of diplopia caused by dysfunction of the abducens nerve.[58] These series reinforce the classical presentation of chordomas: unilateral abducens nerve paresis, followed by bilateral cranial nerve signs, followed by bulbar signs.

Although histologically benign and slow-growing, chordomas are locally invasive. Even though they appear to be well localized, these tumors often involve and infiltrate surrounding bone. For this reason, recurrence after surgery has been the rule. Untreated, however, the average period of survival after onset of symptoms is about 1 year.[39]

It was this dismal natural history and poor surgical track record that established intratumoral decompression followed by radiation therapy as the standard treatment for cranial chordomas.[13] The report by Heffelfinger et al reinforced this standard by reporting median survival rates of 1.5 years after surgery alone, 4.8 years after radiation therapy alone, and 5.2 years after surgery and radiation therapy.[23]

Although this form of management occasionally has resulted in long-term survival, the mean survival of treated patients is 50-60 months, with 5-year survival rates near 50%, and 10-year survival rates at 28%.[12] Proton-beam radiation therapy reportedly has resulted in a 5-year actuarial local control rate of 82% and a 10-year rate of 58%. The 5-year and 10-year actuarial disease-free rates, however,

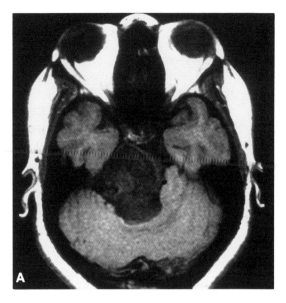

Figure 5. *A large epidermoid tumor is present in the right cerebellopontine angle and middle fossa, resulting in marked distortion of the brain stem. The patient was studied for complex partial seizures, but there were no brain stem findings. Note the non-homogeneous but mostly decreased signal intensity. (A) Axial MRI. (B) Sagittal MRI.*

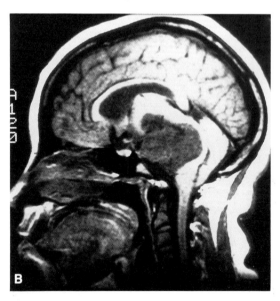

are lower—at 76% and 53%, respectively.[7] Stereotactic radiosurgical treatment has been used successfully, but follow-up periods remain short.[32] In the past decade, refined approaches to the skull base have facilitated radical re-

TABLE 8
**Differential Radiologic Features of Cholesterol Granulomas
and Epidermoid Tumors of the Petrous Apex**

Tumor	CT		MRI		
	Noncontrast-enhanced	Contrast-enhanced	T1-weighted	T2-weighted	Contrast-enhanced
Epidermoid tumor	Hypodense*	No change	Hypointense	Hyperintense	No change
Cholesterol granuloma	Isodense	No change	Hyperintense	Hyperintense	No change

*With respect to brain tissue.

moval of chordomas.[58] The goal of these approaches is complete tumor removal, which necessitates removal of visually abnormal bone as well as a margin of normal bone. Radical removal has been suggested to result in an improved quality of survival.[45]

Epidermoid Tumors and Cholesterol Granulomas

Somewhat more common than chordomas, epidermoid tumors have a predilection for the posterior fossa, especially the CPA, where they are the third most common tumors

encountered[14] (Figure 5A). Epidermoids constitute 5% of the tumors encountered in the CPA.[14] They also are found straddling the tentorium (located both supratentorially and infratentorially) and within the fourth ventricle. A common site also is extradurally in the petrous apex.[49] Tumors in this location also have been called congenital cholesteatomas and have been confused with cholesterol granulomas, which also are found in this region. With the use of magnetic resonance imaging (MRI), these lesions now can be diagnosed properly before surgery[21] (Table 8).

Although many combinations of cranial neuropathies may ensue from the growth of an

TABLE 9
Cranial Nerve Involvement by Epidermoid Tumors of the CPA

Cranial Nerve Involvement	Sabin et al[49] (n = 10)	Yasargil et al[64] (n = 22)	Yamakawa et al[63] (n = 15)	Totals (n = 47)
III, IV, VI				
Diplopia	6	5	4	15
V	4	7	11	22
Pain	(1)	(4)	(2)	(7)
Numbness/ paresthesias	(3)	(3)	(9)	(15)
VII	1	3	12	16
Spasm	(0)	(2)	(2)	(4)
Weakness	(1)	(1)	(10)	(12)
VIII	10	7	23	40
Hypoacusis	(5)	(7)	(14)	(26)
Tinnitus	(5)	(0)	(9)	(14)
IX, X	2	5	7	14
Cerebellar signs	9	10	12	31

TABLE 10
Differential Radiologic Features
of the Three Most Common Neoplasms of the CPA

Tumor	CT		MRI		
	Noncontrast-enhanced	Contrast-enhanced	T1-weighted	T2-weighted	Contrast-enhanced
Epidermoid tumor	Hypodense*	No change	Hypointense*	Hyperintense	No change
Acoustic neuroma	Isodense	Moderate uptake	Isointense	Hyperintense	Marked uptake
Meningioma	Isodense or hyperdense	Intense uptake	Isointense	Isointense	Marked uptake

*With respect to brain tissue.

epidermoid tumor in the CPA, this tumor's association with facial pain has been strong.[24,35,44] Symptoms of patients from three recent series are listed in Table 9. Abnormalities of hearing, vertigo, and cerebellar symptomatology are most often associated with epidermoid tumors in the CPA.[8]

Although epidermoid tumors commonly involve the trigeminal nerve, this phenomenon does not occur often enough to allow these tumors to be distinguished clinically from other pathologic processes in the CPA. The typical appearances of epidermoid tumors on both CT and MRI, however, help to quickly exclude acoustic tumors and meningiomas from the possibilities (Table 10).

Epidermoid tumors and cholesterol granulomas of the petrous apex are closely related to the CPA, but remain extradural. Clinically, these two pathologic entities probably are indistinguishable, although facial palsy may be more common with epidermoid tumors[31,36,59] than with cholesterol granulomas. The patient's typical clinical presentation is dull, ipsilateral headache; progressive facial weakness; and hearing loss. Hemifacial spasm is relatively common, tending to precede progressive facial weakness (Figure 6).

CPA tumors usually are extensive (Figure 5B) and may extend from the incisura to the foramen magnum; however, intracapsular debulking is easily performed with suction. The capsule may closely adhere to vital neurovas-

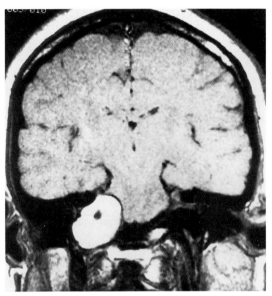

Figure 6. Coronal MRI. This lesion of increased signal intensity in the petrous apex was completely removed through an extended middle fossa approach. The preoperative diagnosis of a cholesterol granuloma was confirmed. The patient's preoperative facial palsy completely resolved, although her hearing loss did not.

cular structures though, foiling attempts at complete removal. Bits of capsule left on the brain stem, basal vessels, or cranial nerves appear to have a benign course with low recurrence rates.[49] Total removal of petrous apex epidermoids also is important to prevent recurrence. Because these lesions are extradural, they are amenable to lateral

extradural approaches such as the infratemporal fossa or transmastoid approaches. Complete removal can be achieved with these
procedures.[16,57] Additionally, many authors
believe that the petrous apex needs to be
exteriorized into an enlarged external auditory meatus.[59]

By contrast, the treatment of cholesterol
granulomas is straightforward. Cyst decompression alone has been quite successful.[31,49]
The consensus in the otolaryngologic literature, however, is that these lesions should be
permanently drained into an air-filled cavity
such as the middle ear,[18] or the sphenoid
sinus.[43] Our experience with removal of the
cyst through an extended middle fossa approach has been rewarding.

Surgical Approaches to Tumors of the Posterior Fossa

Conceptually, each operative procedure can

TABLE 11
Surgical Stages and Goals

Approach
- Wide visualization.
- Minimal working distance.
- Avoidance of brain retraction.
- Preservation of important structures.
- Early interruption of vascular supply.

Resection
- Access and dissect within arachnoid planes.
- Central debulking and then peripheral dissection.
- Removal of all involved dura and bone.

Reconstruction
- Separate intracranial contents from aerodigestive tract, mastoid air cells, and paranasal sinuses.
- Prevent CSF leak.
- Cosmesis.

---

be divided into three portions: approach,
tumor resection, and reconstruction. Each ap-

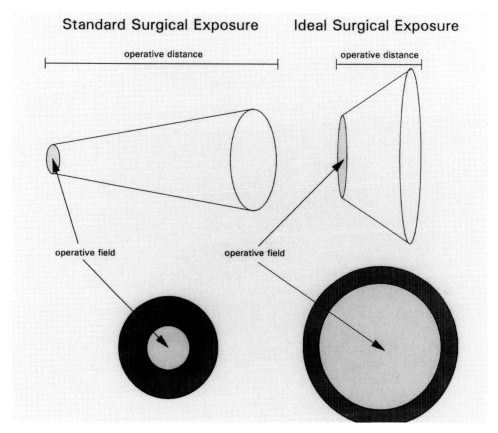

Figure 7. *Diagrammatic representation of the features of an ideal surgical approach: wide exposure and short depth of field.*

proach has its own goals (Table 11). The approach selected should allow excellent visualization, minimize working distance (Figure 7), and avoid brain retraction. All important structures should, of course, be preserved. Sacrifice of these structures (for example, the labyrinth or cochlea) depends on the expectation of total removal and the patient's wishes. Some patients may forgo total removal to retain neurologic function or to avoid possible deficits. The extensive bone removal inherent in an ideal surgical approach to basal posterior fossa tumors also allows the vascular supply from the external carotid branches to be interrupted early and the bone invaded by the tumor to be removed.

Tumor resection begins with the accession and dissection of the arachnoidal plane usually present in patients who have not undergone previous surgery. In patients having undergone previous surgery or radiation, and occasionally in patients who have not undergone surgery, no such plane of dissection exists. In these cases, important neurovascular structures must be identified in areas not involved by tumor and then dissected free. Debulking the tumor allows the walls of the tumor to collapse, facilitating dissection of the capsule without undue traction on surrounding structures. The cranial nerves and blood vessels may course through a basal tumor, and the surgeon should be careful to identify them. Because neither the ultrasonic aspirator nor the laser discriminates between normal and abnormal tissue, great care must be exercised when using these tools. More often than not, the tumor is removed using bipolar cautery and sharp dissection with microscissors.

The goals of reconstruction are to separate the intracranial contents from the aerodigestive tract, paranasal sinuses, and mastoid air cells to prevent CSF leakage and infection. A secondary, but nonetheless important, consideration for the patient is cosmesis. The surgeon should aim for a watertight dural closure if at all possible. A duraplasty with fascia lata may be required. Many times, all that can be achieved at the base is partial

tacking of the fascial graft to the edges of the dural defect. This then is supplemented with fibrin glue. Well-vascularized tissue flaps, such as pericranium, the temporalis muscle, or a free rectus abdominis muscle transfer, reduces the incidence of CSF leakage. This is especially important when the patient has had previous surgery or radiotherapy.

Lateral Approaches to the Posterior Fossa

Traditional neurosurgical approaches to the posterior fossa are well known (retrosigmoid, subtemporal transtentorial, and combined supratentorial and infratentorial). Although they remain useful, these approaches require brain retraction, at times to a significant degree. In addition, the anterior and anterolateral aspects of the brain stem, cranial nerves, and basal vessels are poorly visualized through these approaches. To circumvent these problems, lateral approaches to the posterior fossa have been developed. Each of these approaches increases the exposure of anterior and anterolateral structures with little or no brain retraction. The petrosal, transtemporal, and transcondylar approaches improve exposure of the upper, mid-, and lower petroclival and occipito-clival areas. Together, they allow the surgeon to reach any part of the posterior fossa.

The Petrosal Approach

For the petrosal approach,[2,6] the patient is placed supine. The patient's head is turned 45° away from the side of the tumor, lowered, and tilted toward the opposite side, thus bringing the base of the petrous pyramid to the highest point of the operative field. The ipsilateral shoulder is elevated. A curvilinear incision is made from the base of the zygoma, circling the ear, and descending 1 cm behind the mastoid process (Figure 8). The temporalis muscle and pericranium are elevated to the level of the external ear canal. Four burr holes are placed to straddle the

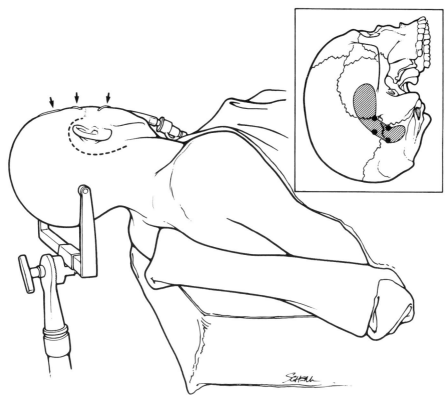

Figure 8. The patient's position and skin incision for a right-sided petrosal approach. EMG needle electrodes are inserted into the facial musculature (arrows). **(Inset)** *Location of burr holes straddling the transverse sinus and the outline of the bone flap. From Al-Mefty.*[4]

transverse sinus. Inferior temporal and sub-occipital bone cuts are made and the bone over the sinus is removed with rongeurs or a high-speed drill. The bone flap is elevated carefully, exposing the transverse and sigmoid sinuses. A mastoidectomy is performed, exposing the sigmoid sinus and the dura anterior to it, the jugular bulb, the lateral and posterior semicircular canals, and the facial nerve in the fallopian canal. The bone overlying the sinodural angle is removed, exposing the superior petrosal sinus (Figure 9).

The dura mater then is opened along the anterior border of the sigmoid sinus and along the floor of the temporal fossa. The vein of Labbé is identified and protected. The superior petrosal sinus is incised between hemoclips (Figure 10); this incision in the tentorium is carried medially to the incisura, avoiding injury to the trochlear nerve and

the superior petrosal vein. Complete sectioning of the tentorium allows the sigmoid sinus, along with the cerebellar hemisphere, to fall back, thus decreasing the need for retraction.

Cranial nerves IV-XII can be visualized by angling the microscope, as can the entire vertebrobasilar system and the anterolateral brain stem (Figure 11).

Transtemporal Approaches (Combined Infratemporal Posterior Fossa Approach)[2,5]

The position of the patient for the transtemporal approaches is similar to that for the petrosal approach. A C-shaped incision is made behind the ear and extended into a convenient skin crease in the neck and up to the temporal area. This flap is elevated ante-

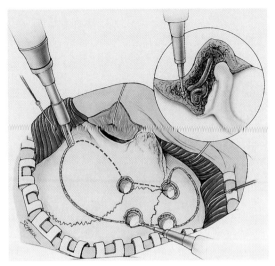

Figure 9. The temporalis and sternocleidomastoid muscles are retracted, as is a triangular pericranial flap, which will later be used to cover the drilled surface of the temporal bone. The burr holes flanking the transverse sinus are interconnected using a drill and a craniotome with a foot attachment. (Inset) After the bone flap is removed, the bone overlying the sigmoid sinus is excised and the petrous bone is drilled extensively to expose the semicircular and facial canals. From Al-Mefty.[4]

riorly in a subcutaneous plane (Figure 12). The external canal is transected at the bony cartilaginous junction. The skin of the external ear canal is everted and closed as a blind sac. A small periosteal flap is rotated and closed over the ear canal (Figure 13).

The pericranium is divided horizontally at the level of the mastoid base. The temporalis and sternocleidomastoid muscles are detached and reflected anteriorly and inferolaterally, respectively. The spinal accessory nerve is identified and preserved. The common, internal, and external carotid arteries are exposed, as are the internal jugular vein and cranial nerves IX-XII.

A mastoidectomy is performed. The facial nerve is skeletonized from the stylomastoid foramen to the geniculate ganglion; it then is transposed anteriorly and secured. The sigmoid sinus is exposed to the jugular bulb and a posterior fossa craniectomy is performed in continuity (Figure 14).

The posterior belly of the digastric muscle and the stylohyoid muscle are transected, and

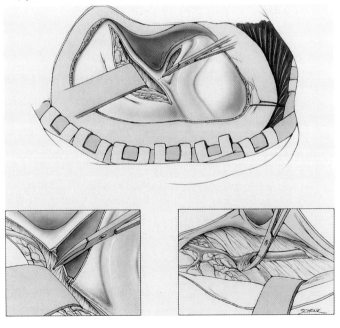

Figure 10. Incisions are made in the temporal dura along the floor of the temporal fossa and in the dura of the posterior fossa anterior to the sigmoid sinus. (Insets) The superior petrosal sinus is divided between clips. The vein of Labbé is dissected free from its arachnoidal bindings to prevent its injury. From Al-Mefty.[4]

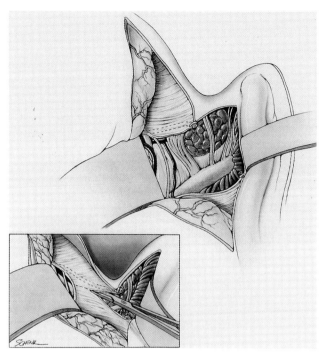

Figure 11 (Inset) *Sectioning of the tentorium continues to the incisura, avoiding injury to the trochlear nerve. The resultant (central image) exposure allows the surgeon to visualize the anterolateral brain stem and vasculature as well as cranial nerves III through XII. From Al-Mefty.*[4]

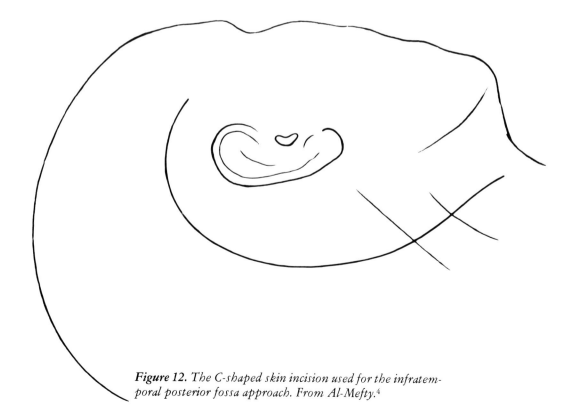

Figure 12. *The C-shaped skin incision used for the infratemporal posterior fossa approach. From Al-Mefty.*[4]

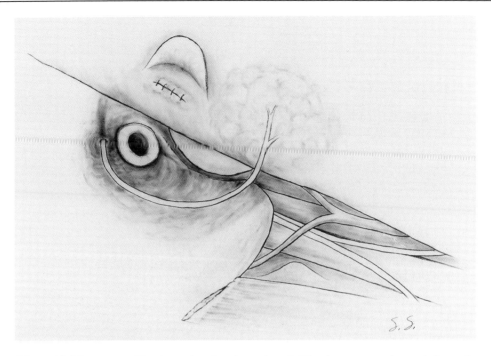

Figure 13. *The ear canal has been closed and a pericranial flap is sewn over it to reinforce the closure. The skeletonized facial nerve is transposed anteriorly. From Al-Mefty.*[5]

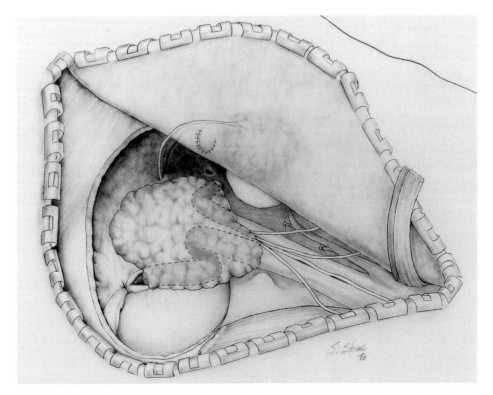

Figure 14. *A total mastoidectomy and posterior fossa craniectomy have been performed, and the facial nerve has been transposed anteriorly. The sigmoid sinus and external carotid branches have been ligated for this glomus tumor. The carotid artery, jugular vein, and lower cranial nerves have been isolated. From Al-Mefty.*[5]

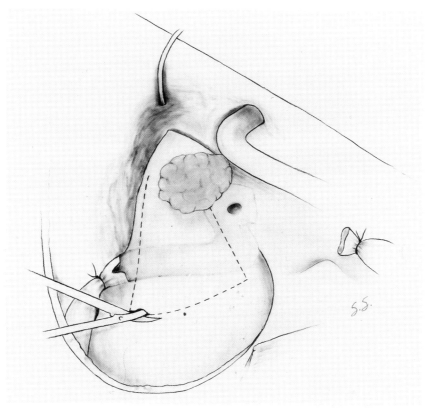

Figure 15. After the lateral wall of the sigmoid sinus and the jugular vein are removed, a trapezoidal durotomy is performed if an intradural extension of the tumor is present. The orifice of the inferior petrosal sinus is identified and packed with oxidized regenerated cellulose. From Al-Mefty.[5]

the stylohyoid process is removed. The sigmoid sinus and the internal jugular vein are ligated. The remnant of skin in the external ear canal and the tympanic membrane are removed, and the internal carotid artery is exposed in the petrous canal. The eustachian tube is obliterated with muscle. The lower cranial nerves are preserved as they emerge from the jugular foramen.

All of these maneuvers are performed without sacrificing the structures of the inner ear by working in the infralabyrinthine space. If involved by the tumor or for increased exposure, the labyrinth and cochlea can be removed, exposing the internal auditory canal and the vertical segment of the petrous carotid artery. The dura is excised in a trapezoid shape, the short side based at the internal auditory canal (Figure 15).

At the end of the intradural portion of the operation, the dura mater is repaired with a graft of fascia lata, and the cavity is obliterated with fat. The temporalis muscle is swung inferiorly and sewn to the sternocleidomastoid muscle. The scalp is then closed in two layers.

Transcondylar Approach

For the transcondylar approach, the patient is placed in the lateral decubitus position. The patient's head is flexed and the ipsilateral shoulder is held caudally with tape. A reversed hockey-stick incision is made; the "heel" of the incision is located at the base of the mastoid process. The incision is extended caudally along the edge of the sternocleidomastoid muscle and posteromedially to expose the suboccipital area. The sternocleidomastoid muscle then is detached from the mastoid

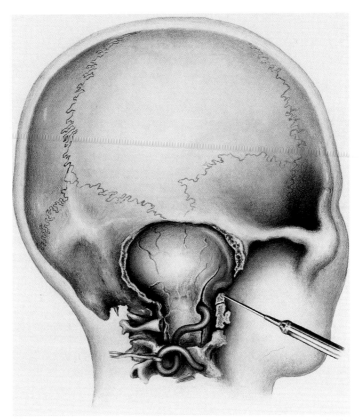

Figure 16. The transcondylar craniotomy. A craniectomy of the lateral posterior fossa exposes the sigmoid sinus. The lamina and the lateral mass of C1 have been removed and the vertebral artery mobilized medially. The occipital condyle is being removed using a high-speed drill. The durotomy, which improves mobilization, circumscribes the vertebral artery at its entrance through the dura.

and retracted inferomedially. Injury to the spinal accessory nerve must be avoided. The lateral mass of C1 is palpated and the muscles are dissected in a subperiosteal plane from the lamina of the first and second vertebrae. As the inferior oblique muscle is detached, the ventral ramus of the second cervical root is identified and followed medially, exposing the vertebral artery between C1 and C2. The transverse foramina of C1 and, if necessary, C2 are opened, and the vertebral artery is mobilized and transposed medially (Figure 16). The periarterial venous plexus in this area may be a source of bleeding. The vertebral artery is followed to its point of entry into the dura, and a lateral posterior fossa craniectomy is fashioned. The sigmoid sinus and jugular bulb are skeletonized with a high-speed drill. If necessary, the lamina of C1 and C2 are removed. The occipital condyle and the lateral mass of C1 are drilled in their posterior and lateral portions (Figure 16). The dura is incised posterior to the sigmoid sinus; this incision is carried inferiorly to the entry of the vertebral artery. The dural ring around the artery is opened fully, and the dural incision continued inferiorly into the lateral aspect of the upper cervical dural sac (Figure 16). After the tumor is removed, the dura is closed tightly, and the muscles are reapproximated in layers.

References

1. Al-Mefty O. Management of glomus jugulare tumors. *Contemp Neurosurg.* 1988;10:1-6.

2. Al-Mefty O. *Surgery of the Cranial Base.* Boston, Ma: Kluwer Academic; 1989.

3. Al-Mefty O. *Meningiomas.* New York, NY: Raven Press; 1991.

4. Al-Mefty O. Petroclival meningiomas. In: Rengachary SS, ed. *Neurosurgical Operative Atlas.* Baltimore, Md: Williams & Wilkins (in press).

5. Al-Mefty O, Fox JL, Rifai A, et al. A combined infratemporal and posterior fossa approach for the removal of giant glomus tumors and chondrosarcomas. *Surg Neurol.* 1987;28:423-431.

6. Al-Mefty O, Fox JL, Smith RR. Petrosal approach for petroclival meningiomas. *Neurosurgery.* 1988; 22:510-517.

7. Austin-Seymour M, Munzenrider J, Goitein M, et al. Fractionated proton radiation therapy of chordoma and low-grade chondrosarcoma of the base of the skull. *J Neurosurg.* 1989;70:13-17.

8. Berger MS, Wilson CB. Epidermoid cysts of the posterior fossa. *J Neurosurg.* 1985;62:214-219.

9. Brackmann DE, House WF, Terry R, et al. Glomus jugulare tumors: effect of irradiation. *Trans Am Acad Ophthalmol Otol.* 1972;76:1423-1431.

10. Castellano F, Ruggiero G. Meningiomas of the posterior fossa. *Acta Radiol (Stockh).* 1953(suppl); 104:1-177.

11. Cherington M, Schneck SA. Clivus meningiomas. *Neurology.* 1966;16:86-92.

12. Cummings BJ, Hodson DI, Bush RS. Chordoma: the results of megavoltage radiation therapy. *Int J Radiat Oncol Biol Phys.* 1983;9:633-642.

13. Dahlin DC, MacCarty CS. Chordoma: a study of 59 cases. *Cancer.* 1952;5:1170-1178.

14. Dubois P. Tumors of the cerebellopontine angle: radiology. In: Wilkins RH, Rengachary SS, eds. *Neurosurgery.* New York, NY: McGraw-Hill Company; 1985;1:704-719.

15. Farrior JB III, Hyams VJ, Benke RH, et al. Carcinoid apudoma arising in a glomus jugulare tumor: review of endocrine activity in glomus jugulare tumors. *Laryngoscope.* 1980;90:110-119.

16. Fisch U, Fagan P, Valavanis A. The infratemporal fossa approach for the lateral skull base. *Otolaryngol Clin North Am.* 1984;17:513-552.

17. Franklin DJ, Moore GF, Fisch U. Jugular foramen peripheral nerve sheath tumors. *Laryngoscope.* 1989; 99:1081-1087.

18. Gacek RR. Evaluation and management of primary petrous apex cholesteatoma. *Otolaryngol Head Neck Surg.* 1980;88:519-523.

19. Givner I. Ophthalmologic features of intracranial chordoma and allied tumors of the clivus. *Arch Ophthalmol.* 1945;33:397-403.

20. Grand W, Bakay L. Posterior fossa meningiomas: a report of 30 cases. *Acta Neurochir (Wien).* 1975; 32:219-233.

21. Greenberg JJ, Oot RF, Wismer GL, et al. Cholesterol granuloma of the petrous apex: MR and CT evaluation. *AJNR.* 1988;9:1205-1214.

22. Hakuba A, Nishimura S. Total removal of clivus meningiomas and the operative results. *Neurol Med Chir (Tokyo).* 1981;21:59-73.

23. Heffelfinger MJ, Dahlin DC, MacCarty CS, et al. Chordomas and cartilaginous tumors at the skull base. *Cancer.* 1973;32:410-420.

24. Hori T, Numata H, Hokama Y, et al. Trigeminal pain caused by a parapontine epidermal cyst. *Surg Neurol.* 1983;19:517-519.

25. Horn KL, House WF, Hitselberger WE. Schwan-

nomas of the jugular foramen. *Laryngoscope.* 1985; 95:761-765.

26. Jackson CG, Cueva RA, Thedinger BA, et al. Cranial nerve preservation in lesions of the jugular fossa. *Otolaryngol Head Neck Surg.* 1991;105:687-693.

27. Jackson CG, Glasscock ME III, Harris PF. Glomus tumors: diagnosis, classification, and management of large lesions. *Arch Otolaryngol.* 1982;108: 401-406.

28. Kamerer DB, Hirsch BE. Paragangliomas ("glomus tumors") of the temporal bone. In: Sekhar LN, Schramm VL Jr, eds. *Tumors of the Cranial Base: Diagnosis and Treatment.* Mount Kisco, NY: Futura Press; 1987:641-654.

29. Kaye AH, Hahn JF, Kinney SE, et al. Jugular foramen schwannomas. *J Neurosurg.* 1984;60:1045-1053.

30. Kendall BE, Lee BCP. Cranial chordomas. *Br J Radiol.* 1977;50:687-698.

31. King TT, Benjamin JC, Morrison AW. Epidermoid and cholesterol cysts in the apex of the petrous bone. *Br J Neurosurg.* 1989;3:451-461.

32. Kondziolka D, Lunsford LD, Flickinger JC. The role of radiosurgery in the management of chordoma and chondrosarcoma of the cranial base. *Neurosurgery.* 1991;29:38-46.

33. Krayenbühl H, Yasargil MG. Cranial chordomas. *Progr Neurol Surg.* 1975;6:380-434.

34. Lang J. *Clinical Anatomy of the Posterior Cranial Fossa and Its Foramina.* New York, NY: Thieme Medical Publishers; 1991:85.

35. Latack JT, Kartush JM, Kemink JL, et al. Epidermoidomas of the cerebellopontine angle and temporal bone: CT and MR aspects. *Radiology.* 1985; 157:361-366.

36. Leonetti JP, Brackmann DE. Glomus vagale tumor: the significance of early vocal cord paralysis. *Otolaryngol Head Neck Surg.* 1989;100:533-537.

37. Leunda G, Vaquero J, Cabezudo J, et al. Schwannoma of the oculomotor nerves: report of four cases. *J Neurosurg.* 1982;57:563-565.

38. Lipkin AF, Coker NJ, Jenkins HA, et al. Intracranial and intratemporal facial neuroma. *Otolaryngol Head Neck Surg.* 1987;96:71-79.

39. Mabrey RE. Chordoma: a study of 150 cases. *Am J Cancer.* 1935;25:501-517.

40. Martinez R, Vaquero J, Areitio E, et al. Meningiomas of the posterior fossa. *Surg Neurol.* 1983;19: 237-243.

41. Mayberg MR, Symon L. Meningiomas of the clivus and apical petrous bone: report of 35 cases. *J Neurosurg.* 1986;65:160-167.

42. McCormick PC, Bello JA, Post KD. Trigeminal schwannoma: surgical series of 14 cases with review of the literature. *J Neurosurg.* 1988;69: 850-860.

43. Montgomery WW. Cystic lesions of the petrous apex: transsphenoidal approach. *Ann Otol Rhinol Laryngol.* 1977;86:429-435.

44. Olivecrona H. Cholesteatomas of the cerebellopontine angle. *Acta Psychiatr Neurol (Copenh).* 1949;24:639-643.

45. Pearlman AW, Friedman M. Radical radiation therapy of chordoma. *Am J Roentgenol.* 1970;108: 333-341.

46. Pluchino F, Crivelli G, Vaghi MA. Intracranial neurinomas of the nerves of the jugular foramen: report of 12 personal cases. *Acta Neurochir. (Wien)* 1975; 31:201-221.

47. Pollack IF, Sekhar LN, Jannetta PJ, et al. Neurile-

momas of the trigeminal nerve. *J Neurosurg.* 1989; 70:737-745.

48. Raffel C, Wright DC, Gutin PH, et al. Cranial chordomas: clinical presentation and results of operative and radiation therapy in twenty-six patients. *Neurosurgery.* 1985;17:703-710.

49. Sabin HI, Bordi LT, Symon L. Epidermoid cysts and cholesterol granulomas centered on the posterior fossa: twenty years of diagnosis and management. *Neurosurgery.* 1987;21:798-805.

50. Samii M, Ammirati M. Cerebellopontine angle meningiomas (posterior pyramid meningiomas) In: Al-Mefty O, ed. *Meningiomas.* New York, NY: Raven Press; 1991:503-515.

51. Samii M, Ammirati M, Mahran A, et al. Surgery of petroclival meningiomas: report of 24 cases. *Neurosurgery.* 1989;24:12-17.

52. Schwaber MK, Gussack GS, Kirkpatrick W. The role of radiation therapy in the management of catecholamine-secreting glomus tumors. *Otolaryngol Head Neck Surg.* 1988;98:150-154.

53. Scott M. The surgical management of meningiomas of the cerebellar fossa. *Surg Gynecol Obstet.* 1972; 135:545-550.

54. Sekhar LN, Jannetta PJ. Cerebellopontine angle meningiomas: microsurgical excision and follow-up results. *J Neurosurg.* 1984;60:500-505.

55. Sekhar LN, Jannetta PJ. Petroclival and medial tentorial meningiomas. In: Sekhar LN, Schramm VL, eds. *Tumors of the Cranial Base: Diagnosis and Treatment.* Mount Kisco, NY: Futura Press; 1987; 623-640.

56. Sekhar LN, Jannetta PJ, Burkhart LE, et al. Meningiomas involving the clivus: a six-year experience with 41 patients. *Neurosurgery.* 1990;27:764-781.

57. Sekhar LN, Schramm VL Jr, Jones NF. Subtemporal-preauricular infratemporal fossa approach to large lateral and posterior cranial base neoplasms. *J Neurosurg.* 1987;67:488-499.

58. Sen CN, Sekhar LN, Schramm VL, et al. Chordoma and chondrosarcoma of the cranial base: an 8-year experience. *Neurosurgery.* 1989;25:931-941.

59. Smith PG, Leonetti JP, Kletzker GR. Differential clinical and radiographic features of cholesterol granulomas and cholesteatomas of the petrous apex. *Ann Otol Rhinol Laryngol.* 1988;97:599-604.

60. Spector GJ, Druck NS, Gado M. Neurologic manifestations of glomus tumors in the head and neck. *Arch Neurol.* 1976;33:270-274.

61. Tung H, Chen T, Weiss MH. Sixth nerve schwannomas: report of two cases. *J Neurosurg.* 1991; 75:638-641.

62. Ulsø C, Sehested P, Overgaard J. Intracranial hypoglossal neurinoma: diagnosis and postoperative care. *Surg Neurol.* 1981;16:65-68.

63. Yamakawa K, Shitara N, Genka S, et al. Clinical course and surgical prognosis of 33 cases of intracranial epidermoid tumors. *Neurosurgery.* 1989;24: 568-573.

64. Yasargil MG, Abernathey CD, Sarioglu AC. Microneurosurgical treatment of intracranial dermoid and epidermoid tumors. *Neurosurgery.* 1989;24:561-567.

65. Yasargil MG, Mortara RW, Curcic M. Meningiomas of basal posterior cranial fossa. In: Krayenbühl H, ed. *Advances and Technical Standards in Neurosurgery.* Vienna, Austria: Springer; 1980;3-115.

CHAPTER 12

Surgical Approaches to Acoustic Neuromas

Steven L. Giannotta, MD

With the renaissance of devising strategies for complex problems involving the cranial base has come the almost inevitable collaboration between certain surgical specialties. Skull base teams have formed from the ranks of neurosurgeons, otologists, plastic surgeons, ophthalmologists, and others to propagate a cross-fertilization of ideas, strategies, and techniques. As a result, intellectual barriers have been broken down, allowing new perspectives in the conceptualization of strategies to expand the horizons of what is possible. Opportunities are available to add unfamiliar but effective concepts and techniques to one's practice, not so much the result of a new breakthrough but through the willingness to borrow on another's expertise.

Thus, regarding surgery for acoustic neuromas, the distinctions between otologic approaches and neurosurgical approaches are beginning to blur as these same strategies become incorporated into the team's overall tactics.[9,19] The following is a catalog of the surgical approaches to acoustic neuromas in contemporary practice, which presents the indications, techniques, drawbacks, and benefits of each approach from the perspective of a team member.

Translabyrinthine Approach

This approach is perhaps the most common strategy in contemporary usage for acoustic tumors because otologists have adopted it as "theirs," and patients with hearing loss naturally gravitate toward "ear doctors." The approach has propagated mainly because of the difficulty in reconciling the conflicting goals of the alternative technique, namely, hearing preservation and a microscopic total removal. The translabyrinthine approach was conceived at the turn of the century, but it was abandoned due to both inadequate techniques for maximizing exposure and poor illumination. With the advent of the operating microscope in the early 1960s, the pioneering efforts of William House and colleagues were rewarded with an effective and accepted technique.[8-12,31,33,35,36]

Technique

General endotracheal anesthesia is utilized with appropriate physiologic monitoring and bladder catheterization. The patient is positioned supine on the operating table with the head resting on soft pads and turned to the side opposite the tumor. Pin headrest fixation is not necessary. Muscle relaxants are used only at the time of induction and endotracheal intubation to allow electromyographic (EMG) monitoring of facial (VII) nerve function during the procedure. EMG needles are placed in the frontalis, orbicularis oculi, and in the orbicularis oris musculature and taped securely after final positioning.[14,22,25] The hair is shaved above and behind the ear and the mastoid process and, along with an area in the lower abdomen, is prepared with an antiseptic solution. The surgeon is seated at the side of the table facing the mastoid and retromastoid area. Following the injection of a local anesthetic with epinephrine, a 5-cm postauricular incision is made 1 inch behind the postauricular crease extending from the mastoid tip, curving forward to end just above the pinna. A separate incision in the temporalis fascia and muscle is performed to fashion a musculofascial flap that will be important at the time of closure.

Self-retaining retractors are placed to maintain the external ear in a forward position. By using the high-speed drill with a large cutting burr and continuous suction irrigation, the cortex over the mastoid bone is removed. Bone removal is begun behind the external auditory canal and along the temporal line. The junction of these two bone incisions generally marks the region of the mastoid antrum and the lateral semicircular canal. This landmark provides the surgeon with a concept of the depth and the three-dimensional relationship of the facial nerve to the posterior and superior semicircular canals. Bone removal continues superiorly to the middle fossa plate, inferiorly to the jugular bulb, posteriorly to the sigmoid sinus, and anteriorly just short of the external auditory canal (Figure 1). For large tumors, bone removal is continued over and posterior to the sigmoid sinus, allowing the gentle retraction of the sinus if necessary. Emissary veins are controlled with bipolar electrocautery and/or cellulose packing.

The operating microscope is brought into position, and the lateral and posterior semicircular canals are progressively removed. The facial nerve, which lies anterior to those structures, is carefully approached, again with the lateral semicircular canal used as the landmark. The facial nerve is skeletonized by using the diamond burr from the external genu inferiorly to the stylomastoid foramen. Acoustically enhanced EMG monitoring allows immediate feedback to the surgeon during this delicate part of the procedure. Care is taken not to remove totally the thin bone around the facial nerve. Once the course of

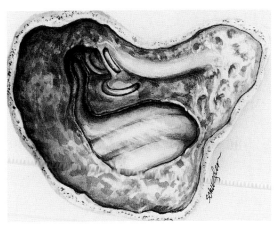

Figure 1. Completed mastoidectomy with exposure of the labyrinth, facial nerve in the fallopian canal, and sigmoid sinus preliminary to translabyrinthine removal of acoustic tumor.

the facial nerve has been ascertained, the vestibule is opened, and the bone around the internal auditory canal is carefully removed. The internal arcuate artery and the cochlear aqueduct generally mark the superior and inferior extent of the internal auditory canal. The bone in the region of the porus acusticus is removed first, with the bone over the lateralmost end of the internal auditory canal saved for last. The superior lip of the porus generally is the most difficult to manage because of its very close proximity to the facial nerve. However, it is important to remove bone superiorly and inferiorly, so that the anteriormost extent of the canal is accessible (Figure 2).

For large tumors, the dural incision is begun just medial to the sigmoid sinus and is carried in a line toward the midportion of the internal auditory canal. At the region of the porus, the dural incision is extended superiorly and inferiorly. Following the identification and opening of the appropriate arachnoid plane separating the cerebellum from the surface of the tumor, intracapsular removal begins with the identification and the electrocautery of accessible feeding vasculature. With acoustic neuromas, the likelihood of the facial nerve occupying the lateral and posterior aspect of the tumor mass is small. Facial nerve monitoring and close

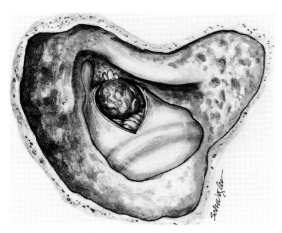

Figure 2. Translabyrinthine exposure of acoustic tumor with detail of lateral end of the internal canal depicting the relationship of the facial nerve to vestibular nerve components.

scrutiny of the tumor capsule will help to avoid injury. With meningiomas or other lesions in the cerebellopontine angle, however, it is important, prior to opening the tumor capsule, to focus attention on the lateral end of the internal auditory canal to positively identify the facial nerve and its course with respect to the surface of the tumor.

With large tumors, only a limited dissection and exploration of the anterior and medial boundaries of the lesion is performed prior to internal decompression. This will help avoid undue traction on the facial nerve and undue compression of the underlying brain stem. With successive attempts at internal decompression, the tumor capsule can be progressively infolded away from the cerebellum, the lower cranial nerves, the trigeminal (V) nerve, and, subsequently, the brain stem. With the progressive removal of the capsule, the tumor can be reduced to a size that will allow safe facial nerve dissection.

Attention then is turned to the lateral end of the internal auditory canal. The transverse and vertical crests of the internal auditory canal are identified. The facial nerve will lie anterior to the vertical crest, and its course can be traced to its junction with the tumor. The facial nerve will adhere more to the tumor at the level of the porus. If difficulty in maintaining the appropriate plane between

the nerve and the tumor is experienced at this juncture, it generally is beneficial to identify the facial nerve at the brain stem, thus allowing dissection of the facial nerve from two directions. This is expedited by further removal of tumor tissue followed by the identification and division of the vestibulocochlear (VIII) nerve at the brain stem. The nerve stimulator and facial nerve monitor can be used for positive identification of the facial nerve at its junction with the brain stem. The postoperative function of the facial nerve is enhanced by continuous saline irrigation during facial nerve dissection. Traction on the nerve is minimized as much as possible, and on occasion, it is important to provide laterally directed traction on the tumor either with a suction tip or with microforceps during the dissection. Any medially directed traction on the tumor will, of necessity, stretch the facial nerve. Once the nerve is completely free of the tumor, the remaining tumor remnants can be removed.

Once hemostasis is complete, the incus is removed and a piece of the temporalis muscle is harvested and placed carefully through the epitympanum into the origin of the eustachian tube. This will form a temporary seal against cerebrospinal fluid (CSF) leakage. Autologous fat then is taken from the lower abdomen. The dural incision is closed up to the internal auditory canal, and strips of autologous fat are placed just through the dural defect to fashion a seal. It is important to perform this maneuver while facial nerve monitoring continues so that the adipose graft does not put undue pressure on the exposed facial nerve. The previously fashioned musculofascial flap is closed tightly over the adipose graft, and the postauricular incision is closed in two layers. A small ear dressing provides satisfactory protection.

Exposure Enhancement

Traditionally, the translabyrinthine approach was believed to be most appropriate for small and medium-sized acoustic neuromas. With increasing experience with the approach and attention to certain details, however, rather sizable lesions can be removed. Lesions 6 cm in diameter and larger have been successfully removed through the translabyrinthine approach without resorting to combining supratentorial or retrosigmoid strategies.[8-10,35,36] The key to the maximization of exposure is the wide skeletonization of dural surfaces bordering the mastoidectomy. The ability to gently retract the underlying structures, including the sigmoid sinus, widens the angle of attack toward the poles of the tumor. Opening of the cochlear aqueduct allows for gradual and early removal of CSF while the drilling and early exposure are completed.

Integral to the management of large tumors, of course, is the progressive radical internal decompression of the tumor mass to facilitate brain stem and cranial nerve dissection. The temptation to begin any brain stem or cranial nerve dissection prior to an exaggerated effort to decompress the tumor mass from the inside should be resisted. This will obviate any transmission of compressive forces to the brain stem and the facial nerve at its exit through the porus acusticus. A number of automated and mechanical measures can be effectively used for the cytoreduction of the bulk of these large masses. Which technique is used is based on personal preference and on the ability to manipulate such instrumentation through a relatively restricted portal.

During the process of internal decompression, it is important to attempt to decompress the portion of the tumor that resides just outside the porus acusticus. This will reduce tissue pressure against the facial nerve as it angles around the porus and will facilitate the identification and dissection of the most tenuous part of the nerve. Also, radical internal decompression along with the facial nerve monitor and stimulator allows the facial nerve to be identified at both the lateral end of the internal auditory canal and its exit zone at the brain stem. Thus, with large tumors with marked attenuation of the facial nerve, the dissection plane can be picked up

and developed in both a lateral and a medial direction to maximize facial nerve anatomic integrity.

Benefits

One of the advantages of the translabyrinthine approach is that it is the most direct with the shortest trajectory from the surface to the tumor. As a result, the entry point through the dura is adjacent to the porus acusticus in front of the cerebellar hemisphere. In effect, cerebellar retraction is replaced by bone removal much in the same way as the pterional approach accomplishes this in aneurysm surgery. Because the entire internal auditory canal is exposed with the initial drilling, microscopic total removal is readily accomplished. Facial nerve preservation is maximized because at the lateral end of the internal auditory canal, the nerve is adjacent to a constant bony landmark, the vertical crest (Bill's bar). Because this portion of the nerve can be identified early in the procedure, facial nerve dissection can proceed alternately in either lateral-to-medial or medial-to-lateral directions. Exposure of the facial nerve in the fallopian canal provides an added benefit. Should facial nerve continuity become compromised, the length of the distal segment can be augmented by removing the segment from the canal for the purposes of end-to-end repair.[1,3,16]

For those very large or complex lesions, the translabyrinthine approach offers the capability of effecting a radical internal decompression without the need for retraction. If such a strategy is insufficient to accomplish complete exposure and removal, a combined supratentorial or retrosigmoid attack can be added easily with the additional benefit of exposure of the facial nerve early in the procedure.[31] Positioning of the patient is simplified and the need for pin headrest fixation is obviated since self-retaining retractor systems are unnecessary. The seated surgeon's arms are held at a comfortable attitude, thus reducing the fatigue factor. In many centers,

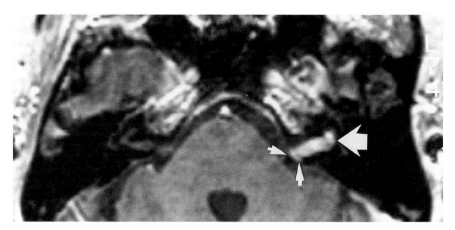

Figure 3. Enhanced MRI of a predominantly intracanalicular acoustic tumor. Poor hearing, impaction in the lateral end of the auditory canal (large arrow), and slight protuberance through the porus acusticus (small arrows) make this an ideal candidate for the translabyrinthine approach.

a team approach is taken with the neurosurgeon and the otologist assuming different responsibilities, which is another factor in reducing fatigue.[9,19]

Drawbacks

The most critical drawback with the translabyrinthine approach is the sacrifice of hearing. Although this is frequently well accepted by patients and may even be preferable to the distraction that attends a poorly functioning ear with no speech discrimination, certainly some professions and activities demand binaural hearing. Thus, in cases of patients with a single hearing ear or with the need for binaural hearing, either an alternative approach should be selected or treatment should be delayed. The unfamiliar anatomy and somewhat restricted access to the posterior fossa can be considered as drawbacks to some surgeons. With the availability of skull base symposia and practical courses, the opportunity to learn the anatomy is unparalleled. Practice and judicious use of cytoreductive technologies and intraoperative monitoring will improve one's ability to resect larger lesions through smaller portals.

CSF leakage has been associated specifically with the translabyrinthine approach, although studies would suggest a similar incidence with the retrosigmoid approach. Autologous adipose grafts and fibrin glue should reduce the incidence of this complication to less than 5%.[5,6,15,28,34]

Indications

In simplest terms, the indication for the translabyrinthine approach is the unlikeliness of serviceable hearing preservation. A number of factors govern this possibility, and all must be taken into consideration. Perhaps the most important is the surgeon's or team's track record on preserving auditory function. If preservation is accomplished rarely, it is unreasonable to apply a hearing preservation strategy for a 3-cm lesion with 50% speech discrimination. As a starting point, lesions greater than 2 cm with more than a 20-dB hearing loss and less than 80% speech discrimination should be considered for the translabyrinthine approach (Figure 3). As experience grows with hearing preservation techniques, such guidelines can be further refined.[11]

Recurrent tumors are ideal for the translabyrinthine approach because hearing preservation is rarely an issue and because the origin of the recurrence usually is within the internal canal—a region that is maximally exposed with this approach.[33] The translabyrinthine approach should be considered with extremely large lesions or with those in which facial nerve preservation may be problematic, as in cases where there is preoperative facial weakness. The ability to repair the facial nerve primarily or with a cable graft, as well as the ability to combine the translabyrinthine approach with others, make such a strategy effective in dealing with those lesions that surpass the boundaries of the cerebellopontine angle.

The translabyrinthine approach is ideal for small tumors in patients with poor hearing. Such cases provide opportunities to become familiar with the requisite anatomy in preparing for the removal of progressively larger lesions. Given the small incision and the lack of any brain retraction, we have found that older individuals seem to tolerate this approach better than the retrosigmoid approach. Also, the lack of dissection or incision into the paravertebral musculature makes postoperative pain control easier and obviates the use of narcotics.

Middle Fossa

The middle fossa approach traditionally has been considered an otologic procedure despite the fact that neurosurgeons were instrumental in its development, and indeed a neurosurgeon coauthored one of the original descriptions.[7,11,17,18,20,29] Its use in acoustic tumors is limited to intracanalicular tumors with preservable hearing, and in that sense, it competes with the retrosigmoid approach. Although there are specific instances where the middle fossa approach has an advantage over the retrosigmoid approach, the greatest value in understanding this technique is that it can form the basis of many other sophisticated cranial base exposures to the anterior and posterior cavernous sinus, the petrous apex, the upper and middle clivus, and the infratemporal fossa.

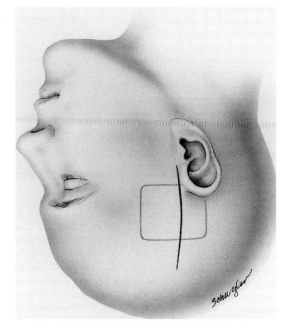

Figure 4. Incision and position of craniotomy for the middle fossa approach to an acoustic tumor.

Technique

The patient is positioned supine with the head turned so the appropriate ear faces up toward the surgeon. Elevation of the shoulder on a pad is optional if head turning is in any way restricted. Once appropriate cranial nerve monitoring and depth of anesthesia have been obtained, a vertical incision is made from the zygoma to the temporal line in front of the ear. The subgaleal space is developed by undermining and a retractor is put in place (Figure 4). The temporalis muscle can be dealt with either by a simple vertical incision, or its origin at the superior temporal line can be identified and an incision made parallel and below. This allows the majority of the muscle to be stripped inferiorly to the zygoma. In the unlikely event that the facial nerve is injured or a facial nerve neuroma is discovered, a well-preserved temporalis muscle can be transposed to reanimate the facial musculature.

A free craniotomy flap is positioned two-thirds anterior to and one-third posterior to the external auditory canal so that the inferior edge is adjacent to the middle fossa floor. Osmotic diuretics are administered for brain relaxation, and, under the operating microscope, the dura is elevated from the floor of the middle fossa. A self-retaining retractor helps in this regard. Hemostasis is accomplished in a variety of ways, including monopolar and bipolar cautery as well as the judicious use of the diamond drill. The middle meningeal artery and foramen spinosum provide the first landmarks, and medially and posteriorly, the foramen ovale the next. The greater superficial petrosal nerve will be seen coursing along the middle fossa floor in an anteroposterior direction. Parts may be covered by a thin shell of bone that can be removed by gentle brushing with the diamond drill bit. As the nerve joins with the geniculate ganglion, it begins to turn medially and dives to enter the lateralmost end of the internal auditory canal. The canal is bounded rostrally by the cochlea, which has no superficial landmark, so the dura covering the course of the facial nerve must serve as the rostral extent of the bone removal. Posteriorly, the arcuate eminence covering the superior semicircular canal serves as an adequate external landmark. Bone is removed from the roof of the canal medially to the edge of the tentorium. Entering the posterior fossa would necessitate dividing the superior petrosal sinus and is not required for the removal of intracanalicular lesions. Complete removal of the roof of the canal at its lateral end will uncover the vertical crest of bone separating the facial nerve anteriorly from the superior vestibular nerve posteriorly (Figure 5).

Avulsing the superior vestibular nerve with a hook also will give direction to the dural opening. Tumors situated on the superior vestibular nerve will push the facial nerve anterior and slightly inferior in the canal and, thus, can be more easily dissected. The cochlear nerve, because of its inferior position in the canal, will not be apparent until the tumor is mobilized and almost entirely dissected. Inferior vestibular nerve tumors can be problematic because the facial nerve and the cochlear nerve may be in a more vulnerable position with respect to the surface of

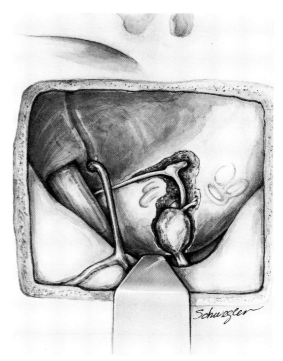

Figure 5. *Completed middle fossa approach to an acoustic tumor depicting the relationship of tumor to the facial and the superior vestibular nerves.*

the tumor. Facial nerve monitoring and brain stem auditory-evoked responses (BAERs) can provide an extra margin of safety. Tumors are best removed in one piece, although piecemeal dissection may be warranted in the interest of protecting the cochlear nerve. Prior to closure, a small piece of autologous fat is positioned over the dural opening and supplemented with fibrin glue. As the retractor is removed, the dura covering the temporal lobe moves back into position, covering the adipose graft. The bone flap is replaced and the temporalis muscle is reattached. The scalp is closed in layers and an ear dressing is applied.

Benefits

The middle fossa approach combines the benefits of a hearing preservation procedure with that of maximal safety to the facial nerve. Hearing preservation with this tech-

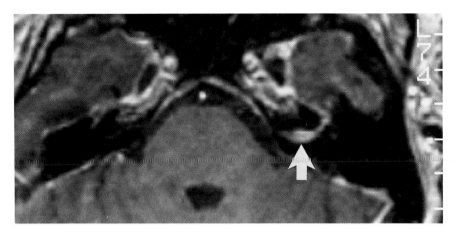

Figure 6. Enhanced MRI demonstrating a totally intracanalicular acoustic tumor. Serviceable hearing and speech discrimination make this case appropriate for a middle fossa approach.

nique ranges from 30% to 50%.[7,11,17,18,20,29] The author, in a small series of 31 cases, preserved functional hearing in 52%. An additional 13% of patients had hearing preserved at a low level at early followup.

Although this approach requires temporal lobe retraction, it benefits from the fact that it is an extradural procedure. This minimizes retractor forces on neural tissue and avoids the potential for compromising the venous drainage of the temporal lobe.

The most important benefit of the middle fossa approach relates to the ability to reliably expose the lateral end of the internal canal without entering the labyrinth. Tumors thus can be removed in one piece because their boundaries are more clearly defined. There is little chance of leaving residual tumor that can potentially serve as a source for recurrence.

Drawbacks and Complications

The middle fossa approach is limited to a narrow range of clinical situations, namely, intracanicular tumors in patients with good hearing. As a result, gaining facility with this procedure is problematic. The anatomy can be easily learned in the skull base laboratory, but a team approach with a neurosurgeon and neuro-otologist working in conjunction may be the best way to proceed initially.

Although temporal lobe edema from retraction is a theoretical complication, it is a rare occurrence. In the one case witnessed by the author, 24 hours of fluid restriction and osmotic dehydrating agents were all that was necessary to manage the problem successfully.

CSF rhinorrhea can occur in rare circumstances and is best treated with several days of lumbar drainage. On one occasion, reoperation was necessary to close the eustachian tube. The etiology of such a leak is invariably an unrecognized opening in an aberrantly positioned air cell.

Indications

Intracanalicular tumors with preservable hearing (20-50 dB loss and 50% to 80% speech discrimination) serve as the foremost indications for this procedure. Those tumors that extend beyond the porus acusticus into the posterior fossa are best approached by a retrosigmoid trajectory if hearing is intact. Tumors that extend to the lateral limit of the internal canal are a subcategory of intracanalicular tumors for which the middle fossa technique is preferred (Figure 6). The maximal chance of microscopic total removal is combined with heightened safety for both the facial and cochlear nerves.

Retrosigmoid Approach

The retrosigmoid, or suboccipital, approach for acoustic neuromas evolved from the venerable but obsolescent posterior fossa exploration, the principles of which emphasized maximal exposure of posterior fossa contents in the interests of localization and diagnosis of the pathologic process. Happily, as preoperative imaging has improved, this approach for acoustic tumors has taken a more lateralized trajectory. Bony removal has become more focused, although the luxurious exposure afforded by unilateral removal of the suboccipital bone still is touted as the major appeal of this technique.[2,21,23,24,26,27,30,32] Microsurgical techniques and earlier diagnoses have altered the goals of the procedure from decompression to maximal preservation of function with minimal operative trauma and microscopic total removal. As a result, "exposure" is governed more by magnification, illumination, and technique facility spawned by experience rather than by widened portals. The following discussion relates to the use of this technique as a hearing preservation tool. Subtle modifications of the standard technique described here are not claimed to be original or unique, but have evolved from ideas and suggestions from colleagues and mentors. Identification of all of the originators is not attempted.

Technique

The patient is positioned supine with the head comfortably turned away from the side of the tumor. Pin headrest fixation is optional and relates only to the anticipated need for self-retaining retractor systems that may be fixed to the headrest. As experience has grown and the approach has taken on a more lateral orientation, the extra time and complexity of the "park bench" position has been largely abandoned. Simply tilting the

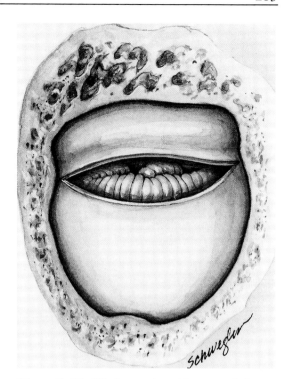

Figure 7. Modified retrosigmoid approach for an acoustic tumor depicting decompression of the sigmoid and a dural incision.

operating table will afford the appropriate trajectories needed during the various procedural steps. Any putative benefits of the sitting position are outweighed by the potential risks and complexities involved. Once appropriate anesthetic and monitoring functions have been performed, including facial nerve EMG and BAERs, a curvilinear incision is made behind the ear similar to that for the translabyrinthine approach.[13] A separate musculofascial flap is developed, and, using one's preferred drilling technology, a partial mastoidectomy skeletonizing the sigmoid sinus, posterior fossa dura anterior to the sinus, posterior semicircular canal, and endolymphatic duct and sinus is accomplished (Figure 7).

A separate free bone flap is turned posterior to the sigmoid sinus. Removal of the rim of the foramen magnum is unnecessary except in the most massive tumors. Osmotic agents are administered and the dura is opened based on the posterior border of the

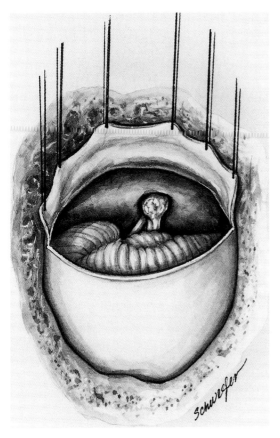

Figure 8. Completed exposure of an acoustic tumor using the retrosigmoid approach showing the elevation of the sigmoid and the relation of the tumor to the facial and vestibulocochlear nerves.

sigmoid sinus. Multiple stay sutures placed adjacent to the sinodural junction slightly elevate and anteriorly displace the sinus. The cerebellar hemisphere is gently retracted enough to expose the arachnoid of the cisterna magna, which is punctured. With the egress of CSF, combined with osmotically activated diuresis and sigmoid sinus decompression, the cerebellum can be retracted with a suction tip placed on a patty enough to expose tumors of the size consistent with an attempt at hearing preservation. In cases with tumors less than 2 cm in diameter, the vestibulocochlear nerve should be identified near its junction with the brain stem, and an assessment made of the position of the cochlear component with respect to vestibular

fibers (Figure 8). Tumors of the superior vestibular nerve will deflect the cochlear nerve inferiorly and medially. The facial nerve will be further medial and occasionally caudal to the cochlear nerve and is confirmed with the stimulator electrode. Vestibular fibers over the tumor's surface can be divided and an internal decompression effected as the next step based on the surgeon's judgment and experience. Alternatively, the lip of the porus is removed by first assessing the tumor's extent within the canal. The posterior semicircular canal is palpated through the decompressed posterior fossa dura anterior to the sigmoid sinus. It, along with the endolymphatic duct, identified during the mastoid drilling, marks the extreme limit of the internal auditory canal removal to prevent entering the labyrinth. Drilling proceeds, alternating appropriate-sized cutting and diamond burrs, until the contour and lack of fullness of the canal dura suggests that the lateral border of the tumor has been reached. For tumors that reach the lateral end of the internal canal, drilling continues to the lateral crest of bone just short of the labyrinth. The canal dura is opened and the superior vestibular and facial nerves are identified. Limited internal decompression of the intracanalicular portion of the tumor, in conjunction with the stimulating electrode, aids in this maneuver. Cranial nerve dissection is completed with fine dissectors, hooks, or scissors, with care taken to preserve the requisite vascularity.

Prior to closure, a search is made for air cells that may have been opened during the drilling of the porus. Wax and a small autologous adipose graft will help to form a temporary and permanent seal, respectively. The posterior fossa dura is closed in a watertight fashion with a fascial graft if necessary, and autologous fat is placed in the mastoid defect and over the dural incision. The bone flap is replaced to reduce muscular adhesions to the dura, a potential cause of long-term postoperative headache. The temporalis muscle and fascia are closed as a separate layer to maintain pressure against the adipose graft. Following skin closure, an ear dressing is placed.

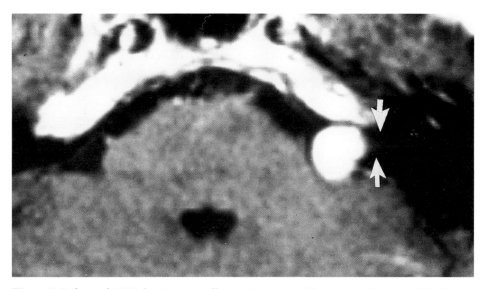

Figure 9. Enhanced MRI showing a small acoustic tumor with no extension toward the lateral end of the internal auditory canal. Excellent hearing in this patient provides an indication for a retrosigmoid approach.

Benefits

Perhaps the greatest benefit of the retrosigmoid approach for acoustic neuromas is the familiarity that most neurosurgeons have with this technique. Variations of the approach are used to treat a myriad of pathologic processes that are strongly lateralized within the posterior fossa. As a technical strategy, the retrosigmoid approach also enjoys versatility as one of its main benefits. It can be used both for large and small tumors of the VIII nerve complex. We prefer the technique for use in hearing preservation procedures, especially in those where the intracanalicular portion of the tumor is not severely impacted in the lateral end of the internal auditory canal. With judicious case selection, auditory function can be preserved in 30% to 50% of cases. The most widely acknowledged benefit of the retrosigmoid approach is the panoramic exposure of the cerebellopontine angle and the surrounding environs. However, as sophisticated microsurgical techniques mandated by hearing preservation operations become more widely utilized, such luxurious exposures of regions unaffected by the primary pathologic process seem less important.

Drawbacks and Complications

There are very few significant drawbacks related to the retrosigmoid approach. It, perhaps, is less desirable with those tumors that are laterally impacted in the internal auditory canal. Drilling the posterior lip of the internal acoustic meatus enough to expose the lateral end of the canal occasionally can cause entry into the vestibule or the posterior semicircular canal.[4] Failure to completely expose the lateral end of the canal will increase the possibility of leaving residual tumor.[33]

The intraoperative use of microscopic mirrors to explore the lateral end of the canal not infrequently identifies a residual fragment of tumor, even when a clean dissection plane has been developed and complete microscopic removal has been felt to have been accomplished. The temptation to retract the cerebellar hemisphere with self-retaining retractors occasionally can lead to excessive forces that go unrecognized during a long surgical procedure. With the suboccipital or retrosigmoid approach, we attempt to perform the majority of the procedure without the use of self-retaining retractors, as this can obviate retractor damage.

Indications

We have reserved the retrosigmoid approach for tumors that require a hearing preservation operation. Patients with lesions smaller than 2.5 cm and with hearing thresholds of 50 dB or less and speech discrimination of 50% or better are considered ideal for this approach. Great weight is placed on preoperative magnetic resonance imaging (MRI) in terms of assessing the amount of tumor impacted in the internal auditory canal. Those lesions in which the tumors do not extend past the medial two-thirds of the canal are considered excellent candidates for hearing preservation in conjunction with complete microscopic removal (Figure 9). With larger tumors, the retrosigmoid approach is used if the only hearing ear is involved or a subtotal removal is to be accomplished in order to preserve functional hearing on that side.

Conclusion

The current excitement over the development of aggressive strategies to deal with complex lesions of the cranial base has spawned a new sense of collaboration between otologists and neurosurgeons. As a result, neurosurgeons have become more comfortable with the anatomy of the temporal bone. This has allowed a greater willingness to view certain strategies in a more generic sense rather than as a possession of a particular discipline. Thus, the approaches to acoustic neuromas described in this chapter should be looked upon as a menu of techniques to be selected based on the individual characteristics of the patient and the tumor.

References

1. Barrs DM, Brackmann DE, Hitselberger WE. Facial nerve anastomosis in the cerebellopontine angle: a review of 24 cases. *Am J Otol.* 1984;5: 269-272.
2. Bentivoglio P, Cheeseman AD, Symon L. Surgical management of acoustic neuromas during the last five years, II: results for facial and cochlear nerve function. *Surg Neurol.* 1988;29:205-209.
3. Brackmann DE, Hitselberger WE, Robinson JV. Repair of the facial nerve in the cerebellopontine angle. In: Graham MD, House WF, eds. *Disorders of the Facial Nerve.* New York, NY: Raven Press; 1982:379-385.
4. Domb GH, Chole RA. Anatomical studies of the posterior petrous apex with regard to hearing preservation in acoustic neuroma removal. *Laryngoscope.* 1980;90:1769-1777.
5. Epstein GH, Weisman RA, Zwillenberg S, et al. A new autologous-based adhesive for otologic surgery. *Ann Otol Rhinol Laryngol.* 1986;95:40-45.
6. Ferrante L, Palatinsky E, Acqui M, et al. Endaural extracranial repair for cerebrospinal otorrhea with human fibrin glue: technical note. *J Neurol Neurosurg Psychiatry.* 1988;51:1438-1440.
7. Gantz BJ, Parnes LS, Harker LA, et al. Middle cranial fossa acoustic neuroma excision: results and complications. *Ann Otol Rhinol Laryngol.* 1986;95: 454-459.
8. Giannotta SL. Translabyrinthine approach for removal of medium and large tumors of the cerebellopontine angle. *Clin Neurosurg.* 1991;38:589-602.
9. Giannotta SL, Pulec JL. Tumors of the cerebellopontine angle: combined mangement by neurological and otological surgeons. *Clin Neurosurg.* 1987;34: 457-466.
10. Glasscock ME, Hayes JW. The translabyrinthine removal of acoustic and other cerebellopontine angle tumors. *Ann Otol.* 1973;82:415-427.
11. Glasscock ME III, Kyeton JF, Jackson CG, et al. A systematic approach to the surgical management of acoustic neuroma. *Laryngoscope.* 1986;96:1088-1094.
12. Hardy DG, MacFarlane R, Baguley D, et al. Surgery for acoustic neurinoma: an analysis of 100 translabyrinthine operations. *J Neurosurg.* 1989;71:799-804.
13. Hardy RW Jr, Kinney SE, Lueders H, et al. Preservation of cochlear nerve function with the aid of brain stem auditory evoked potentials. *Neurosurgery.* 1982;11:16-19.
14. Harner SG, Daube JR, Ebersold MJ, et al. Improved preservation of facial nerve function with use of electrical monitoring during removal of acoustic neuromas. *Mayo Clin Proc.* 1987;62:92-102.
15. Harner SG, Laws ER Jr. Translabyrinthine repair of cerebrospinal fluid otorhinorrhea. *J Neurosurg.* 1982;57:258-261.
16. House JW, Brackmann DE. Facial nerve grading system. *Otolaryngol Head Neck Surg.* 1985;93: 146-147.
17. House WF, Gardner G, Hughes RL. Middle cranial fossa approach to acoustic tumor surgery. *Arch Otolaryng.* 1968;88:631-641.
18. House WF, Hitselberger WE. The middle fossa approach for removal of small acoustic tumors. *Acta Otolaryngol (Stockh).* 1969;67:413-427.
19. Kelly DL Jr, Britton BH, Branch CL Jr. Cooperative neuro-otologic management of acoustic neuromas and other cerebellopontine angle tumors. *Southern Med J.* 1988;81:557-561.
20. Kurze T, Doyle JB Jr. Extradural intracranial (middle fossa) approach to the internal auditory canal. *J Neurosurg.* 1962;19:1033-1037.
21. Lye RH, Dutton J, Ramsden RT, et al. Facial nerve preservation during surgery for removal of acoustic nerve tumors. *J Neurosurg.* 1982;57:739-746.
22. Møller AR, Jannetta PJ. Preservation of facial func-

tion during removal of acoustic neuromas: use of monopolar constant-voltage stimulation and EMG. *J Neurosurg.* 1984;61:757-760.

23. Neely JG. Is it possible to totally resect an acoustic tumor and conserve hearing? *Otolaryngol Head Neck Surg.* 1984;92:162-167.

24. Ojemann RG, Levine RA, Montgomery WM, et al. Use of intraoperative auditory evoked potentials to preserve hearing in unilateral acoustic neuroma removal. *J Neurosurg.* 1984;61:938-948.

25. Prass RL, Lüders H. Acoustic (loudspeaker) facial electromyographic monitoring, I: evoked electromyographic activity during acoustic neuroma resection. *Neurosurgery.* 1986;19:392-400.

26. Rand RW, Kurze TL. Facial nerve preservation by posterior fossa transmeatal microdissection in total removal of acoustic tumors. *J Neurol Neurosurg Psychiatry.* 1965;28:311-316.

27. Rhoton AL Jr. Microsurgery of the internal acoustic meatus. *Surg Neurol.* 1974;2:311-318.

28. Rossitch E Jr, Wilkins RH. The use of fibrin glue in neurosurgery. In: Wilkins RH, Rengachary SS, eds. *Neurosurgery Update I: Diagnosis, Operative Technique, and Neurooncology.* 1990:195-197.

29. Shelton C, Hitselberger WE, House WF, et al. Hearing preservation after acoustic tumor removal: long-term results. *Laryngoscope.* 1990;100:115-119.

30. Sugita K, Koboyashi S. Technical and instrumental improvements in the surgical management of acoustic neurinomas. *J Neurosurg.* 1982;57:747-752.

31. Tator CH, Nedzelski JM. Facial nerve preservation in patients with large acoustic neuromas treated by combined middle fossa and transtentorial translabyrinthine approach. *J Neurosurg.* 1982;57:1-7.

32. Tator CH, Nedzelski JM. Preservation of hearing in patients undergoing excision of acoustic neuromas and other cerebellopontine angle tumors. *J Neurosurg.* 1985;63:168-174.

33. Thedinger BS, Whittaker CK, Luetje CM. Recurrent acoustic tumor after a suboccipital removal. *Neurosurgery.* 1991;29:681-687.

34. Tos M, Thomsen J. Cerebrospinal fluid leak after translabyrinthine surgery for acoustic neuroma. *Laryngoscope.* 1984;95:351-354.

35. Tos M, Thomsen J, Harmsen A. Results of translabyrinthine removal of 300 acoustic neuromas related to tumour size. *Acta Otolaryngol (Stockh).* 1988;452:38-51. Suppl.

36. Whittaker CK, Luetje CM. Translabyrinthine removal of large acoustic tumors. *Am J Otol.* 1985;5 (suppl):155-160.

CHAPTER 13

Surgical Approaches to Tumors of the Posterior Fossa Cranial Nerves (Excluding Acoustic Neuromas)

Fred G. Barker II, MD, and Robert G. Ojemann, MD

A remarkable variety of tumors may affect the cranial nerves of the posterior fossa* (Table 1). In this chapter, we discuss trigeminal and facial neuromas, meningiomas of the posterior pyramid of the petrous bone, epidermoid tumors, lipomas, glial tumors, choroid plexus papillomas, miscellaneous mass lesions of the cerebellopontine angle (CPA), and tumors of the jugular and hypoglossal foramina. We exclude tumors primarily located in the cavernous sinus, the clivus, and the foramen magnum, any of which may extend secondarily into the posterior fossa.

Trigeminal Neuroma

These rare tumors (approximately 250 cases have been reported) have been the subject of classic monographs,[44,103] as well as other reports by several authors.[9,64,69,80,92,124] They usually are benign nerve sheath tumors, arising most frequently between the ages of 40 and 60, without predilection for sex, and they grow slowly. The majority of cases have not been associated with neurofibromatosis. A handful of examples with malignant histology have been reported.[35,80]

The earliest symptom is usually a sensory disturbance on the face. There may be trophic change of the ipsilateral cornea (neurolytic keratitis) from involvement of the

ophthalmic branch of the trigeminal nerve (V_2). Larger tumors may compress adjacent cranial nerves, including the trochlear (IV) and the abducens (VI) nerves, giving rise to diplopia, and the facial (VII), vestibulocochlear (VIII) nerve complex, causing facial weakness and/or unilateral deafness. Eventually, signs of brain stem compression develop.[80] Occasionally, there is a decrease in hearing due to tumor occlusion of the eustachian tube.

These tumors are hyperdense on plain computed tomography (CT) and with bone windowing frequently are seen to have eroded the bone of the petrous apex, with a smooth sharp margin. Enhancement is dense and homogeneous. Magnetic resonance imaging (MRI) is helpful in delineating the exact anatomic extent of the tumor and its relationships to surrounding structures. The lesions show decreased signal on T1-weighted images, increased signal on T2-weighted images, and enhance densely with gadolinium (Figure 1).

The critical location of these tumors, which can arise anywhere from the nerve root in the posterior fossa to its extracranial branches, is responsible for the formidable challenge associated with their removal. Jefferson[44] proposed a grading system of three classes based on the location of the main bulk of the tumor. Class A tumors are located primarily within the posterior fossa, Class B primarily within the middle fossa, and Class C tumors have significant masses in both posterior and middle fossae with a thin "hourglass" bridge

*References 12, 34, 71, 76, 90, 114

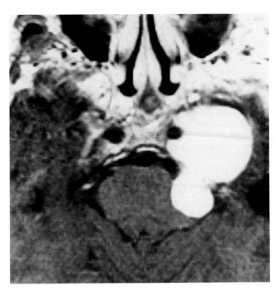

Figure 1. Trigeminal neuroma. Axial MRI with gadolinium enhancement. (TR 550 ms, TE 20 ms, first echo, 1.5 T field.)

around the petrous apex. Additional schemes of classification have been suggested to denote those tumors that are centered further forward in the cavernous sinus or extracranially, but these tumors are unusual, accounting for perhaps 5% of the total. The majority of tumors arise from the region of the gasserian ganglion.[80] The precise extent of the tumor is important when selecting an operative approach from the many advocated by various authors.

Class A tumors (20% of the total), located primarily within the posterior fossa, usually are removed through a retrosigmoid suboccipital craniotomy. This operative approach is described under the section entitled "Cerebellopontine Angle Meningiomas." The tumors tend to extend somewhat beyond the tentorium, but when the extension is not massive, the entire tumor can be removed through this approach. The technique resembles that for removing an acoustic tumor, with initial central debulking preceding the separation of the capsule from the brain stem and the cranial nerves. Electrophysiologic monitoring of the trigeminal and facial nerves is essential, and others may be monitored as needed.

When additional exposure is necessary, the operation may be converted into a combined infratentorial and supratentorial approach, with optional splitting of the tentorium. This approach will be described below.

Class B tumors (50% of the total), which are confined to the middle fossa with the frequent exception of a small extension below the tentorium, may be excised through a subtemporal intradural approach. A lumbar drain, in addition to the use of furosemide and mannitol, aids the exposure and minimizes complications from temporal lobe retraction. If the tumor is quite small, an extradural approach may suffice.

Class C tumors (25% of the total) present the most serious surgical challenge, and authors differ on the preferred operative approach. These authors prefer a craniotomy combining the exposure needed for a subtemporal approach with that required for a suboccipital retrosigmoid approach. The tentorium is split. The principles of tumor removal are the same. The various cranial nerves will be splayed over the tumor capsule: oculomotor and abducens medially, trochlear superiorly, facial and vestibulocochlear inferiorly. In general, a complete tumor removal can be achieved, but some pieces of the capsule may not be safe to remove (e.g. when tightly stuck to the brain stem). The regrowth of residual tumor usually has been slow.[9,69,124] Although trigeminal deficits present before removal generally remain unchanged or are worsened postoperatively, new deficits of other cranial nerves are unusual.

Facial Nerve Neuromas

About 300 cases of these neuromas have been reported.[68,83] There is no sex preference and patients are usually middle-aged. The most common symptom is facial weakness (73% of patients).[68] Facial paralysis is seen in one-half of the patients at presentation, often preceded by facial twitching. There is usually a history of relentless progression of

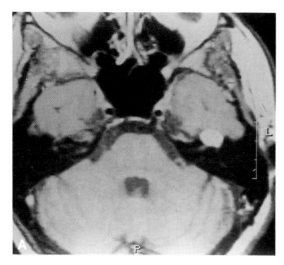

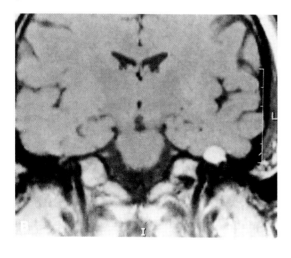

Figure 2. Facial nerve neuroma. MRI with gadolinium enhancement. (T1-weighted image, 1.5 T field.) The tumor is located at the geniculate ganglion. (A) Axial. (B) Coronal.

facial weakness over time. Presentation with sudden paralysis of the nerve was noted only once in a series of 48 patients.[83] The next most common symptom was hearing loss (in half of the patients).[68] Any portion of the nerve may be affected, with perhaps a slight predilection for the region of the geniculate ganglion. Only three cases of malignant histology have been seen.[77] MRI offers the most advantageous mode of imaging[89] (Figure 2). When the tumor occurs in the internal auditory canal, it cannot be distinguished from an acoustic neuroma.

When the bulk of the tumor is located in the posterior fossa, an operative approach similar to that used for acoustic tumors is selected. Good results have been achieved with either the translabyrinthine or the retrosigmoid suboccipital approach; the latter may be preferred if there is useful hearing in the ipsilateral ear. If the tumor extends significantly beyond the fundus of the internal auditory meatus however, the translabyrinthine approach is clearly preferable, allowing the petrous portion of the nerve to be exposed, as well as giving access to both proximal and distal stumps of the nerve should transection and a nerve graft be required, as in 75% of the cases.

In another common situation, the tumor presents its main mass into the middle fossa. A subtemporal extradural approach is well suited for these tumors.[21,83,94,113] If necessary, the tegmen tympani is drilled off to expose the intratemporal portion of the tumor. Reconstruction of the nerve from this approach is difficult, but hearing may be preserved.

Those facial nerve tumors centered in the horizontal portion of the nerve, or more distally, usually are removed through a transmastoid or other extracranial approach.[83]

When the tumor is small, it may be possible to separate it from the trunk of the nerve.[61] The involved portion of the nerve, however, usually requires resection, and a sural or greater auricular nerve graft is used to bridge the gap in the nerve.[51,83,102] House Grade III (moderate facial weakness) function may result from such reconstruction,[68] with worse results if the facial paralysis is long-standing.[83]

The most important immediate postoperative concern when facial paralysis is present is management of the ipsilateral eye, which is at risk for damage from corneal exposure. The eye is immediately taped shut, and at an early opportunity, an oculoplastic procedure is performed (tarsorrhaphy or gold-weight implantation). Some surgeons recommend a temporalis transposition graft, which is designed to improve symmetry in the appearance of the lower face within weeks. This

TABLE 1
Frequency of Cerebellopontine Angle Tumors*

Acoustic neuroma	87.2%
Meningioma	4.0%
Epidermoid tumor	2.5%
Facial nerve neuroma	1.5%
Glial tumors (all types combined)	0.9%
Trigeminal neuroma	0.4%
Arachnoid cyst	0.3%
All others combined	3.2%

*Three pooled series (12, 76, 90); total 2,012 patients.

procedure does not interfere with the results of later facial nerve regeneration. If there is no recovery of facial nerve function, or a facial nerve interposition graft is impossible for technical reasons, a partial hypoglossal-facial anastomosis is performed.[70]

Not all facial nerve neuromas require surgery. When the patient presents with a long-standing facial paralysis and deaf ear from a small tumor, observation may be indicated, particularly if the patient is elderly.[51] Similarly, an ipsilateral only-hearing ear may be a relative contraindication to surgery. Some authors feel that preoperative facial function better than House Grade III constitutes a contraindication as well.[68]

Cerebellopontine Angle Meningiomas

The most common tumor after acoustic neuroma in most large series of CPA mass lesions is the meningioma, constituting about 4% of tumors in this location (Table 1). Some authors prefer the term *meningioma of the posterior pyramid,* a description that also would embrace tumors of the jugular foramen.[55,98] Another term used for these tumors, particularly those that extend into the clivus, is *petroclival.*[2,4,99] Several series have been reported.[25,56,104,112,123] These benign CPA tumors share the same characteristics of slow growth and female preponderance as meningiomas in other intracranial locations. Symptoms usually are present for many years before the tumor is discovered. Otologic signs

and symptoms are slightly less prominent than in acoustic neuroma patients, with complete unilateral hearing loss uncommon. This probably is because the tumor usually does not grow to any extent into the internal auditory canal. The degree of involvement of other cranial nerves depends on the location of the tumor on the petrous bone.

The differential diagnosis rests on radiologic criteria. Despite subtle differences in enhancement characteristics on CT[120] and MRI,[119] both acoustic tumors and meningiomas may enhance densely (Figure 3). Their distinction relies on several characteristics.[75] Acoustic tumors commonly erode the internal auditory meatus, whereas meningiomas only rarely do. The meningioma forms an obtuse angle with the uninvolved adjacent face of the petrous bone, the acoustic neuromas form an acute angle. Meningiomas more commonly extend through the tentorial incisura, or have a broad base on the tentorium and rarely extend in the internal auditory meatus; the acoustic tumor nearly always extends into the internal auditory meatus. The meningioma is more likely to show calcification on CT, and occasionally may cause hyperostosis of the petrous bone, which is not seen with acoustic neuromas. The most important criterion is the location of the epicenter of the tumor on the petrous bone, which is always the internal auditory meatus for an acoustic neuroma, but rarely so for a meningioma. Three-dimensional CT reconstructions are of great help in visualizing the anatomic relationships of the tumor, as are MRI cuts in axial, coronal, and sagittal planes. With large meningiomas, angiography can be valuable in determining the relationships of the tumor to major branches of the basilar artery,[82] or for consideration of preoperative embolization. While angiography may demonstrate a vascular blush or feeding vessels characteristic for meningiomas, it is not needed for smaller tumors (under 3 cm), and overall it is not so accurate as MRI in predicting the correct diagnosis preoperatively.[25,112]

The operative approach is selected with the anatomic relations of the tumor in mind. We generally use a suboccipital craniotomy.[86,87]

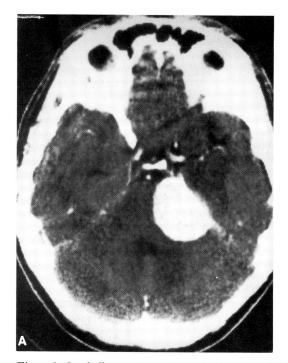 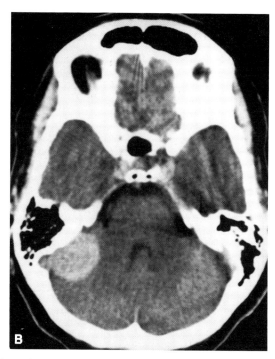

Figure 3. Cerebellopontine angle meningiomas. Axial CTs, with intravenous contrast enhancement. *(A)* Tumor centered anterior to internal auditory meatus. *(B)* Tumor centered posterior to internal auditory meatus.

The patient is placed in the lateral position with a pad under the ipsilateral shoulder. The head is positioned with the falx parallel to the floor and slightly elevated. The vertical incision, 2 cm posterior to the tip of the mastoid, starts 2 cm above the top of the pinna and extends slightly below the hairline. A pericranial tissue graft is taken from the superior portion of the incision for later dural closure. Bone is exposed over the lateral two-thirds of the cerebellar hemisphere and is removed with a high-speed craniotome. If necessary, further bone is removed to expose the transverse sinus and its junction with the sigmoid sinus. The dura is opened in a stellate fashion to the margins of the sinuses. Self-retaining retractors are placed on the cerebellum after cerebrospinal fluid (CSF) drainage from the lateral cisterns. If the tumor is large (3 cm), lateral cerebellar tissue is removed to minimize retraction. If visible, the petrosal vein is cauterized and divided. The cerebellum now is separated from the tumor capsule. Retractors gradually are placed deeper as the dissection proceeds. The glossopharyngeal (IX), vagus (X), spinal

accessory (XI), and hypoglossal (XII) nerves are identified if possible, separated from the capsule if necessary, and protected with a rubber dam. The displacement of the facial and vestibulocochlear nerves depends on the site of tumor origin on the petrous bone.

The tumor capsule now is stimulated, seeking the facial nerve, and the capsule is opened in a safe location. An intracapsular decompression is carried out with an ultrasonic aspirator or bipolar electrocautery and microscissors. If possible, the tumor's attachments to the dura and petrous bone are divided to interrupt the blood supply. Brisk bleeding from bone may require bone wax, monopolar cautery with a coated instrument, or use of a diamond bit on a high-speed drill for control. As the capsule is hollowed out, it is generally dissected free from the cerebellum and the brain stem, as well as from the cranial nerves, which usually are covered with a rubber pledget as soon as they are separated from the tumor mass. Occasionally, the tumor may envelop cranial nerves or critical vessels, which must be spared. When the internal auditory meatus is reached, its posterior wall is drilled off as required for removal of the tumor from the canal. Once the facial and vestibulocochlear nerves are identified both proximally and distally, the tumor capsule can be carefully separated from the nerve complex, with facial nerve stimulation acting as a means to identify the margins of an often-attenuated nerve. When tumor removal is complete, the remaining involved dura is excised if possible. When the internal auditory canal has been exposed by drilling the posterior margin of the internal auditory meatus, wax is used to occlude any exposed mastoid air cells and a fat graft is placed in the internal auditory meatus to avoid CSF leak. The pericranial graft is used to close the dura in a watertight fashion and the bone flap is replaced with wires. The wound then is closed in layers.

A major determinant of ease of complete tumor removal is the relation of the tumor to the internal auditory meatus. When the base of the tumor is anterior to the internal auditory meatus, an attempt at complete removal through the suboccipital approach carries a significant risk of postoperative facial nerve dysfunction and hearing loss, because the facial/vestibulocochlear complex is between the surgeon and the tumor. About a third of posterior pyramid meningiomas fall into this category.[55] In addition, tumors arising anterior to the internal auditory meatus more frequently contain an *en plaque* component,[98] often with intrafascicular tumor growth within the cranial nerves. Several other surgical approaches have been described for these anterior tumors. Yasargil and colleagues described a frontotemporal transsylvian approach,[123] and House et al a similar subtemporal extradural approach with resection of the petrous tip,[38] giving exposure of the portions of the tumor near the tentorial notch and the upper brain stem, basilar artery, and oculomotor nerve. Kawase et al[47,48] have discussed a similar anterior approach to the portion of the posterior pyramid medial to the dural entrance of the trigeminal nerve, achieved by drilling off the anterior petrous bone through an extradural

subtemporal exposure. The superior petrosal sinus is clipped and divided between the trigeminal and facial nerves, and the tentorium is incised medially until the tentorial notch is reached. An extension of the exposure more anteriorly, into the posterior cavernous sinus, also may be performed. Finally, a removal of the petrous tip via a subtemporal approach forms part of the "combined retroauricular and preauricular transpetrosal-transtentorial approach" reported by Hakuba et al,[30] which will be described below. The same group has used only the subtemporal removal of the petrous tip to access the CPA.[28]

Another portion of the posterior aspect of the petrous bone that is difficult to access through the suboccipital presigmoid or retrosigmoid approaches is the area ventral to the insertions of the trigeminal, facial, and vestibulocochlear nerves. An approach exposing this dural surface through the anterior petrous bone has been described that also may be a useful adjunct for tumors in this difficult region.[105] This approach uses a preauricular skin incision with a frontotemporal craniotomy, a neck dissection, and resection of the mandibular condyle, followed by removal of the inferior portion of the petrous apex with a drill. Exposure from Dorello's canal to the hypoglossal foramen, medial to the trigeminal, abducens, facial, and vestibulocochlear nerves, is afforded. The exposure of the petrous tip, medial to the insertion of the trigeminal nerve, is reported to be superior to that achieved with the House or Kawase exposures described previously,[38,48] because of further drilling medial to the petrous internal carotid artery. However, the actual insertions of the trigeminal, facial, and vestibulocochlear nerves, as well as the CPA itself, are poorly visualized. This approach has been used primarily in combination with other approaches to complete the resection of a tumor that was incompletely removed at the first operation.[105]

Various modifications of the suboccipital approach involving more lateral bony removal include the presigmoid approach described by Al-Mefty[1,2,4] and by Samii et al,[97,99] which does not require division of the sigmoid sinus. The posterior portion of the petrous bone is drilled off without entering the labyrinth or exposing the facial nerve. The dura then is incised along the lateral margin of the sigmoid sinus, and the superior petrosal sinus is divided. The tentorium is transected anteriorly, toward the petrous apex, as well as with a second incision toward the incisura. This allows wide exposure of the region anterior to the brain stem from the parasellar region posteriorly as far as the internal auditory meatus. Hearing is not destroyed, and the approach may be extended inferiorly to expose the occipital condyle and jugular foramen. A "combined retroauricular and preauricular transpetrosal-transtentorial approach," reported by Hakuba and colleagues,[30] combines the far lateral bony removal anterior to the sigmoid sinus of the "presigmoid approaches" with removal of the petrous tip via a subtemporal route. This exposes the entire dural triangle bounded by the sigmoid sinus and the superior and inferior petrosal sinuses. These approaches are advantageous when a significant portion of the tumor is located ventral to the brain stem, or when the tumor arises from the clivus.

Tumors that extend further than the internal auditory meatus toward the jugular foramen cannot be totally removed through these approaches, with the exception of the presigmoid approaches when extended inferiorly to unroof the jugular foramen. A combination of the retrosigmoid and subtemporal exposures, splitting the tentorium and transverse sinus, in either one or two stages, may be required.

We do not use the translabyrinthine approach for CPA meningiomas, although this may be quite suitable for small tumors centered on the internal auditory meatus.[60] In such cases, however, the preoperative diagnosis is more likely to be acoustic tumor rather than meningioma.

Using modern techniques, complete excision of these challenging tumors often is achieved. When we are required to leave residual tumor, we use serial CT or MRI to monitor for recurrence, rather than proceeding directly to radiation therapy, unless the tumor shows histologic features of aggressiveness, such as "sheeting" of cells, focal necrosis, or an abnormally high incidence of mitotic figures.[18] Standard external-beam radiotherapy has been used. Such therapy has been shown to decrease recurrence rates in some series,[29] although these studies addressed all meningiomas and not specifically those in the CPA. The place of radiosurgical techniques in treating these tumors has yet to be solidly defined, but early reports[53,109] suggest that results will be favorable. In a group of meningiomas primarily located at the skull base that were treated with the cobalt 60 Gamma Knife, more than half showed a decrease in size following treatment, and actuarial 2-year tumor growth control was achieved in 96% of these patients. Cranial nerve palsies were few (4%).[53] Another small series found no new neurologic deficits in a series of skull base meningiomas treated with the Gamma Knife, and some patients experienced improvement in cranial nerve deficits.[109] Both of these tumor series, however, comprised meningiomas primarily located outside the CPA. Experience with acoustic tumors has suggested a 30% risk of at least temporary palsy of the trigeminal or facial nerve.[53] The complication rate for irradiation of CPA meningiomas may be more closely reflected by this number, but sufficient experience has not yet been acquired for accurate estimation. In addition, the protracted natural history of these tumors will require longer follow-up than currently is available for an accurate assessment of the benefits of this treatment. At present, this modality offers only an intriguing adjunct to surgery, which remains the primary treatment.

Epidermoid Tumors

The epidermoid tumor is the third most common neoplastic occupant of the CPA (Table 1). Exquisitely slow-growing, this tumor infiltrates the posterior fossa, surrounding cranial nerves and vessels. It produces symptoms of trigeminal neuralgia or hemifacial spasm in a higher proportion of cases than do either acoustic tumors or meningiomas.[6,8,85] The mechanism of these symptoms is poorly understood. Otherwise, the tumor causes a typical, slowly progressive CPA syndrome. Occasionally, recurrent attacks of aseptic meningitis have been noted, due to the release of the intensely irritating cyst contents into the subarachnoid space.[7]

CT may reveal a low-density mass (attenuation slightly greater than 0 Hounsfield units), which is nonenhancing. Occasionally, high-density cyst contents or calcification within the mass can be seen. Bone windows may show erosion of adjacent bone with sharp margins. MRI demonstrates the mass well as low-signal on T1-weighted images (slightly greater than CSF) and high-signal on T2-weighted images. The tumor may be seen best on the first-echo T2-weighted image[5] (Figure 4).

The tumor is approached through a standard retrosigmoid suboccipital craniotomy, unless the tumor is centered anterior to the internal auditory meatus in the petrous apex or involves both the posterior and middle cranial fossae when a subtemporal approach is used.[50] Once the tumor is exposed, the thin capsule is opened and the pearly-white contents are removed with suction and cautious use of ring curets. The tumor may surround cranial nerves and/or important blood vessels. Yasargil and colleagues have emphasized the "artificial surgical channel" created by the tumor itself, which is exploited by cyst content removal. This allows dissection to proceed far anterior through the retrosigmoid exposure, even through the incisura.[122] Portions of the capsule that are not adherent to the brain stem or other critical structures are removed. The extreme slow growth of the tumor lends support to a philosophy of leaving the tumor capsule in place when it is adherent to cranial nerves, important blood vessels, or the brain stem, since regrowth is likely to be very slow.[8,96]

At the conclusion of the resection, copious

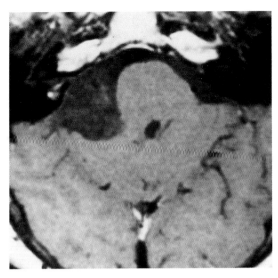

Figure 4. Epidermoid tumor. Axial MRI with gadolinium enhancement. (TR 600 ms, TE 25 ms, first echo, 1.5 T field.)

saline irrigation is used, and the patient is maintained on high-dose steroids, tapered slowly to avoid postoperative aseptic meningitis.[13] Late followup usually demonstrates improvement in preoperative cranial nerve deficits.[5,96] Degeneration of an epidermoid into primary intracranial squamous cell carcinoma has been reported, but is exceedingly rare (about 20 cases reported[81]). The regrowth of the tumor may be monitored with MRI, but reoperation is deferred until the patient's symptoms become troublesome. An average of 5-10 years may elapse between operations in patients whose tumors recur.[5,121] Reoperation usually is accompanied by the same benign postoperative course as the first procedure. A 20-year survival rate of 92% was found in one study.[121]

Lipomas

The lipoma of the CPA is a rare tumor with a slow, insinuating growth pattern that is reminiscent of the epidermoid. It may cause a typical progressive CPA syndrome,[63] or unusual symptoms such as fluctuating hearing loss[52] or hemifacial spasm.[66] Typical symptoms of trigeminal neuralgia also have

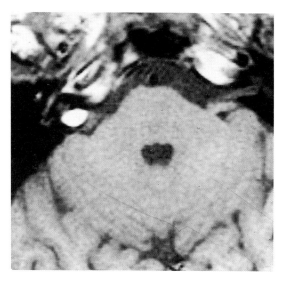

Figure 5. Cerebellopontine angle lipoma. Axial MRI without gadolinium enhancement. (TR 600 ms, TE 12 ms, first echo, 1.5 T field.)

been reported.[26]

CT scan shows a nonenhancing mass with fat density (-25 to -100 Hounsfield units), which may erode the internal auditory meatus. Calcification within the tumor suggests the possibility of a teratoma. MRI shows a lesion which is high-signal on T1-weighted sequences, with the signal diminishing with increased T2-weighting[115] (Figure 5). Fat-suppression techniques would be expected to extinguish this signal, but their use has not yet been reported.

Attempts have been made to resect such tumors, but characteristically at operation, the facial and vestibulocochlear nerves are surrounded or infiltrated by the tumor, which may extend into the internal auditory meatus. Despite the use of lasers and other microsurgical techniques, an incomplete removal is nearly always the result. Attempts at extensive removal almost invariably cause an increase in neurologic deficit. In one case, this included palsies of the facial and vagus nerves.[63] The reason would appear to be that the cranial nerves passing through the tumor split into fascicles and individual nerve fibers that run through the fatty parenchyma. As the surgeon attempts to debulk the tumor, these fibers are unintentionally resected.[15] In some cases, the partial resections that have been achieved have relieved the patient's symptoms, but unless these are sufficiently troubling (such as severe hemifacial spasm or disabling pain) that the risk of deficit is acceptable, an expectant course is indicated. The suggestion that these tumors are really "malformations" resulting from maldifferentiation of primitive meningeal tissue into fat, rather than undergoing the normal process of attenuation, would indicate that the fatty parenchyma of these masses may be under similar regulation to that of the remainder of the body's fat.[115] If this is so, simple weight loss might suffice to relieve early symptoms.

Gliomas

Glial tumors presenting in the CPA include the extension of a brain stem astrocytoma or medulloblastoma,[37] an ependymoma protruding through the foramen of Luschka, and, rarely, a subependymoma. Development of a CPA or jugular foramen syndrome, which may be rapid, and often is accompanied by symptoms indicating brain stem compromise, is the usual presentation. The connection between the CPA mass and the actual intra-axial epicenter of the tumor may not be apparent on preoperative imaging studies, although this probably will be less frequent since the introduction of MRI. Treatment is subtotal resection and adjuvant therapy selected with regard to histology. Shunting of the ventricular system may be necessary.

Choroid Plexus Papillomas

Papillomas of the choroid plexus that arise from the tuft of plexus outside the foramen of Luschka ("Bochdalek's flower basket") project into the CPA, resulting in a clinical syndrome similar to that seen in other CPA tumors. When there is significant extension into the fourth ventricle, there is nearly always hydrocephalus. About 20 cases have been recorded, some with malignant histology.[22,45,48]

Imaging studies frequently demonstrate calcification, enhancement, and sometimes a cyst. MRI shows a mass with a low signal on T1 and a high signal on T2, and may delineate a portion of the tumor extending through the foramen of Luschka into the fourth ventricle.[22] Arteriography may demonstrate blood supply from the anterior inferior cerebellar artery (AICA). The AICA forms the normal blood supply for this portion of the choroid plexus, and AICA supply to other CPA tumors is unusual.[118]

At surgery, the tumor usually is soft and vascular. Removal is difficult because the tumor may surround cranial nerves IX and X, as well as AICA branches. A complete removal is the goal but is not always possible. When incomplete removal has been performed, and the histology is malignant, radiotherapy is indicated.

Miscellaneous Mass Lesions of the Cerebellopontine Angle

Cystic Lesions

A variety of cystic lesions of the CPA have been reported, with various names to denote the histologic nature of the cyst wall: arachnoid,[71,95] epithelial,[65] neuroepithelial,[16] respiratory epithelial,[62,78] and enterogenous cysts.[117] Some are incidental findings on CT or MRI, and some present with characteristic syndromes of the CPA.

When the cyst is symptomatic, regardless of histology, treatment consists, when possible, of complete excision of the cyst wall, and when this is not possible (as with arachnoid cysts), of fenestration and shunting of the cyst. Shunting into nearby subarachnoid cisterns is convenient and avoids the necessity of a catheter to the peritoneum.

Vascular Malformations

Vascular malformations occasionally are encountered in the CPA. The most common variety is the cavernous malformation, sometimes referred to as a "cavernous angioma" or "hemangioma."[67,73,88] About 20 cases have

been reported. The lesions are situated most often within the internal auditory meatus, although quite large lesions occupying the CPA, with an associated cyst, also have been seen,[40] as have lesions in the geniculate ganglion.[73] The clinical hallmark is deficit of facial or auditory function that seems out of proportion to the small size of the lesion, which usually is wholly intracanalicular.

CT may show calcification within the lesion, and MRI shows a high-signal intensity on both T1- and T2-weighted pulse sequences. There is dense enhancement with gadolinium. The lesion usually is closely applied to the nerves in the canal, and in some patients the nerves may be entirely engulfed, requiring resection of both nerves to achieve removal of the lesion. In other cases, the lesion does not contain the nerves and may be removed with little or no postoperative deficit.

Even rarer is the CPA arteriovenous malformation,[67] which has a similar clinical and radiologic presentation. Presumably, this lesion might be detected by preoperative arteriography, but MRI does not establish the diagnosis, and the preoperative diagnosis usually is intracanalicular acoustic neuroma. Treatment is surgical removal. The natural history of this lesion, and of the cavernous malformation of the internal auditory canal, both seem to progress toward deafness and facial palsy, but so far the number of cases reported is very small, and no such lesion has been prospectively followed with conservative treatment.

CPA Masses Secondary to Systemic Diseases

Systemic diseases that may cause mass lesions in the CPA include metastatic tumors and granulomatous diseases, such as syphilis, sarcoidosis, and Lyme disease.[71,74] The primary diagnosis usually has not been made preoperatively. Even when a systemic tumor has been previously noted, CPA metastasis is sufficiently rare that the possibility of acoustic tumor or another typical CPA mass should be seriously entertained. When the primary tumor is a breast carcinoma, the higher incidence of meningioma that has been reported in association with breast cancer[32] must be borne in mind, although this association has not been specifically confirmed for CPA lesions. Treatment of granulomas and metastases in the CPA usually is subtotal or total excision, with postoperative therapy guided by the primary diagnosis.

Tumors of the Jugular Foramen

The jugular foramen, containing the glossopharyngeal nerve in its anteromedial pars nervosa and the vagus and spinal accessory nerves, and the jugular bulb in its posterolateral pars venosa,[58,93] is an uncommon location for tumors. When tumors arise in this location, however, they pose a special surgical challenge because of the proximity of a number of vital structures. The majority of tumors in this location are neuromas or glomus tumors, but meningiomas, inflammatory masses, metastatic or primary malignancies, and other types of pathology may be found here as well.

Neuromas of the Nerves of the Jugular Foramen

A neuroma can arise from any of the three cranial nerves that pass through the jugular foramen. Roughly 100 cases have been reported.[36] The great majority originate in the glossopharyngeal and vagus nerves, with only 12 cases of spinal accessory nerve neuromas found in one review.[41] At this point in their course, all three nerves contain peripheral myelin,[59] and the tumors are schwannomas. Patients usually do not suffer from neurofibromatosis. There is no clear sex preference.

The clinical presentation of these tumors is diverse, and a complete "jugular foramen syndrome," or palsies of the glossopharyngeal, vagus, and spinal accessory nerves, is seen only occasionally.[23,36,41,49,111] Depending on the site of origin of the tumor, three main patterns of growth are seen, influencing the type

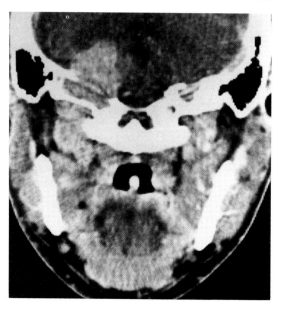

Figure 6. Jugular foramen meningioma. Direct coronal CT with intravenous contrast enhancement. The extracranial extension of the tumor is visible.

of clinical presentation. When the tumor arises intracranially, and grows into the CPA, hearing loss is seen, followed by signs of compression of the brain stem and/or cerebellum. Some of these patients have no clinically discernable deficit of the lower cranial nerves.[49] Tumors arising either at the point of passage of the nerve through the skull, causing expansion of the foramen, or extracranially, expanding as an infratemporal fossa mass, usually give rise to deficits of nerves IX to XI.[36] A presentation with large masses both intracranially and extracranially with a narrow bridge through the foramen also may be seen.[91]

Radiographic studies show a mass centered on the jugular foramen, with imaging characteristics similar to those of an acoustic tumor. CT is particularly helpful in delineating bony erosion, which is smooth and has a regular border that sometimes is sclerotic. MRI is preferable in establishing precise anatomical relationships to soft tissue structures and vessels[72] (Figure 6). The two studies are complementary, and neither has entirely supplanted the other. Arteriography serves to exclude a glomus tumor and to define the status of the ipsilateral and contralateral venous drainage system.

The surgical approach is selected to suit the extent of the tumor. Tumors located primarily within the posterior fossa, with a slight extension into the foramen, are approached in the same way as described for CPA meningiomas, through a standard suboccipital retrosigmoid craniotomy. When the tumor extends significantly into the extracranial space, a neck dissection will be required. This is performed in conjunction with an otolaryngologist. The intracranial portion of the tumor usually is amenable to resection through a suboccipital retrosigmoid approach; bony removal may be extended anteroinferiorly until the jugular foramen is reached. The incision described for the suboccipital craniotomy is extended along the anterior border of the sternocleidomastoid muscle to the level of the hyoid bone. The cranial attachments of the sternocleidomastoid muscle, the posterior belly of the digastric, and the styloid muscles are mobilized. Care is taken to identify and preserve the facial nerve at its exit from the skull at the stylomastoid foramen. Next, the lower cranial nerves are identified in the neck and traced proximally to their entrance into the lower pole of the tumor.

The suboccipital portion of the procedure is conducted as described previously, with further bony removal over the sigmoid sinus until its entry into the foramen. The mastoid is drilled out, with further removal of petrous bone to expose the facial nerve for anterior translocation if necessary. The tumor removal follows the principles described previously, with the dural opening extending inferiorly as necessary for exposure. Particular care is necessary when separating lower cranial nerves from the tumor capsule. The involved cranial nerve will almost certainly need to be resected, but this may be limited to only a few of the nerve's rootlets in some cases. After tumor removal, a watertight dural closure is essential; we use a pericranial graft, with fine Prolene™ sutures for difficult portions of the closure deep in the wound. A lumbar drain is not routinely used.

Other authors prefer a presigmoid approach (described previously, under "Cerebellopontine Angle Meningiomas"), an extended infratemporal approach,[20,23,43] a translabyrinthine or infralabyrinthine approach,[49,57] a "transjugular-transpetrosal" approach,[29] or a "widened transcochlear approach" (combining the transcochlear and infratemporal approaches[91]) for tumors extending through the base of the skull, sometimes in combination with the full suboccipital exposure. Extracranially, the jugular vein may need to be ligated and divided, and similarly the lateral sinus. A special consideration for tumors of the spinal accessory nerve is the potential extension of the tumor into the spinal root of the nerve, which may necessitate a laminectomy of C1 and C2 for total removal.[46]

Whatever approach is used, there is a very high incidence of postoperative deficits of cranial nerves IX to XI,[36] with essentially no preoperative deficits resolving and, usually, new deficits present. One group stated that "complete removal of neuromas involving the jugular foramen is usually synonymous with paralysis of cranial nerves IX, X, and XI,"[36] and results of other groups would reinforce this conclusion.[23,49] If the lower cranial nerves show good preoperative function, we prefer to leave in place any tumor capsule that adheres to them, accepting a subtotal removal rather than risking a postoperative deficit with frequently serious sequelae, such as difficulty swallowing and aspiration pneumonia. When cranial nerve X has been lost prior to surgery, as is often the case, the additional deficit postoperatively is likely to be minimal, and we seek a total removal. Tracheostomy and gastrostomy are not routinely necessary when there has been a gradual loss of function preoperatively. A thin-walled feeding tube may be useful in the early postoperative course, but if there is severe acute disability of the lower cranial nerves, a tracheostomy and/or feeding gastrostomy may be required. Positioning the patient with the "good side" down in the immediate postoperative period may help to avoid early aspiration pneumonia.

Otolaryngologic procedures have been developed for treatment of these disabilities.[116] Symptoms resulting from compression of the brain stem or cerebellum generally have been relieved. When removal has been incomplete the tumor usually recurs, although it may not be symptomatic for many years.[110,111]

Glomus Jugulare Tumors

Glomus jugulare tumors are thought to arise from chemoreceptor cells situated in the adventitia of the jugular bulb within the jugular foramen. They are a subclass of the paraganglioma group of tumors. They usually are benign, but their rate of growth is variable. Some secrete catecholamines or other substances.[43] An association with carotid body tumors has been noted.

Clinically, the tumors present with variable components of the jugular foramen syndrome, with the addition of frequent hearing impairment, facial palsy, and headache.[101] There often is a red, pulsating mass in the ear canal. The tumor may be quite large on presentation, extending even from the cavernous sinus to the parapharyngeal space. The tumors are identified and anatomic boundaries are defined by CT or MRI, with angiography revealing the characteristic, extremely vascular pattern almost unique to this tumor. Two classifications based on anatomic criteria, described by Fisch and Mattox[20] and Glassock and Jackson et al,[43] are widely used. A review of clinical aspects, diagnostic protocols, and surgical principles is available.[43] (See Chapter 11.)

The variable natural history, infiltrative growth into a sensitive area, high vascularity, and benign histology have made radiation a popular choice of treatment, and experiences with a variety of radiotherapy techniques have been reported.[11,17,31,54] The results have been good, with one group[17] reporting 3 instances of tumor progression or recurrence in 45 treated patients,[3] with one fatality from miscalculated dosage. A comprehensive review[108] found identical rates of local control for radiation and surgery, with far fewer cranial

nerve palsies in the radiation-treated group. Our own preference for treatment of glomus tumors has been radiation, with only rare requirement for surgery.

This is by no means a universal preference, and many groups have reported results of surgical series.[3,14,20,42,43,100] The approaches favored are identical to those mentioned for jugular foramen neuromas. Every effort should be made to interrupt the arterial supply to the tumor as completely as possible before beginning tumor resection. This supply will arise from the ipsilateral vertebral artery as well as from the external carotid artery, particularly the ascending pharyngeal branch. Interruption of the sigmoid sinus upstream from the tumor also is said to be an advantage.[91] The sigmoid and inferior petrosal sinuses and jugular vein will need to be resected in most cases. An additional option is preoperative embolization, which has been shown to decrease blood loss and operative time, but without beneficial effect on the frequency of cranial nerve injury.[79] Indeed, cranial nerve palsies may occur as a complication of embolization. The neuroanesthesiologist should be aware of the catecholamine-secreting status of the tumor. Additional lower cranial nerve palsies postoperatively are the rule when the tumor extends intracranially or into the infratemporal fossa, and are not infrequent even in smaller tumors.[14,42] Many of the approaches mentioned destroy hearing in the ipsilateral ear, and temporary facial palsy may be expected if an approach involving anterior translocation of the facial nerve is used. Postoperative CSF leaks are another possible complication.

Meningiomas of the Jugular Foramen

Konovalov et al[55] found 9% of the meningiomas of the posterior surface of the petrous pyramid to extend to the jugular foramen, and one review found only 12 cases that appeared to have originated there.[39] These tumors have a predilection for younger patients and tend to extend extracranially along or within the lumen of the jugular vein, sometimes extending as far as the level of C3.[39] They are removed using surgical techniques similar to those discussed for jugular foramen neuromas or glomus tumors, usually requiring an extracranial neck dissection.

Tumors of the Hypoglossal Foramen

Neuromas of the hypoglossal nerve are extremely rare lesions. About 40 have been recorded. Patients are middle-aged, and three-quarters are women.[10,84] Excluding five cases of neurofibromatosis, the remainder of the tumors usually have been entirely intracranial, with the main tumor mass most often ventral to the brain stem. Seven cases of the "dumbbell" type, with masses both intracranially and extracranially, have been reported. Wholly extracranial tumors, outside the range of this chapter, present as parapharyngeal masses.

There is nearly always a complete palsy of the hypoglossal nerve. Additional symptoms have included pareses of cranial nerves V through XI as well as signs of cerebellar and brain stem compression. Imaging techniques show a tumor whose absorption or signal characteristics resemble those of jugular foramen neuromas, but extending through the hypoglossal foramen. In one case, extracranial extension was well delineated with MRI, and this would seem to be the radiologic procedure of choice, with gadolinium contrast enhancement.

Surgical approaches for this tumor have not been systematically explored by any single group of authors; nearly all reports having been of a single case because of the rarity of the tumor. In general, a suboccipital retrosigmoid approach has been used in attempts to remove those tumors that have been entirely intracranial. This approach has met with limited success. The extracranial portion of the tumor is left in place perforce when this approach is used for dumbbell tumors.

A number of approaches recently have been developed for removal of masses ante-

rior to the caudal brain stem.[24,33,106,107] These approaches share removal of the anterolateral rim of the foramen magnum, as far as the occipital condyle. Even further anterior bony removal is possible with the addition of an occiput-to-C2 fusion.[107] The lateral portion of the laminae of C1 and C2 may be removed if necessary for tumor extension below the foramen magnum.[24,106,107] These approaches afford excellent exposure of the intradural aspect of the hypoglossal foramen. Odake used a similar approach, with division of the sigmoid sinus and additional lateral bony resection to include the posterior wall of the hypoglossal canal, as well as resection of the lateral mass of C1, for a one-stage removal of a hypoglossal neuroma with both intradural and extradural components.[84] The extracranial portion of these tumors occupies a space with the jugular vein and internal carotid artery as its lateral border. A firm grasp of the anatomy of the structures inferomedial to the jugular foramen—an area rarely entered—thus is necessary for safe surgery in this region.[19] These approaches also can be used for other intradural lesions of the anterior foramen magnum and clivus, subjects beyond the range of this discussion.

In addition to neuromas of the hypoglossal nerve, a variety of other lesions, such as granulomas and meningiomas, have been reported in this same area. These lesions are too rare for extensive experience to have been accumulated. Their exposure for surgical removal is effected using the same techniques as described previously.

References

1. Al-Mefty O. Surgery of the posterior cranial base. In: *Surgery of the Cranial Base.* Boston, Mass: Kluwer Academic Publishers; 1989:259-274.
2. Al-Mefty O. Surgical exposure of petroclival tumors. In: Wilkins RH, Rengachary SS, eds. *Neurosurgery Update, I.* New York, NY: McGraw Hill; 1990: 409-414.
3. Al-Mefty O, Fox JL, Rifai A, et al. A combined infratemporal and posterior fossa approach for the removal of giant glomus tumors and chondrosarcomas. *Surg Neurol.* 1987;28:423-431.
4. Al-Mefty O, Fox JL, Smith RR. Petrosal approach for petroclival meningiomas. *Neurosurgery.* 1988; 22:510-517.

5. Altschuler EM, Jungreis CA, Sekhar LN, et al. Operative treatment of intracranial epidermoid cysts and cholesterol granulomas: report of 21 cases. *Neurosurgery.* 1990;26:606-614.

6. Auger RG, Piepgras DG. Hemifacial spasm associated with epidermoid tumors of the cerebellopontine angle. *Neurology.* 1989;39:577-580.

7. Becker WJ, Watters GV, de Chadarevian JP, et al. Recurrent aseptic meningitis secondary to intracranial epidermoids. *Can J Neurol Sci.* 1984;11: 387-389.

8. Berger MS, Wilson CB. Epidermoid cysts of the posterior fossa. *J Neurosurg.* 1985;62:214-219.

9. Bordi L, Compton J, and Symon L. Trigeminal neuroma: a report of eleven cases. *Surg Neurol.* 1989; 31:272-276.

10. Bordi L, Symon L, Cheesman AD. Hypoglossal neuroma following excision of a huge recurrent acoustic neuroma and facio-hypoglossal anastomosis: a complex management problem. *Acta Neurochir (Wien).* 1990;104:143-146.

11. Boyle JO, Shimm DS, Coulthard SW. Radiation therapy for paragangliomas of the temporal bone. *Laryngoscope.* 1990;100:896-901.

12. Brackmann DE, Bartels LJ. Rare tumors of the cerebellopontine angle. *Otolaryngol Head Neck Surg.* 1980;88:555-559.

13. Cantu RC, Ojemann RG. Glucosteroid treatment of keratin meningitis following removal of a fourth ventricle epidermoid tumour. *J Neurol Neurosurg Psychiatry.* 1968;31:73-75.

14. Cece JA, Lawson W, Biller HF, et al. Complications in the management of large glomus jugulare tumors. *Laryngoscope.* 1987;97:152-157.

15. Christensen WN, Long DM, Epstein JI. Cerebellopontine angle lipoma. *Human Pathol.* 1986;17: 739-743.

16. Ciricillo SF, Davis RL, Wilson CB. Neuroepithelial cysts of the posterior fossa: case report. *J Neurosurg.* 1990;72:302-305.

17. Cummings BJ, Beale FA, Garrett PG, et al. The treatment of glomus tumors in the temporal bone by megavoltage radiation. *Cancer.* 1984;53:2635-2640.

18. de la Monte SM, Flickinger J, Linggood RM. Histopathologic features predicting recurrence of meningiomas following subtotal resection. *Am J Surg Pathol.* 1986;10:836-843.

19. de Oliveira E, Rhoton AL Jr, Peace D. Microsurgical anatomy of the region of the foramen magnum. *Surg Neurol.* 1985;24:293-352.

20. Fisch U, Mattox D. Infratemporal fossa approach type A. In: Fisch U, Mattox D. *Microsurgery of the Skull Base.* New York, NY: Thieme Medical Publishers; 1988:133-281.

21. Fisch U, Mattox D. Transtemporal supralabyrinthine approach. In: Fisch U, Mattox D. *Microsurgery of the Skull Base.* New York, NY: Thieme Medical Publishers; 1988:417-542.

22. Ford WJ, Brooks BS, El Gammal T, et al. Adult cerebellopontine angle choroid plexus papilloma: MR evaluation. *AJNR.* 1988;9:611.

23. Franklin DF, Moore GF, Fisch U. Jugular foramen peripheral nerve sheath tumors. *Laryngoscope.* 1989;99:1081-1087.

24. George B, Dematons C, Cophignon J. Lateral approach to the anterior portion of the foramen magnum: application to surgical removal of 14 benign tumors: technical note. *Surg Neurol.* 1988; 29:484-490.

25. Granick MS, Martuza RL, Parker SW, et al. Cerebellopontine angle meningiomas: clinical manifestations and diagnosis. *Ann Otol Rhinol Laryngol.* 1985;94:34-38.

26. Graves VB, Schemm GW. Clinical characteristics and CT findings in lipoma of the cerebellopontine angle: case report. *J Neurosurg.* 1982;57:839-841.

27. Guthrie BL, Carabell C, Laws ER Jr. Radiation therapy for intracranial meningiomas. In: Al-Mefty O, ed. *Meningiomas.* New York, NY: Raven Press; 1991:255-262.

28. Hakuba A. [Total removal of cerebellopontine angle tumors with a combined transpetrosal-transtentorial approach.] *No Shinkei Geka.* 1978; 6:347-354. [Japanese]

29. Hakuba A. [An anatomical and technical note for neurosurgery of the jugular foramen tumor.] *No Shinkei Geka.* 1982;10:359-367. (Jpn) English abstract.

30. Hakuba A, Nishimura S, Jang BJ. A combined retroauricular and preauricular transpetrosal-transtentorial approach to clivus meningiomas. *Surg Neurol.* 1988;30:108-116.

31. Hansen HS, Thomsen KA. Radiotherapy in glomus tumors (paragangliomas): a 25 year-review. *Acta Otolaryngol (Stockh).* 1988;suppl 449:151-154.

32. Helseth A, Mork SJ, Glattre E. Neoplasms of the central nervous system in Norway; V: meningioma and cancer of other sites: an analysis of the occurrence of multiple primary neoplasms in meningioma patients in Norway from 1955 through 1986. *APMIS.* 1989;97:738-744.

33. Heros RC. Lateral suboccipital approach for vertebral and vertebrobasilar artery lesions. *J Neurosurg.* 1986;64:559-562.

34. Hitselberger WE, Gardner G Jr. Other tumors of the cerebellopontine angle. *Arch Otolaryngol.* 1968; 88:712-714.

35. Horie Y, Akagi S, Taguchi K, et al. Malignant schwannoma arising in the intracranial trigeminal nerve: a report of an autopsy case and a review of the literature. *Acta Pathol Jpn.* 1990;40:219-225.

36. Horn KL, House WF, Hitselberger WE. Schwannomas of the jugular foramen. *Laryngoscope.* 1985; 95:761-765.

37. House JL, Burt MR. Primary CNS tumors presenting as cerebellopontine angle tumors. *Am J Otol.* 1985;6 (Suppl):147-153.

38. House WF, Hitselberger WE, Horn KL. The middle fossa transpetrous approach to the anterior-superior cerebellopontine angle. *Am J Otol.* 1986; 7:1-4.

39. Inagawa T, Kamiya K, Hosoda I, et al. Jugular foramen meningioma. *Surg Neurol.* 1989;31:295-299.

40. Iplikcioglu AC, Benli K, Bertan V, et al. Cystic cavernous hemangioma of the cerebellopontine angle: case report. *Neurosurgery.* 1986;19:641-642.

41. Iwasaki K, Kondo A. Accessory neurinoma manifesting with typical jugular foramen syndrome. *Neurosurgery.* 1991;29:455-459.

42. Jackson CG, Cueva RA, Thedinger BA, et al. Conservation surgery for glomus jugulare tumors: the value of early diagnosis. *Laryngoscope.* 1990;100: 1031-1036.

43. Jackson CG, Johnson GD, Poe DS. Lateral trans-temporal approaches to the skull base. In: Jackson CG, ed. *Surgery of Skull Base Tumors.* New York, NY: Churchill Livingstone; 1991;141-196.

44. Jefferson G. The trigeminal neurinomas with some remarks on malignant invasion of the gasserian ganglion. *Clin Neurosurg.* 1955;1:11-54.

45. Kalangu K, Reznik M, Bonnal J. Papillome du plexus choroïde de l'angle ponto-cérébelleux: présentation d'un cas et revue de la littérature. *Neurochirurgie.* 1986;32:242-247. English abstract.

46. Kawaguchi S, Ohnishi H, Yuasa T, et al. Spinal accessory nerve neurinoma in the C2 spinal canal. *Neurol Med Chir (Tokyo).* 1987;27:1190-1194.

47. Kawase T, Shiobara R, Toya S. Anterior trans-petrosal-transtentorial approach for sphenopetro-clival meningiomas: surgical method and results in 10 patients. *Neurosurgery.* 1991;28:869-876.

48. Kawase T, Toya S, Shiobara R, et al. Transpetrosal approach for aneurysms of the lower basilar artery. *J Neurosurg.* 1985;63:857-861.

49. Kaye AH, Hahn JF, Kinney SE, et al. Jugular foramen schwannomas. *J Neurosurg.* 1984;60:1045-1053.

50. King TT, Benjamin JC, Morrison AW. Epidermoid and cholesterol cysts in the apex of the petrous bone. *Br J Neurosurg.* 1989;3:451-461.

51. King TT, Morrison AW. Primary facial nerve tumors within the skull. *J Neurosurg.* 1990;72:1-8.

52. Kitamura K, Futaki T, Miyoshi S. Fluctuating hearing loss in lipoma of the cerebellopontine angle. *ORL J Otorhinolaryngol Relat Spec.* 1990;52:335-339.

53. Kondziolka D, Lunsford LD, Coffey RJ, et al. Stereotactic radiosurgery of meningiomas. *J Neurosurg.* 1991;74:552-559.

54. Konefal JB, Pilepich MV, Spector GJ, et al. Radiation therapy in the treatment of chemodectomas. *Laryngoscope.* 1987;97:1331-1335.

55. Konovalov AN, Makhmudov UB, Koposov AS. [Surgery of meningiomas of the posterior surface of the pyramid of the temporal bone.] *Zh Vopr Neirokhir.* 1988:14-19. Russian.

56. Laird FJ, Harner SG, Laws ER Jr, et al. Meningiomas of the cerebellopontine angle. *Otolaryngol Head Neck Surg.* 1985;93:163-167.

57. Lambert PR, Johns ME, Winn RH. Infralabyrinthine approach to skull-base lesions. *Otolaryngol Head Neck Surg.* 1985;93:250-258.

58. Lang J. Anatomy in and on the jugular foramen. *Adv Neurosurgery.* 1989;17:125-132.

59. Lang J, Reiter U. Uber die intrazisternale Länge der Hirnnerven VII-XII. *Neurochirurgia (Stuttg).* 1985;28:153-157.

60. Langman AW, Jackler RK, Althaus SR. Meningioma of the internal auditory canal. *Am J Otol.* 1990;11:201-204.

61. Lee KS, Britton BH, Kelly DL Jr. Schwannoma of the facial nerve in the cerebellopontine angle presenting with hearing loss. *Surg Neurol.* 1989;32:231-234.

62. Lee ST, Huang CC. Respiratory epithelial cyst in the cerebellopontine angle. *Surg Neurol.* 1989;32:418-420.

63. Leibrock LG, Deans WR, Bloch S, et al. Cerebellopontine angle lipoma: a review. *Neurosurgery.* 1983;12:697-699.

64. Lesoin F, Rousseaux M, Villette L, et al. Neurinomas

of the trigeminal nerve. *Acta Neurochir (Wien).* 1986;82:118-122.

65. Leung SY, Ng THK, Fung CF, et al. An epithelial cyst in the cerebellopontine angle: case report. *J Neurosurg.* 1991;74:278-282.

66. Levin JM, Lee JE. Hemifacial spasm due to cerebellopontine angle lipoma: case report. *Neurology.* 1987;37:337-339.

67. Linskey ME, Jannetta PJ, Martinez AJ. A vascular malformation mimicking an intracanalicular acoustic neurilemoma: case report. *J Neurosurg.* 1991;74:516-519.

68. Lipkin AF, Coker NJ, Jenkins HA, et al. Intracranial and intratemporal facial neuroma. *Otolaryngol Head Neck Surg.* 1987;96:71-79.

69. McCormack PC, Bello JA, Post KD. Trigeminal schwannoma: surgical series of 14 cases with review of the literature. *J Neurosurg.* 1988;69:850-860.

70. McKenna MJ, Cheney ML, Borodic G, et al. Management of facial paralysis after intracranial surgery. *Contemporary Neurosurgery,* 1991:13:1-7.

71. Martuza RL, Parker SW, Nadol JB Jr, et al. Diagnosis of cerebellopontine angle tumors. *Clin Neurosurg.* 1985;32:177-213.

72. Matsushima T, Hasuo K, Yasumori K, et al. Magnetic resonance imaging of jugular foramen neurinomas. *Acta Neurochir (Wien).* 1989;96:83-87.

73. Mazzoni A, Pareschi R, Calabrese V. Intratemporal vascular tumours. *J Laryng Otol.* 1988;102:353-356.

74. Mokry M, Flaschka G, Kleinert G, et al. Chronic Lyme disease with an expansive granulomatous lesion in the cerebellopontine angle. *Neurosurgery.* 1990;27:446-451.

75. Möller A, Hatam A, Olivecrona H. The differential diagnosis of pontine angle meningioma and acoustic neuroma with computed tomography. *Neuroradiology.* 1978;17:21-23.

76. Morrison AW, King TT. Space-occupying lesions of the internal auditory meatus and cerebellopontine angle. *Adv Otorhinolaryngol.* 1984;34:121-142.

77. Muhlbauer MS, Clark WC, Robertson JH, et al. Malignant nerve sheath tumor of the facial nerve: case report and discussion. *Neurosurgery.* 1987;21:68-73.

78. Muller J, Voelker JL, Campbell RL. Respiratory epithelial cyst of the cerebellopontine angle. *Neurosurgery.* 1989;24:936-939.

79. Murphy TP, Brackmann DE. Effects of preoperative embolization on glomus jugulare tumors. *Laryngoscope.* 1989;99:1244-1247.

80. Nager GT. Neurinomas of the trigeminal nerve. *Am J Otolaryngol.* 1984;5:301-333.

81. Nishiura I, Koyama T, Handa J, et al. Primary intracranial epidermoid carcinoma: case report. *Neurol Med Chir (Tokyo).* 1989;29:600-605.

82. Numaguchi Y, Kishikawa T, Ikeda J, et al. Angiographic diagnosis of acoustic neurinomas and meningiomas in the cerebellopontine angle: a reappraisal. *Neuroradiology.* 1980;19:73-80.

83. O'Donoghue Gm, Brackmann DE, House JW, et al. Neuromas of the facial nerve. *Am J Otol.* 1989;10:49-54.

84. Odake G. Intracranial hypoglossal neurinoma with extracranial extension: review and case report. *Neurosurgery.* 1989;24:583-587.

85. Ogleznev KYa, Grigoryan YuA, Slavin KV. Parapontine epidermoid tumours presenting as trigeminal neuralgias: anatomical findings and operative results.

Acta Neurochir (Wien). 1991;110:116-119.

86. Ojemann RG. Meningiomas: clinical features and surgical management. In: Wilkins RH, Rengachary SS, eds. *Neurosurgery, I.* New York, NY: McGraw-Hill Inc.; 1985:635-661.

87. Ojemann RG, Martuza RL. Acoustic neuroma. In: Youmans JR, ed.: *Neurological Surgery, IV.* Philadelphia, Pa.: Saunders; 1990:3316-3350.

88. Pappas DG, Schneiderman TS, Brackmann DE, et al. Cavernous hemangiomas of the internal auditory canal. *Otolaryngol Head Neck Surg.* 1989;101:27-32.

89. Parnes LS, Lee DH, Peerless SJ. Magnetic resonance imaging of facial nerve neuromas. *Laryngoscope.* 1991;101:31-35.

90. Pech A, Cannoni M, Pellet W, et al. Les tumeurs de l'angle ponto-cérébelleux a l'exception des neurinomes de l'acoustique. *Ann Oto-laryng (Paris).* 1986; 103:293-301. English abstract.

91. Pellet W, Cannoni M, Pech A. The widened transcochlear approach to jugular foramen tumors. *J Neurosurg.* 1988;69:887-894.

92. Pollack IF, Sekhar LN, Jannetta PJ, et al. Neurilemomas of the trigeminal nerve. *J Neurosurg.* 1989; 70:737-745.

93. Rhoton AL, Buza R. Microsurgical anatomy of the jugular foramen. *J Neurosurg.* 1975;42:541-550.

94. Rosenblum B, Davis R, Camins M. Middle fossa facial schwannoma removed via the intracranial extradural approach: case report and review of the literature. *Neurosurgery.* 1987;21:739-741.

95. Rousseaux M, Lesoin F, Petit H, et al. Les kystes arachnoïdiens de l'angle ponto-cérébelleux. *Neurochirurgie.* 1984;30:119-124.

96. Sabin HI, Bordi LT, Symon L. Epidermoid cysts and cholesterol granulomas centered on the posterior fossa: twenty years of diagnosis and management. *Neurosurgery.* 1987;21:798-805.

97. Samii M, Ammirati M. The combined supra-infratentorial pre-sigmoid sinus avenue to the petroclival region: surgical technique and clinical applications. *Acta Neurochir (Wien).* 1988;95:6-12.

98. Samii M, Ammirati M. Cerebellopontine angle meningiomas (Posterior pyramid meningiomas). In: Al-Mefty O, ed. *Meningiomas.* New York, NY: Raven Press; 1991:503-515.

99. Samii M, Ammirati M, Mahran A, et al. Surgery of petroclival meningiomas: report of 24 cases. *Neurosurgery.* 1989;24:12-17.

100. Samii M, Draf W. Surgery of tumors of the lateral posterior skull base and petrous bone. In: Samii M, Draf W, eds. *Surgery of the Skull Base: an Interdisciplinary Approach.* New York, NY: Springer-Verlag; 1989:410-425.

101. Samii M, Sephernia A, Mahran A, et al. Surgery of the jugular foramen. *Adv Neurosurgery.* 1989;17: 140-152.

102. Samii M, Turel KE, Penkert G. Management of seventh and eighth nerve involvement by cerebellopontine angle tumors. *Clin Neurosurg.* 1985;32: 242-272.

103. Schisano G, Olivecrona H. Neurinomas of the gasserian ganglion and trigeminal root. *J Neurosurg.* 1960;17:306-322.

104. Sekhar LN, Jannetta PJ. Cerebellopontine angle meningiomas: microsurgical excision and follow-up results. *J Neurosurg.* 1984;60:500-505.

105. Sen CN, Sekhar LN. The subtemporal and preauricular infratemporal approach to intradural structures ventral to the brain stem. *J Neurosurg.* 1990;73: 345-354.

106. Sen CN, Sekhar LN. An extreme lateral approach to intradural lesions of the cervical spine and foramen magnum. *Neurosurgery.* 1990;27:197-204.

107. Sen CN, Sekhar LN. Surgical management of anteriorly placed lesions at the craniocervical junction: an alternative approach. *Acta Neurochir (Wien).* 1991; 108:70-77.

108. Springate SC, Weichselbaum RR. Radiation or surgery for chemodectoma of the temporal bone: a review of local control and complications. *Head Neck.* 1990;12:303-307.

109. Steiner L. Lindquist C, Steiner M. Meningiomas and gamma knife radiosurgery. In: Al-Mefty O, ed. *Meningiomas.* New York, NY: Raven Press; 1991: 263-272.

110. Sweasey TA, Edelstein SR, Hoff JT. Glossopharyngeal schwannoma: review of five cases and the literature. *Surg Neurol.* 1991;35:127-130.

111. Tan LC, Bordi L, Symon L, et al. Jugular foramen neuromas: a review of 14 cases. *Surg Neurol.* 1990; 34:205-211.

112. Tator CH, Duncan EG, Chrales D. Comparisons of the clinical and radiological features and surgical management of posterior fossa meningiomas and acoustic neuromas. *Can J Neurol Sci.* 1990;17: 170-176.

113. Tew JM Jr, Yeh HS, Miller GW, et al. Intratemporal schwannoma of the facial nerve. *Neurosurgery.* 1982; 13:186-188.

114. Thomsen J. Cerebellopontine angle tumors, other than acoustic neuromas: a report on 34 cases; a presentation of 7 bilateral acoustic neuromas. *Acta Otolaryngol (Stockh).* 1976;82:106-111.

115. Truwit CL, Barkovich AJ. Pathogenesis of intracranial lipoma: an MR study in 42 patients. *AJNR.* 1990; 11:665-674.

116. Tucker HM. Postoperative management and rehabilitation of cranial nerve deficits. In: Jackson CG, ed. *Surgery of Skull Base Tumors.* New York, NY: Churchill Livingstone; 1991:273-286.

117. Umezu H, Aiba T, Unakami M. Enterogenous cyst of the cerebellopontine angle cistern: case report. *Neurosurgery.* 1991;28:462-466.

118. van Swieten JC, Thomeer RTWM, Vielvoye GJ, et al. Choroid plexus papilloma in the posterior fossa. *Surg Neurol.* 1987;28:129-134.

119. Watabe T, Azuma T. T_1 and T_2 measurements of meningiomas and neuromas before and after Gd-DTPA. *AJNR.* 1989;10:463-470.

120. Wu E, Tang Y, Zhang Y, et al. CT in diagnosis of acoustic neuromas. *AJNR.* 1986;7:645-650.

121. Yamakawa K, Shitara N, Genka S, et al. Clinical course and surgical prognosis of 33 cases of intracranial epidermoid tumors. *Neurosurgery.* 1989;24: 568-573.

122. Yasargil MG, Abernathey CD, Sarioglu AC. Microneurosurgical treatment of intracranial dermoid and epidermoid tumors. *Neurosurgery.* 1989;24:561-567.

123. Yasargil MG, Mortara RW, Curcic M. Meningiomas of basal posterior cranial fossa. *Adv Tech Stand Neurosurg.* 1980;7:3-115.

124. Yasui T, Hakuba A, Kim SH, et al. Trigeminal neurinomas: operative approach in eight cases. *J Neurosurg.* 1989;71:506-511.

Index

Page numbers for tables, figures, and illustrations are in *boldface italics*.

Previously Published Books in the *Neurosurgical Topics* Series

For order information call (708) 692-9500.